Leading

Managing

Healthcare

Leading *and* Managing Healthcare

Neil Gopee

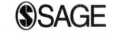

Los Angeles | London | New Delhi
Singapore | Washington DC | Melbourne

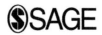

Los Angeles | London | New Delhi
Singapore | Washington DC | Melbourne

SAGE Publications Ltd
1 Oliver's Yard
55 City Road
London EC1Y 1SP

SAGE Publications Inc.
2455 Teller Road
Thousand Oaks, California 91320

SAGE Publications India Pvt Ltd
B 1/I 1 Mohan Cooperative Industrial Area
Mathura Road
New Delhi 110 044

SAGE Publications Asia-Pacific Pte Ltd
3 Church Street
#10-04 Samsung Hub
Singapore 049483

Editor: Alex Clabburn
Senior assistant editor: Ruth Lilly
Production editor: Katherine Haw
Copyeditor: Clare Weaver
Proofreader: Neil Dowden
Indexer: Neil Gopee
Cover design: Sheila Tong
Typeset by: Knowledgeworks Global Ltd.
Printed in the UK

Library of Congress Control Number: 2021945521

British Library Cataloguing in Publication data

A catalogue record for this book is available from the British Library

ISBN 978-1-5297-3300-6
ISBN 978-1-5297-3299-3 (pbk)

At SAGE we take sustainability seriously. Most of our products are printed in the UK using responsibly sourced papers and boards. When we print overseas we ensure sustainable papers are used as measured by the PREPS grading system. We undertake an annual audit to monitor our sustainability.

Contents

List of Figures

List of Tables

List of Abbreviations

A&E – accident and emergency (departments)
ACL – action-centred leadership
ACP – advanced clinical practice/practitioner
AHP – Allied Health Profession
BACP – British Association for Counselling and Psychotherapy
BEICHMM – buildings, equipment, information technology, consumables, human resources, methods and money
CCG – Clinical Commissioning Group
CIPD – Chartered Institute of Personnel and Development
CMI – Chartered Management Institute
CODH – Council of Deans of Health
CPD – continuing professional development
CQC – Care Quality Commission
DH – Department of Health
DHSC – Department of Health and Social Care
DTOC – delayed transfers of care
EBP – evidence-based practice (evidence-informed practice)
EBMgt – evidence-based management
EHR – electronic health records
EI – emotional intelligence
FHM – frontline healthcare manager
FTE – full-time equivalent
FYFV – Five Year Forward View
GMC – General Medical Council
GP – general practitioner
HCPC – Health and Care Professions Council
HEE – Health Education England
HRM – human resource management
HSCA – Health and Social Care Act 2012
HSW – Healthcare Support Worker (includes NSW – Nursing Support Worker)
ICB – Integrated Care Board

ICP – integrated care pathway
ICS – Integrated Care System
IDPR – Individual Development and Performance Review (also known as
Appraisal)
IHI – Institute for Healthcare Improvement
IPE – inter-professional education
JSNA – Joint Strategic Needs Assessment
LA – local authority
LETB – Local Education and Training Board
MBO – management by objectives
MDT – multi-disciplinary team
NAO – National Audit Office
NEWS2 – National Early Warning Score (2nd edition)
NHS – National Health Service
NHSE – NHS England
NHSESCC – NHS England Survey Co-ordination Centre
NHSE+I – NHS England and NHS Improvement
NHSI – NHS Improvement
NHS KSF – NHS Knowledge and Skills Framework
NHS LTP – NHS Long Term Plan
NICE – National Institute for Health and Care Excellence
NMC – Nursing and Midwifery Council
NRHP – Newly Registered Healthcare Professional
NRN – Newly Registered Nurse
ONS – Office for National Statistics
PALS – Patient Advice and Liaison Service
PCN – Primary Care Network
PDP – personal development plan
PDSA – Plan–Do–Study–Act cycle
PESTLE – political–economic–social–technological–legal–ethical/
environmental
PHE – Public Health England
PSI – patient safety incidents
QI – quality improvement
RCN – Royal College of Nursing
RCT – randomised controlled trial
RCA – root cause analysis
RNA – Registered Nursing Associate
SDEC – same day emergency care
SIGN – Scottish Intercollegiate Guidelines Network
SMART – (refers to objectives being) specific, measurable, achievable, realistic
(or relevant) and time-bound
SOP – standards of proficiency

STP – Sustainability and Transformation Partnership
SWOT – strengths, weaknesses, opportunities and threats
TQM – total quality management
UCC – urgent care centre
UKHSA – UK Health Security Agency
UTC – urgent treatment centre
WBL – work-based learning
WHO – World Health Organization

About the Author

Neil Gopee is Lecturer at Coventry University in the Faculty of Health and Life Sciences teaching mainly research and evidence-informed practice, principles of teaching, learning and assessment, and leadership and management in healthcare. Previously, Neil was Course Director for the mentorship and practice teacher courses at Coventry University, and for the MBA Public Health Management programme in addition to several other academic duties. He has also worked as external examiner at a number of UK universities in relation to the above-named topic areas, as well as for the post-graduate certificate in higher education (lecturer preparation) programme. Work as a reviewer for various peer-reviewed journals has also been a useful dimension of Neil's work.

Neil is a NMC Registered Nurse, having worked in general intensive care nursing, in primary care and as a mental health nurse. Through his nursing career, this combination of clinical experiences has been supplemented by attendance at numerous professional development short and long courses, including various workshops on writing for publication, and also completing his doctorate in continuing professional education at the University of Warwick. Neil's first textbook entitled *Mentoring and Supervision in Healthcare* was published in 2007, which in its fourth edition is entitled *Supervision and Mentoring in Healthcare* (published 2018). Along the way, he also wrote *Practice Teaching in Healthcare* and co-authored *Leadership and Management in Healthcare* (up to its third edition).

Acknowledgements

I would like to thank Alex Clabburn, Senior Editor at SAGE Publications, for ongoing support with my work on this book.

I also thank Claire Pahal, Resuscitation Officer and Advanced Life Support Instructor at South Warwickshire NHS Foundation Trust and European Paediatric Advanced Life Support Instructor, for her support in constructing Figure 7.1 in relation to micro-decisions that need to be made in the event of a cardiopulmonary resuscitation being required by an individual who has just collapsed.

Introduction

The daily duties that frontline healthcare managers perform are pivotal for the delivery of safe, effective and compassionate care. Be it in acute hospital wards, in community care services, or in care home settings, care interventions are always expected to be of high standard, and are performed by knowledgeable and competent healthcare staff.

With becoming a registered practitioner (or registrant) comes responsibility and accountability towards service users and towards colleagues, and towards all learners in the care setting. Consequently, managing and leading competently are essential skills that all newly qualified healthcare professionals have to equip themselves with for managing everyday practice in delivering care.

This textbook is aimed at newly registered healthcare professionals (NRHPs) who take on the duties and responsibilities of frontline healthcare managers (FHMs), and aims to address the knowledge base and skills required to enable FHMs to manage effectively and efficiently. It has been developed as an essential resource on leadership and management that can be utilised by care professionals working at Bands 5 and 6, or their equivalent levels, to support their everyday practice. More senior frontline healthcare staff may also find the content useful as a baseline that their frontline teams can work from.

A range of generic books on leadership and management that cuts across all organisations is available for FHMs to consult, and this textbook harnesses the generic knowledge on leadership and management and demonstrates how to apply appropriate ones to healthcare. It also draws on my personal experience of management of care in the frontline in a variety of care settings and on teaching leadership and management within higher education over numerous years.

There is a range of similarities and some differences in the ways in which care is delivered and managed throughout the world, and yet the ways in which the core tasks of management of human and materials resources and healthcare work are conducted have fundamental similarities. Consequently, the theories and their application addressed in this textbook should be easily adaptable to healthcare systems and management of care delivery methods and issues in most countries outside the UK as well.

Integrating theory and practice is important, and therefore the book uses Action points related to some of the key concepts to enable healthcare professionals to reflect on ways in which the theories and guidance discussed can be applied to day-to-day practice in care settings.

Acquisition of new knowledge and skills should be an enjoyable journey and it is hoped that the easy-to-follow layout of this book will capture your attention and prove to be an essential resource that supports your everyday management and leadership practice that results in high-quality, person-centred care delivery as competent frontline healthcare managers.

Organisation of the Book

Chapter 1

To begin to put the content of this book in context, Chapter 1 starts with a brief exploration of the place and importance of management and leadership at the care delivery end of healthcare. It then refers to the nature of the population that health and care services provide for, followed by socio-economic and governmental contexts of care provision and care delivery. This is then followed by a deeper exploration of current healthcare strategies, policy and legislation that affect daily care, and new and evolving modes of care provision such as Sustainability and Transformation Partnerships and Integrated Care Systems. The role of professional regulation, of royal colleges and professional bodies as well as Chief Professions Officers are also highlighted.

As with the remaining chapters, Chapter 1 also endeavours to examine the significance of the national and regional policies to your practice setting and your role through Action points; and provides guidance on related good practice just before the chapter summary.

Chapter 2

The focus of Chapter 2 is very much on the experiences of newly qualified healthcare professionals' evolving responsibilities as team members and towards service users. In relation to their management duties, the chapter examines relevant methods of organising and communicating daily care, frontline managers' accountability and ethical practice, teaching and practice supervision duties towards students' and team members' learning, ending with a detailed exploration of the challenges and competing priorities that frontline care professionals encounter, and the personal resources that should enable them to manage those challenges.

Chapter 3

With leadership being one of the most prominent features of FHMs' duties, this chapter seeks to enable the reader to gain (or revisit) a deep understanding of the nature of leadership as a relatively elusive concept, which is followed by the reasons for effective leadership in health services, who provides leadership in healthcare along with leadership influence and power, and styles of leadership. The chapter then delves into a number of ways in which healthcare professionals provide leadership, starting with earlier theories but exploring in further detail the current more informed healthcare leadership theories and leadership frameworks to enable more systematic development and application of leadership skills. The chapter ends with the self-assessment of leadership skills and action plan for further leadership skill development for FHMs.

Chapter 4

As the principal focus of Chapter 4, the day-to-day management duties and activities of frontline managers is first ascertained, which is followed by an examination of the definitions of managers and management, and then of healthcare providers as organisations, and how organisations are structured and function. Subsequently, there is a close examination of well-established research-driven theories of management, and how they can be applied to healthcare settings. Styles of management that frontline managers can adopt is then explored, followed by ways in which FHMs ensure effective communication in care settings in the form of, for example, delegation of work, and accurate documentation and record-keeping.

Chapter 5

The very essence of management is the management of resources, and this chapter in particular examines the whole range of resources that are required for effective care delivery, and then explores why resources have to be managed. The chapter then delves into ways of managing non-human resources such as budgets effectively, beginning with the sources of funding for health services, and ways in which budgets are managed with good effect. It then looks at management of other non-human resources such as buildings, equipment, consumables, devices and care protocols and guidelines. Finally, the chapter examines management of human resources in the workplace, including recruitment and retention of staff, safe staffing and skill mix, and then employers' and employees' expectations of each other, including gauging staff satisfaction with their work, all of which are aimed at delivery of high-quality care. It also emphasises ensuring best value for money and working within a set budget, and therefore developing budget management skills.

Chapter 6

Moving on to teamwork, Chapter 6 explores the nature of teamwork in healthcare, what constitutes effective inter-disciplinary healthcare teams and their characteristics, the reasons for teamwork in care settings, how teams are formed, team roles, effective inter-disciplinary teams and leading inter-professional teams. The chapter then examines the role of staff motivation, the various approaches, theories and research on staff motivation, and then how team performance can be monitored and maximised, and team learning.

Chapter 7

Multiple decisions are made by frontline managers during the course of any shift at work, and problems dealt with. The range of care decisions made by frontline healthcare professionals is quite remarkable. This chapter starts by clarifying the terms decision-making and problem-solving and differentiates between them, before exploring ways of making decisions systematically, including whether decisions should be based on knowledge or intuition, and then examines the various ways of solving problems systematically, and includes root cause analysis. Finally, the chapter examines the nature of conflict in care settings, why they occur, and how we respond to conflict and resolve them.

Chapter 8

Enhancing and monitoring quality of care is of utmost importance, and a crucial component of FHMs' duties. Why there is so much emphasis and scrutiny of quality in health services is explored first in this chapter, followed by asking what is high-quality healthcare, which is then followed by exploring patient safety as a component of high-quality care, other components being clinical effectiveness and service users' experience of health services. Then a number of ways in which healthcare quality can be improved is discussed, going beyond service improvement and service transformation, and delving into the most prominent models and frameworks for quality improvement, as well as a number of contributory quality improvement techniques or tools. Issues related to quality improvement, such as clinical negligence claims and their implications, are also addressed.

Chapter 9

The management of change and innovations is yet another component of FHMs' duties. After identifying a range of recent changes in treatment and care delivery, including digitalisation in health services, the reasons for continuing changes are ascertained, followed by the systematic management of change which includes project management, and are discussed under the aegis of models of change management that can be applied. Users' perspective and sub-organisational culture are analysed as well as ways in which the change leader and their team carefully plan and lead the change, including applying strategies for implementing change, and evaluating and sustaining the change.

Chapter 10

The management of healthcare professionals' continuing learning is also a component of FHMs' duties. Chapter 10 firstly briefly re-examines the FHM's role in managing structured preceptorship development programmes, followed by discussion on revalidation requirements of team members, as well as career-long continuing learning, and management training and development programmes for frontline managers. Funding for staff development is also briefly explored. The management of students' practice learning is also analysed, as is the learning culture of practice settings and healthcare organisations. The management of issues related to learning and development such as managing poor practice and learning from patient safety incidents are also addressed. It includes self-assessment of management skills by FHMs, together with action planning.

How to Use the Book

A variety of features have been integrated into this textbook to make the text easy to follow and to enable application of the theories and concepts to care settings. This includes *Action points* within every chapter to trigger reflection on current practice and to learn from events and experiences in care settings. These are always followed by some commentary.

Guidance on good practice related to the content of each chapter features near the end of the chapters. Guidance for ensuring high-quality care, and Guidance for effective change management, for example, endeavour to highlight the key messages that have been constituted within the text of the chapter with the aim of informing your practice and for you to apply them to day-to-day practice.

Chapter summaries are provided at the end of each chapter as an aide-mémoire of the areas covered, some of which you might wish to relocate and revisit.

The relatively short *Further Reading* list at the end of each chapter comprise suggestions for follow-up reading that provides more detail on implementation of particular concepts and theories.

A *Glossary* of terms has been incorporated at the end of the book as a reminder of the meaning of a number of key concepts that are inherent within leadership and management.

In the References list some of the references may look old, but they include only the most defining management research, e.g. Hawthorne experiments, and cutting-edge management researchers. e.g. Drucker, Stewart, McGregor, etc.

Terminology

The following terminology is used throughout the book.

The terms 'care setting' and 'practice setting' are used interchangeably, and represent all healthcare sites where service users access health services, including acute hospital wards, care homes and nursing homes, GP surgeries, outpatients clinics, social care settings, the patient's own home, day centres for vulnerable adults, or for adults with learning disabilities or autism, etc.

The term 'service users' and 'patient' are also used interchangeably and in the wider sense. There is a subtle difference in these terms in that service users arrive and stay in care settings for a short or longer period of time, while patients are those who are very ill and may not even be aware they are ill and in an acute hospital accessing healthcare.

'Care' is used as a generic term that includes nursing care, but also represents therapy and treatment, although currently government documents use the word care when referring to social care.

The terms 'healthcare professional', 'care professional' and 'registrant' are used interchangeably to refer to qualified nurses, midwives and allied health or social care professionals (e.g. physiotherapist, dietitian), who are registered with their respective professional regulatory bodies.

'Healthcare organisation' refers to any organisation specifically set up for healthcare provision and delivery, e.g. Acute NHS trusts, Foundation trust, Teaching NHS trust, GP practice, nursing home, primary healthcare centre, etc.

Frontline healthcare managers (FHMs) is the term applied throughout the book to refer to healthcare professionals who have frontline management responsibilities for a designated group of patients, a team of staff or a practice setting. This responsibility may be for the duration of a span of duty (e.g. managing the practice setting) or may be more permanent in nature (e.g. managing a team of staff or a group of patients). The term is used as a way of differentiating between the role and responsibilities of the first-line manager from those of middle and senior managers.

See Glossary for definitions of various management and leadership terminologies at the back of this book.

1

Leadership and Management in Contemporary Healthcare

Chapter Objectives

The chapter objectives for frontline healthcare managers in relation to leadership and management in contemporary healthcare are:

- Identify the significance of effective leadership and management in healthcare, and the pre-registration education that newly qualified healthcare professionals will have received for leading and managing care delivery;
- Stipulate the wide range of roles and duties undertaken by FHMs specifically in relation to their leadership and management responsibilities in practice settings;
- Articulate the contemporary demographic, social, economic, technological and political contexts in which health services are currently provided;
- Explain the current legislation, policies and strategies that underpin care delivery and their relevance for FHMs in their leadership and management roles;
- Analyse workforce requirements, and the issues they pose in relation to health and social care provision and delivery; and
- Appreciate the role of professional regulation of care professions and codes of practice that care professionals must abide by, for compassionate, competent, safe and effective care delivery.

Introduction

With almost 20% of the UK government's total annual expenditure being spent on healthcare, just under half of which is spent on the workforce of well over one million 'full-time equivalent' employees just in England (King's Fund, 2019a), the ways in which the money allocated to each NHS trust annually is spent simply have to be 'managed' carefully and with accountability, while ensuring that the goals of the NHS are achieved in full. For England, these goals are declared mostly in the *NHS Constitution for England* (Department of Health and Social Care [DHSC], 2019a), and the *NHS Long Term Plan for England* (NHS England, 2019a), as well as in several other associated UK policy documents.

The *NHS Constitution* indicates, for example, that the NHS provides a comprehensive service, available to everyone in England, irrespective of gender, race, disability, age, sexual orientation, religion, belief, or marital or civil partnership status; and that it has a duty to each and every individual whom it serves, and must respect their human rights. It includes the statement that leadership is essential to ensure that money allocated for health and social care services achieve maximum standards of care, and that the money is spent efficiently.

Thus, management and leadership form the foundation for ensuring safe, effective and highest standards of care delivery, and for healthcare resources to be distributed equitably. It could be argued that all healthcare employees need to exercise effective management and leadership regarding healthcare resources, which includes personnel all the way from the Secretary of State for Health to senior healthcare managers, and to frontline healthcare managers (FHMs), as well as healthcare departments not directly involved in patient care. It involves not just management of funds, it also involves management of all human and non-human resources (e.g. equipment, salaries, etc.) with their associated costs.

As with all healthcare managers, the FHM's day-to-day duties span a wide range of activities, which in effect can be grouped largely under six main areas, namely:

- Organising care for the span of duty and beyond;
- Care and treatment activities;
- Managing staff and other resources within their areas of responsibility;
- Teaching and educating colleagues, students and patients;
- Engaging with research and the evidence base for practice; and
- Leadership.

These duties and roles are also grouped as 'the four pillars' of advanced clinical practice for health and social care professionals which are: (i) clinical practice; (ii) leadership and management; (iii) education; and (iv) research (Health Education England, NHS Improvement [NHSI] and NHSE, 2017: 8; NHS Employers, 2019a). Since this book focuses predominantly on the leadership and management duties of FHMs, this first chapter starts by highlighting the significance of leadership and management in today's care provision and delivery, and briefly the pre-registration educational preparation for the responsibilities and duties that newly registered healthcare professionals (NRHPs) and FHMs will collaboratively engage in through being part of an inter-disciplinary healthcare workforce.

Subsequently, the chapter concentrates on the prevailing demographic and social context of the UK that determines healthcare needs and services, including healthcare policies, strategies and legislation that influence treatment and care of health problems that healthcare professionals and frontline managers manage in their daily duties. It thereby contextualises the FHM's duties vis-à-vis the current aims and principles of the National Health Service (NHS), and considers the requirements and impact of the *Health and Social Care Act 2012* (HSCA), and the *NHS Long Term Plan for England* (NHS LTP) and subsequent strategy and guidelines.

The chapter also considers briefly the role of care professions regulators, professional bodies and codes of practice that healthcare professionals must abide by.

The Significance of Effective Leadership and Management in Healthcare

Leadership for high-quality care delivery has always been of utmost importance as effective leaders of healthcare professions have shown the ways for best practice over the years. Effective organisation and management of care signifies a satisfied workforce and content service users. Educational preparation for these roles aims to enhance the effectiveness of both leadership and management in healthcare.

The *Healthcare Leadership Model's* (NHS Leadership Academy, 2021) nine-dimensioned framework of the key characteristics, attitudes and behaviours of effective healthcare leaders provides guidance on ways in which leadership should be applied in care delivery settings. Several other leadership frameworks and models can be found in the general literature: for example, Kouzes and Posner's (2017) research-based 'Five Practices of Exemplary Leadership' model, which also identifies the top four characteristics that followers believe good leaders should have – see Figure 1.1.

Following an analysis of clinical leadership in relation to sub-optimal care in healthcare settings, Whitby (2018) concludes that the leadership of frontline nurses is a major determinant of patients' experience of healthcare and their perception of the quality of care they receive, and that nurses and other healthcare professionals are well placed to improve organisational cultures if the appropriate support and training is available.

Furthermore, research by various other parties on, for example, clinical leadership, often more focused on specific disciplines, is continuously being conducted

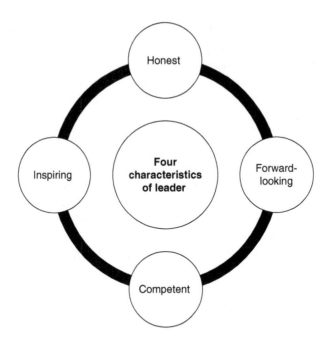

Figure 1.1   Top four characteristics that followers believe each leader should have

and their findings published. For instance, a cross-sectional survey of a randomly selected sample of 378 registered nurses working in direct patient care in acute care hospitals found that transformational clinical leadership by staff nurses is significantly associated with decreased adverse patient incidents (Boamah, 2018).

Several systematic reviews of literature have also been published. For example, one review conducted by Sfantou et al. (2017) to examine the effects of leadership styles on quality of healthcare revealed that leadership is a core element for enabling well-co-ordinated and integrated provision of care, from both patients' and healthcare professionals' points of view.

On the other hand, there have been several instances of poor leadership in health and care services over the last two decades, which have resulted in harm to service users. One instance is of extensive patient neglect at a UK hospital (Francis, 2013), another is the abuse of people with learning disabilities at other UK hospitals (BBC One *Panorama*, 2019), and yet another is failures of clinical care in a UK maternity unit (Wise, 2015). Often, poor leadership is the reason for such malpractice.

External monitoring of quality of care and treatment in all health and social care settings is regularly formally conducted by the Care Quality Commission (CQC), which also publishes details of instances of poor practice and thereby risk of harm to service users. Furthermore, in line with care profession regulators' fitness to practise duties, the Nursing and Midwifery Council (NMC), General

Medical Council (GMC) and other professional regulators publish proceedings of instances of neglect or other types of professional malpractice by individual registrants that have been reported to them.

When malpractice surfaces, effective management and leadership entails instantly resolving the situation, and learning from each incident so that appropriate safety measures are instituted to prevent recurrence, both locally and nationally, as discussed in some detail in Chapter 10 of this book.

Effective leadership in contemporary care delivery is often based on the principles of collective leadership, which put simply entails all team members endorsing and participating in leadership activities; and is also referred to as 'shared leadership'. Leadership in healthcare is examined in extensive detail in Chapter 3 of this book.

What Is Effective Care Management?

Having considered the significance of effective leadership, the next area to consider is effective organisation and management of care, which is of course the main role fulfilled by FHMs in the course of their daily duties. Frontline managers' responsibilities and duties include planning and prioritising, organising, delegating, guiding and supervising clinical activities, as they apply their management expertise to ensure service user outcomes are achieved through the delivery of high-quality care, whereby they also achieve the organisation's operational objectives.

ACTION POINT 1.1
Duties and roles of care setting managers

Focus on the day-to-day 'real life' management duties that FHMs in your workplace perform, and the issues that they deal with. Then, drawing on your own professional experience, make a comprehensive list of many of the professional activities that FHMs engage in over a number of spans of duty (or shifts). Consider also the components stated in Figure 1.1 and identify those activities undertaken over:

- a particular shift
- a 24-hour period
- a one-week period
- a period of one month, or a year.

Consider their duties in relation to dealing with routine as well as with unexpected events during different spans of duty. You can undertake this activity individually, or with colleagues, or in small groups.

You should have been able to identify several managerial duties that FHMs engage in regularly and, given ample time, you should be able to add to the list that you have compiled in response to Action point 1.1, especially when considering the less frequent activities that managers engage in during a whole week, a month, or a year. From the point in time when FHMs start their span of duty, they engage in multiple care activities, such as receiving reports on service users' progress and care needs; and allocation of individual service users to team members. Out of a long list of frontline health and care setting managers' managerial activities identified by RNs and finalist pre-registration student nurses, a random list of ten of these are:

- ensuring everyone in the care setting follows health and safety rules for staff, patients and visitors;
- managing resources – human and material;
- hands-on clinical interventions and evaluating care delivery;
- co-ordinating care and motivating inter-disciplinary team members;
- participation in management initiatives;
- supervision of learning, preceptoring, training and education;
- managing duty roster, identifying annual leave;
- ensuring all abide by code of practice, e.g. confidentiality;
- checking individual monitors, handheld devices, computers, etc. are functioning correctly;
- involvement in clinical governance activities, e.g. audits, collecting statistics.

Your answers to Action point 1.1 naturally will have indicated that the FHM is both a care practitioner and a care manager–leader. Groups of roles and activities of FHMs are addressed by the main areas covered within the chapters of this book, as illustrated in Figure 1.2.

Managerial role components and a range of perspectives on effective management in practice settings are analysed in extensive detail in Chapter 4 of this book, and in the context of training in management skills in Chapter 10.

ACTION POINT 1.2
Developing your own management and leadership knowledge and competence

Having had some knowledge and experience of management and leadership development during your pre-registration programme, as well as since accessing your current post, consider which of the day-to-day activities and responsibilities that you engage with as a registrant will enable you to enhance your management and leadership capabilities, particularly in relation to teamwork, delegation, etc.

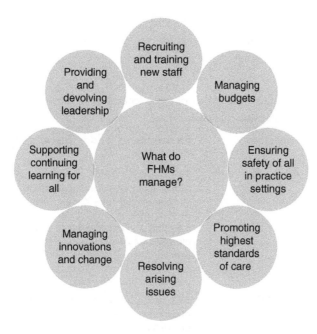

Figure 1.2   Grouping the management roles and activities of frontline healthcare managers

It is recognised that healthcare professionals careers take different forms, in that while some professionals choose increasing responsibility in care settings, others choose a more lateral career journey, moving to different specialism or care settings (HEE, 2015: 53). The HEE also recognises professional development into management and leadership as one of the career pathways in its 'nursing career framework' for healthcare professionals.

Pre-registration Education for Leading and Managing Care Delivery

Pre-registration nursing, midwifery and AHP education programmes incorporate knowledge and competence in leadership and management that students have to develop during their preparatory programme. For example, in the NMC's (2018a) *Standards of proficiency for registered nurses* under the 'platform' 'Leading and managing nursing care and working in teams', a number of knowledge and competence areas are identified, examples of which are presented in Table 1.1 below. There are 12 outcomes specified under this 'platform', and there are further leadership- and management-related outcomes under other platforms, such as under 'Improving safety and quality of care' and 'Co-ordinating care'.

The HCPC (2018) standards of proficiency (SOP) for all AHPs are based around 15 generic statements; and those for midwifery under six domains; and those for nursing under seven platforms.

Table 1.1   Examples of standards of proficiencies across healthcare professions that address leadership and management

Healthcare professions	Examples of leadership and management outcomes
Nursing (under platform 5) (NMC, 2018a)	5.1 understand the principles of effective leadership, management, group and organisational dynamics and culture and apply these to team working and decision-making 5.5 safely and effectively lead and manage the nursing care of a group of people, demonstrating appropriate prioritisation, delegation and assignment of care responsibilities to others involved in providing care
Midwifery SOP (under Domain 5) (NMC, 2019)	5.19 safely and effectively lead and manage midwifery care, demonstrating appropriate prioritising, delegation and assignment of care responsibilities to others involved in providing care 5.20 demonstrate positive leadership and role modelling, including the ability to guide, support, motivate, and interact with other members of the interdisciplinary team
AHPs: Dietitian (under generic statements 1 & 13) (HCPC, 2013 [being reviewed])	1.2 recognise the need to manage their own workload and resources effectively and be able to practise accordingly 13.3 understand the concept of leadership and its application to practice

---

ACTION POINT 1.3
Leadership competencies for your profession

Check the SOP for your profession to see for yourself that they do indeed include leadership development, and what else they say in addition to the outcomes and competencies mentioned in Table 1.1.

Check also the specialist practice skills, such as Advanced Clinical Practice (NHS Employers, 2019a) to identify the outcomes and competencies related to leadership included in the role.

Both pre-registration and specialist/advanced practice competencies are easily available on the internet.

Learning to lead and manage care occurs through students taking mandatory theory modules on these activities at university, as well as through practice learning during practice placements with the support of practice learning supervisors. In practice learning, students are exposed to management and leadership activities when they are asked to be responsible for managing the care of a bay of four patients on an acute ward, for example, or by being given a small carefully selected case load to manage in community settings. They do this under direct, then later indirect, supervision, with their supervisors at hand to assist them or for consultation as and when required.

Providing Health Services within the Contemporary Social Context

Having highlighted the importance of leadership and management in care provision, and identified some of the day-to-day duties of FHMs so far in this chapter, this section briefly examines the contemporary social context within which health and social care is provided, which includes the nature of the population (demography) and the incidence of health problems (epidemiology), as well as the expectations of the healthcare employees in the twenty-first century.

The NMC (2018a: 3) reinforces the need to be aware of the social context of care by stating that registered nurses (RN) 'work in the context of continual change, challenging environments, different models of care delivery, shifting demographics, innovation, and rapidly evolving technologies'.

Demographic influences on healthcare needs of the population

The United Kingdom (UK) population for whom the NHS provides care and treatment amounted to approximately 66.4 million in mid-2018 and is projected to be 70.4 million by 2030 (Office for National Statistics [ONS], 2020). The ONS further highlights, for example, that there were 12.2 million people (18.3%, i.e. one in five people) in the UK in the 65 years and over age group in 2018, which is projected to increase to over 14 million people (21.2%) by 2030. It also documents life expectancy for males and females, number of childbirths per woman, how the population density varies across the UK, etc.

As in various parts of the world, population increases also signifies the need for increases in contemporary health and social care provision, and the increase in the number of older people is also associated with an increase in those with long-term health problems, such as cardio-vascular diseases, kidney problems, respiratory problems and lung cancer, diabetes, etc. (NHSE, 2019a), and consequently rising demands on health services. Accordingly, as people live longer, the use of health services by people over 65 also increases exponentially; that is, generally older people use health services more than younger people (NHSE, 2017a).

The population's healthcare needs have to be gauged to determine the nature and amount of care, prevention and treatment required by the population. In addition to illnesses associated with ageing, there are also more demand for services that cater for people with mental health problems, for children and young people with cancer, etc.

Since the UK government provides health services for every UK citizen, it also has to ensure adequacy of health service provision and funding. Paradoxically, there are newer and more effective methods of treatment and cure of health conditions for which there were limited treatment options in the past, or which were deemed untreatable, based on the development of new technologies and innovations in treatment.

Not only does increasing age lead to more use of health services, the availability of newer more effective methods of treatment also increases the cost of care provision. This is further complicated by rising service user expectations and litigation. Thus, there are considerable financial challenges for the NHS, whose annual budget for the UK for 2020/2021 was of approximately £178 billion, and £36 billion for personal social services (HM Treasury, 2020; The Times Budget, 2020: 16).

The healthcare budget equates to almost one-fifth of the government's total spending each year, and to sustain this trend of increasing NHS funding, the NHSE (2014a), for example, indicated that efficiency savings of around £30 billion needed to be made by March 2021. Efficiency savings and efficient management of NHS funds has been a recurring theme within healthcare provision and healthcare delivery for around three decades, and still is, as noted in different parts of this textbook.

However, the NHS LTP (NHSE, 2019a) also recognises that NHS productivity has improved at a faster rate than the overall UK economy (efficiency), which shows that efficiency efforts have been effective (financial management of health and social care will be explored further in Chapter 5 of this book). It asserts that overall, 'For all major conditions (e.g. cancer, cardiovascular disease, male suicide) the quality of care and the outcomes are now measurably better than a decade ago' (p. 44) and forecasts that they will continue to improve. NHS England (2017a) indicates that outcomes of effectiveness, safety, patient satisfaction with healthcare and waiting times are generally good in the UK and have been improving.

The nature of the healthcare workforce in the twenty-first century

New technology tends to affect all types of jobs over the course of time. Moreover, for various reasons, the nature of the healthcare workforce has also been changing with, for example, creation of new roles such as 'lead nurse', clinical nurse specialist, clinical pharmacists, physician associates, nurse/therapy consultant, community matrons, and an increase in the number of healthcare support workers (HSWs) employed as part of workforce redesign. Roles that transcend disciplines and organisational boundaries are increasingly being established with teams that provide both health and social care. There are also changes in shift patterns such as twilight shifts, 12-hour shifts and annualised contracts.

In *We are the NHS: People Plan for 2020/2021 – Action for us all*, NHS England (2020a) indicates that service users across England are served by 1.3 million employees working in the NHS and in NHS-commissioned services, along with millions of employees working in social care and public health services, in addition to individuals in the voluntary sector. Alternatively, the King's Fund (2019a) indicates that the (whole of the) NHS is the largest employer in Europe with a workforce of 1.4 million health-social care staff, which takes approximately 45% of the NHS operational budget.

(Just a note on the word 'operational' to indicate that operational budget or operational planning normally refers to one-year budgets or plans, and 'strategic' normally refers to five-year or ten-year plans or budgets, sometimes two-year.)

However, with 100,000 vacancies unfilled in the health service in early 2020 (Lay, 2020: 2) due to lack of suitable candidates, and also high attrition rate on some undergraduate health profession courses (Jones-Berry, 2018), workforce shortfall presents as a major issue in health services.

Furthermore, the *Next Steps on the NHS Five Year Forward View* (NHSE, 2017a: 55) notes that, 'The NHS in 2020 is going to be looking after more patients, …. We are therefore going to need to continue to improve productivity and grow our frontline workforce, especially in priority areas such as nursing, mental health, urgent and primary care.' It identifies a number of measures for increasing the number of RNs, doctors and AHPs, and particularly identifies shortage of endoscopists, ultrasonographers, radiologists, etc.

Consequently, the government has made a concerted effort to increase staff numbers through further training redesigns (e.g. apprenticeships) and created new and innovative roles (e.g. Registered Nursing Associate [RNA] and physician's assistant).

From health services employers' perspective, employees are expected to contribute to the delivery of the aims of NHS Constitution and the government's annual mandate to NHSE. Conversely, employee expectations from their employers is also gradually changing. Prevailing expectations of new recruits include the following:

- flexible shift patterns;
- part-time working;
- different shift patterns, twilight shifts and 12-hour shifts;
- opportunities for continuing learning and further training;

- career advancement opportunities towards future specialisation and advanced practice;
- a safe place to work (Health & Safety Regulations);
- many prefer a career, others just a job;
- teamworking;
- sufficient pay.

A survey of employers reported by Muller-Heyndyk (2019) reveals that employers believe that top priority for 98% of employees is flexible working hours, and for 89% it is more agile working (flexibility regarding time and place the employee works). Other preferences include consideration of employees' mental health, diversity and inclusion, and parental leave.

Following an examination of the social and demographic contexts of care provision, this next section provides an account of the most influential recent and current legislation and policies that directly influence care provision, along with novel mechanisms and models of care that are unfolding.

Earlier Policies and Strategies that Continue to Influence Care Delivery

Various policies and strategies have markedly influenced the day-to-day duties and responsibilities of FHMs recently, as also does each profession's code of practice, national and local guidelines, government legislation, as well as research and audits. Healthcare policy in the UK often emanates from the governing political party's goals and policies for care provision.

A policy constitutes a set of directives that has been officially agreed by a specified group of people, a business organisation, a government or a political party, along with specific actions that must be taken in particular situations or settings (e.g. no smoking policy). A strategy, on the other hand, comprises a well-designed plan of action related to clear goals and is, therefore, a blueprint of activities for five to ten forthcoming years.

The overarching legislation that currently governs healthcare is the *Health and Social Care Act 2012* (HSCA) (Legislation.gov.uk, 2012), under which various policies and strategies for healthcare are specified. Legislation is another word for an Act of Parliament, a law. Some of the recent legislation, policies and strategies that continue to influence health and social care in UK include the following, details of which can easily be found on the internet.

- *The NHS Plan – A Plan for Investment, a Plan for Reform* (DH, 2000b)
- *Our Health, Our Care, Our Say: A New Direction for Community Services* (DH, 2006)
- *High Quality Care for all – NHS Next Stage Review Final Report* (DH, 2008a)

- *The Equality Act 2010* (Home Office, 2010)
- *Equity and Excellence – Liberating the NHS* (DH, 2010a):
- *The Care Act* (Legislation.gov.uk, 2014; DHSC, 2016a, 2020b)

The Care Act (Legislation.gov.uk, 2014; DHSC, 2016a, 2020b), for example, addresses social care in England. Its main purpose is to specify local authorities' duties in relation to assessing the needs of adults who are at risk of abuse or neglect, and their eligibility for publicly funded care and support, as well as for those who care for them. It aims to subsequently ensure the wellbeing of people at such risk, which is followed by personalisation of care services, thereby putting the person at the centre of the care process. The mechanism is facilitated by local authorities, in collaboration with CQC, HEE and the Health Research Authority.

Government White Papers such as *Integration and Innovation* (DHSC, 2021), are sometimes preceded by a Green Paper or other form of consultation publication, which in turn is usually preceded by a period of verbal consultation within the DHSC. On publication of such Papers, members of the public and professional organisations comment on their content, which are taken into consideration to produce a government Bill, which in turn later becomes an Act of Parliament.

Recent healthcare policy has endeavoured to steer away from healthcare targets, to focus on quality of care (e.g. DH, 2008a). However, even if not explicitly stated, targets for healthcare will remain as they also constitute health service goals, as in the 2019/2028 NHS LTP (NHSE, 2019a). Targets for NHS trusts to achieve include waiting times in accident and emergency (A&E) departments, faster cancer diagnosis, etc. When targets are set, NHS trusts have to report regularly on progress, and the LTP (discussed shortly in this chapter) identifies the issue that 'Key waiting time targets are being consistently missed …' even 20 years after the publication of *The NHS Plan* (DH, 2000b).

ACTION POINT 1.4
NHS Targets for your specialism

Are you aware of targets for care provision and delivery that have been set by the government for your specialist area, and/or for your department at your place of work? Ask a senior colleague if unsure. If there are targets, how well does your department meet those targets?

Despite the comment about targets in the LTP mentioned above, on-and-off reports and policies have suggested a move away from targets, and focus on quality of care, patient involvement and so forth. However, there are benefits and drawbacks related to NHS targets. For example, Smyth (2020) reports that having A&E targets saves 15,000 lives a year, in that the knock-on effect of meeting the

A&E four-hour waiting time target is that patients get admitted to hospital beds, and thereby access treatment. On the other hand, for those patients who are not seen within the four-hour limit, their wait can be even more protracted. Furthermore, targets tend to be aspirations of governments and unscientific, and consistently missing targets suggests that they are unrealistic. As Lacobucci (2019: 1455) identified in the *BMJ*, targets often remain unachieved, and 'they don't work'.

Healthcare organisations and systems then need to translate policies, such as targets, and assess the impact on their day-to-day and longer-term activities, which may include organisational strategies, policies and guidance for employees that the FHM needs to be knowledgeable of, and work within, as both a manager and employee of the organisation. The FHM needs to be able to create space to identify the impact of government health and social care policy and their objectives, and how they will affect their profession and the patients and service users within their practice setting. Four of the most influential current policies and strategies are examined in the next section.

Current Healthcare Strategies, Policy and Legislation that Affect Daily Care

The policies and strategies that will now be examined are those that affect current care provision and delivery directly, with their implementation and impact continuously monitored. Other longer-term documents and policies remain in force, such as the Equality Act 2010, the work of CQC, that of the National Institute for Health and Care Excellence (NICE), etc. This section on current healthcare strategies, policy and legislation focuses on the *NHS Constitution for England, The Health and Social Care Act 2012, Five-Year Forward View* and *The NHS Long Term Plan*.

The NHS Constitution for England

With the purpose of continually reaffirming the philosophy and aims of the NHS, which was established back in 1948, the DHSC (2019a) has published the *NHS Constitution for England* (first published in 2009), which re-asserts that the NHS operates with 'a common set of principles and values' for the UK public, and that the content of the *NHS Constitution* is legally binding. The constitution is reviewed regularly, as all policy documents should be, and essentially re-states the NHS's commitment to its principles and values, and the rights, pledges, duties and responsibilities of the various parties involved. These principles and values include:

- Access to NHS services is based on clinical need, not an individual's ability to pay, and therefore free of charge in the majority of circumstances.

- The NHS works across organisational boundaries in partnership with other organisations in the interest of patients, local communities and the wider population, working jointly with local authorities, other public sector organisations and a wide range of private and voluntary sector organisations.

One of the rights of the public declared in the *NHS Constitution* is the right to receive NHS services free of charge, the right to access NHS services, and the right to receive care and treatment that is appropriate for them, meets their needs and reflects their preferences; and healthcare providers cannot renege on this, and full compliance is expected of them.

Nonetheless, although the NHS caters for healthcare in all four UK countries through NHS England, Health and Social Care in Northern Ireland, NHS Scotland and NHS Wales, funding for provision of healthcare, public health and social services vary to some extent across the four nations. This is because in 1999, the responsibility for these services was devolved to the Northern Ireland, Scotland and Wales governments through their national assemblies, along with the power to decide on their own policy priorities to meet the specific needs of the countries' own populations (NAO, 2012).

On comparing the healthcare needs of the population of the four nations and healthcare provision, the NAO (2012) and Nuffield Trust (2014) observe for example that:

- Prescriptions charges are paid by service users only in England, not in Scotland, Wales and Northern Ireland.
- Average life expectancy at birth, and therefore health needs, varies between the nations, for men in Scotland this being 75.9 years to 78.6 in England, and for women this being 80.4 in Scotland to 82.6 in England.
- Scotland has more GPs per head of population than any of the other three countries.
- England spends less on health services per person than the other three countries.

The Health and Social Care Act 2012

One of the main aims of the Health and Social Care Act 2012 (HSCA) was to build upon reforms that had already been implemented during preceding years, and to launch mechanisms for improving healthcare continuously. The mechanisms in the current structure of the NHS therefore is largely still based on the directives in the 2012 HSCA, which was eventually passed after several adjustments were made to components in the initial *Equity and Excellence* (DH, 2010a) White Paper, and came into effect in 2013.

Subsequent changes include setting up of NHSI in 2016, which replaced five organisations including NHS finance inspector *Monitor*. Almost a decade after the HSCA, further changes were made based on the White Paper *Integration and Innovation* (DHSC, 2021). See Figure 1.3 for a diagrammatic illustration of the current structure of the NHS in England.

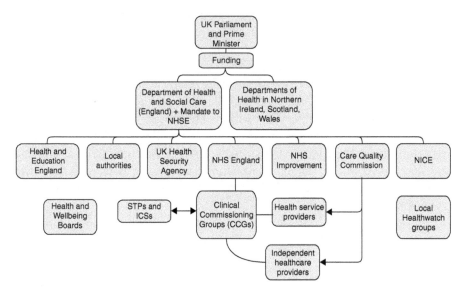

Figure 1.3   Structure of NHS in England

Note: Public Health England was replaced by UK Health Security Agency (UKHSA) in late 2021; CCGs will be dissolved and replaced; and ICSs will become Integrated Care Partnerships.

Overall, the organisational structure of the NHS has changed quite a few times over the seven decades of the NHS so far. More consistent, however, has been the range of service providers which in England include NHS trusts, NHS foundation trusts (163 in total in England), community healthcare NHS trusts, NHS mental health services, ambulance service NHS trusts (all totalling around 230 trusts); and independent providers (private hospitals, care homes, hospices, etc).

As illustrated in Figure 1.3, a number of key mechanisms were established under HSCA, which included the creation of NHS England, the formation of Clinical Commissioning Groups (CCG) (but due to be dissolved and replaced in 2022), and the transfer of public health to local authorities. Other 'executive' organisations instituted subsequently include NHS Resolution, Health Research Authority, NHS Digital and Social Work England. Briefly, the functions of the most prominent mechanisms developed under the Act are as follows.

NHS England (NHSE)

As one of the most prominent organisations that were set up under the HSCA in 2013, NHSE holds the budget for health service provision under the NHS in England. NHSE then distributes approximately 65% of the £130 billion budget for the NHS to the 106 CCGs in England (e.g. NHS Confederation, 2021), and holds healthcare providers to account for spending money effectively and efficiently. The remaining 35% of its budget is divided amongst local authorities and public health, on primary care and on direct commissioning of national level specialised services (provided in relatively few hospitals), for armed forces' serving personnel and their families, etc.

The NHSE combined with NHSI in 2019, and jointly their main purpose is to deliver the goals set out in the *NHS Long Term Plan for England* (NHSE, 2019a) by providing national direction balanced with local autonomy to secure the best outcomes for service users (NHSE, 2020b). The combined NHSE and NHSI (NHSE+I) currently operate through seven regional teams, namely East of England, London, Midlands, North East and Yorkshire, North West, South East and South West, who are responsible for the quality and the financial and operational performance of all NHS organisations in their region. NHSE itself is currently also responsible for ensuring that CCGs meet and maintain standards set out in the HSCA and in the NHS Constitution.

Clinical Commissioning Groups (CCGs)

At the inception of HSCA in 2013, 211 CCGs replaced the 152 primary care trusts who were previously involved in commissioning service user treatment and care, and working with NHSE they took on responsibility for commissioning healthcare across England with the use of the majority of the NHSE budget. Each CCG is led by a Governing Body made up of general practitioners (GPs), a nurse and other healthcare practitioners. They commission care and treatment that is delivered by healthcare providers (i.e. by NHS trusts, NHS Foundation trusts and independent provider groups).

Every one of the 8,000-plus GP practices in England became a member of a CCG, but over the years many CCGs have merged, often in the interest of efficiency, so that in 2021 there were only 106 CCGs (NHS Confederation, 2021). CCGs (also known as clinical commissioners) commission health services including urgent and emergency care (e.g. A&E), maternity and new-born, learning disabilities and autism, community health services, mental health services and elective hospital treatments.

However, CCGs' roles have been evolving to ensure joined-up health and social care, working in close collaboration with local authorities to integrate health-social care. CCGs undergo annual performance assessment by NHSE using 51 indicators which includes financial management, and in 2020, some CCGs were deemed as 'failing' or 'at risk of failing' (NAO, 2018a).

'Commissioning is the process by which health and care services are planned, purchased and monitored' (King's Fund, 2019a). It involves allocation of the finance made available to them to improve the health and wellbeing of their populations. Commissioning takes into consideration the findings of Joint Strategic Needs Assessment (JSNA) of local health and social care needs, which is produced by local HWBs as a 'Joint Health and Wellbeing strategy'. These strategy reports for local communities are generally widely available on the internet, which the reader can access and inspect for themselves to see if the recommendations made reflect local healthcare needs.

An analysis of HWBs' roles is presented by Humphries (2019) whose observations include the deficient assimilation of HWBs' strategies due to the historical health-social care dichotomy, which Sustainability and Transformation Partnerships (STPs) and Integrated Care Systems (ICSs) have been endeavouring to rectify. With the establishment of 42 ICSs covering the whole of England by April 2021, all CCGs will become defunct when the ICSs become fully operational by 2022 (NHS News, 2021), with ICSs taking over CCGs commissioning duties as well.

UK Health Security Agency (UKHSA)

Established under HSCA 2012 as Public Health England (PHE), the UK Health Security Agency (UKHSA) replaced PHE in 2021 apparently because PHE wasn't sufficiently effective in its management of the coronavirus pandemic (*BBC News*, 2020). Public health is about protecting people's health from threats to their health such as epidemics of food poisoning, winter influenza, etc; and it is about health improvement by enabling people to quit smoking, preventing obesity, etc. Understandably, enhancing the health of the public has been on consecutive governments' agendas for several decades. The UKHSA (2022: 1) indicates that it 'is responsible for protecting every member of every community from the impact of infectious diseases, chemical, biological, radiological and nuclear incidents and other health threats.' As with PHE, the UKHSA has replaced several previous public health agencies (including the Health Protection Agency), it provides scientific information and operational leadership at national and local levels, and is answerable to the DHSC.

Health and Wellbeing Boards (HWBs)

In 2013, HWBs were established in all 152 local authorities with adult social care and public heath responsibilities to act as a forum for key leaders from the local health and social care system to work together to improve the health and wellbeing of their local population (King's Fund, 2016a). They also work with CCGs to produce joint strategic needs assessment (JSNA) reports on the health and social care needs of the local population for CCGs and health service providers to consider.

Health Education England (HEE)

Education and training are fundamental for equipping the healthcare workforce with the appropriate set of knowledge, competence and attributes. HEE was established to fund professional education for health services and, therefore, to ensure 'that the workforce of today and tomorrow has the right numbers, skills, values and behaviours, at the right time and in the right place' (HEE, 2020b: 4). It functions as a 'Non-Departmental Public Body' under the provisions of the Care Act 2014 with the aim of providing the 'right workforce' to support the delivery of high-quality healthcare and health improvement to service users.

With more than 160,000 students studying on healthcare profession courses at any one time, and a workforce of well over one million people in the NHS in over 300 different types of jobs with continuing learning needs, HEE's roles are explored further in Chapter 10 in relation to funding of learning for healthcare professionals.

Service providers

One of the most vital components in Figure 1.3 comprise the service providers, namely NHS trusts and independent providers. Another type of NHS trust is *NHS Foundation trusts*, which were first established in 2004 (Nuffield Trust, 2020), and entailed NHS trusts applying for NHS Foundation trust status which would give them more autonomy over management of their allocated finances with minimal interference from government (Legislation.gov.uk, 2012; Gov.uk, 2016).

Other vital mechanisms that form part of the NHS are NHS Improvement (NHSI), Care Quality Commission (CQC), National Institute for Health and Care Excellence (NICE), Health and Wellbeing Boards, Healthwatch, and others identified in Figure 1.3.

NHS Improvement is responsible for overseeing the financial sustainability of NHS trusts and NHS Foundation trusts, as well as independent providers of NHS-funded care, and for offering strategic leadership and practical help to all healthcare providers. Collectively, the NHSE+I utilise their combined resources to ensure best outcomes for service users, through strong governance (quality of care and leadership) and accountability (NHSI, 2020a).

The *Care Quality Commission* (CQC) (2020a) is an organisation that was established before the HSCA, and became operational in 2010 to scrutinise the quality of care in all health and social care services in England, across NHS providers, local authorities, private companies and voluntary organisations. It therefore regulates health and care services such as hospitals, care homes, dentists, care and support in the community, clinics, mental health services, walk-in centres and GP practices by doing spot-checks on whether they meet fundamental standards of quality and safety; that is by inspecting if they are safe, effective, caring, responsive and well-led.

The health of the nation and healthcare have featured as high priorities for most subsequent political parties in government. Numerous short- and long-term strategies for specific aspects of healthcare are issued periodically. For example, two years after the *Health and Social Care Act 2012* (Legislation.gov.uk, 2012), NHSE's (2014a) strategy entitled *Five Year Forward View* was published, followed by a number of subsequent 'forward view' publications.

The 'Five Year Forward View'

As noted already in this chapter, the nature and extent of healthcare services in the UK is determined by a variety of factors, and from different directions. It is influenced by contemporary and anticipated demographic and epidemiological developments, by new government policies, NICE guidelines, patient surveys, major paradigm shifts and research. Accordingly, NHSE (2014a) published the landmark document the *Five Year Forward View* (FYFV), which was also endorsed by CQC, HEE and other significant organisations, to address the anticipated healthcare needs during the subsequent five years. It foresaw major health problems to include those resulting from smoking, being overweight or obese, over-indulgence in alcohol, etc. with an increasing number of people with complex and long-term conditions such as Type 2 Diabetes, mental health problems and cancer.

Specific health issues that NHSE was required to address were published in government's mandate for healthcare provision by NHSE (e.g. DH, 2016), and then annually (DHSC, 2020a). The 2016 mandate included the provision of a seven-day health service, access to a GP on evenings and weekends (coincides with out-of-hospital care), new models of care programmes, etc. It required operational plans to address:

- 62-day cancer waiting standard;
- mental health access standards related to 'Improved Access to Psychological Therapies' (IAPT), and dementia diagnosis;
- publication of avoidable mortality rates.

NHS trusts and NHS Foundation trusts were also required to produce a five-year Sustainability and Transformation Plan (STP) (changed to Sustainability and Transformation Partnerships two years later) to drive the FYFV (NHSE, 2014a: 3) aspirations. The annual mandate was replaced by *The Government's 2019-20*

Accountability Framework with NHS England and NHS Improvement from 2019 (DHSC, 2020a – revised).

However, the focus of FYFV was very much on the 'triple aims' of care provision that STPs were designed to achieve, and has been re-enforced in NHS LTP (NHSE, 2019a). The triple aims (also known as 'national challenges') are: (1) better health and wellbeing for everyone, (2) transformed quality of care delivery for all patients, and (3) sustainability of finances intertwined with efficiency savings (NHSE, 2015a: 17). The concept 'triple aims' is widely adopted in USA healthcare as well (Institute for Healthcare Improvement [IHI], 2020a), and similarly comprise:

- improving the patient experience of care (including quality and satisfaction);
- improving the health of populations; and
- reducing the per capita cost of healthcare.

The triple aims of FYFV were to be achieved through new models of care, such as urgent treatment centres (UTCs) and enhanced health in care homes (EHCH), and when they were set up, they were referred to as vanguards (NHSE, 2015b; Ruane, 2019). Some of these models evolved into 'out-of-hospital' care, which features prominently in LTP (NHSE, 2019a). Subsequent FYFV publications document strategic workings in different healthcare specialisms, such as *General Practice Forward View*, *FYFV for Mental Health*, *National Maternity Review – A Five Year Forward View of Maternity Care*, etc.

ACTION POINT 1.5
Progress with FYFV where you work,
or in your specialist area

Explore with one of your managers, or senior colleagues, if any of the above-mentioned care models and triple aims of the FYFV have been implemented at your workplace or healthcare organisation, and the progress made (that is before going on to the *NHS Long Term Plan*).

Subsequent to the 2014 FYFV, various other documents were published to enable implementation of its objectives, including the *Next Steps on the NHS Five Year Forward View* (NHSE, 2017a), which identified the progress made up to then. Furthermore, the NHS LTP (NHSE, 2019a, p. 18, section 1.22) further identifies the achievements made by 2019, which include the following:

- Rolled out evening and weekend GP appointments nationally, so that accessing primary care is easier and more convenient for patients;

- 100% of the population now able to access urgent and emergency care advice through the NHS 111 online service;
- Begun rolling out urgent treatment centres (UTCs) across the country, with the ability to book appointments in UTCs through NHS 111;
- Introduced new standards for ambulance services to ensure that the sickest patients receive the fastest response;
- Introduced comprehensive clinical streaming at the front door of A&E departments, so patients are directed to the service best suited to their needs on arrival;
- Begun implementing same day emergency care (SDEC), thereby increasing the proportion of people who are not admitted overnight in an emergency;
- Reduced the number of people and the length of stay of patients who remain in hospital for more than 21 days, and freeing up nearly 2,000 beds;
- Hospitals have consequently used fewer inpatient bed days for non-elective patients;
- Continued growth in the number of whole-time equivalent A&E consultants, which are up by 30% over the past five years;
- Rolled out the Emergency Care Data Set (ECDS) to all major A&E departments to enable better tracking of the quality and timeliness of care.

The NHS Long Term Plan

Published in early 2019, the *NHS Long Term Plan* (NHS LTP) (NHSE, 2019a) is the current ten-year government strategy for healthcare provision in England that has been constituted to build on the progress made through the preceding five-year FYFV strategies. As can be expected, the NHS LTP addresses wide-ranging care provision matters such as funding, waiting times, workforce matters, etc., and it addresses clinical priorities including managing cardiovascular disease, maternity and neonatal health, mental health, diabetes, etc.

The NHS LTP, together with relevant subsequent documents, obviously needs to be consulted in detail by healthcare professionals to become fully au fait with its ten-year plan for health services in England. Corresponding similar long-term plans have been published by the appropriate departments in Northern Ireland, Wales and Scotland. The areas addressed by the NHS LTP for England include the following:

- 'Out-of-hospital care' is to be enhanced with such facilities as urgent treatment centres (UTCs), same day emergency care (SDEC) and increasing focus on population health, physical and mental, which would reduce pressure on emergency hospital services.
- Further development and outcome improvement of maternity and neonatal services, children and young people's physical and mental health services, and for major health conditions such as cardio-vascular disease, diabetes, etc.

- Increasing the number of nurses, midwives, allied health professionals (AHPs) and doctors, worded as 'A comprehensive new workforce' plan.
- Digitally enabled care, with widespread digital access to services by patients and healthcare professionals, as well as with predictive techniques supporting local ICSs (see also NHSE, 2020c) to plan and optimise care for their populations.
- Additional funding to be made available to implement the plan, and also better use of capital investment (funding) and existing assets.

Although NHS LTP is a 2019–28 plan that includes a range of 'commitments', the document recognises that various improvements will naturally happen well before 2028, such as halving maternity-related deaths by 2025. The NHS LTP, however, also recognises that there are currently funding, workforce and waiting time issues in the NHS, and extra funds are therefore being made available. However, at the launch of the NHS LTP, different perspectives were provided by non-governmental sectors. For example, while supporting the intentions and aims of the NHS LTP, the Royal College of Nursing (RCN) (2019a) asserted that the continuing problem of staffing shortages needs to be addressed urgently if it is to succeed, a concern also voiced by the Nuffield Trust (2020).

Furthermore, the Health Foundation (2019) indicated that while extra money was being made available to implement the plan, funds for social care and public health was being reduced at the same time – the public health grant was reduced by 25% since 2014–15 – which can have a detrimental knock-on effect. Additionally, several NHS trusts are struggling with financial deficits and waiting times in A&E, with delays in cancer diagnosis and routine operations, and trusts are likely to need support with these while endeavouring to implement the plan.

However, further details have been published in two main documents along with several others focusing on specific aspects of the NHS LTP. First, the *NHS Long Term Plan Implementation Framework* (NHSE, 2019b) which addresses the 2019/20 to 2023/24 period for which dedicated funding is to be provided by the government, and that sets out further detail on how the commitments in the LTP will be delivered. Second is the *NHS Operational Planning and Contracting Guidance 2020/21* (NHSE+I, 2020a) which, as the name indicates, provides numerous specific guidance on ways in which, and new mechanisms by which, the components of the NHS LTP ten-year plan are to be enabled and achieved over the year.

Therefore, in addition to the requirements in the ten-year NHS LTP, the five-year implementation framework (NHSE, 2019b), and the one-year operational planning and contracting (NHSE+I, 2020a), the NHS in England also has to deliver the requirements of the DHSC (March 2020a) mandate to NHS England, and the UK government's NHS Constitution (DHSC, 2019a).

Further mechanisms include the setting up of a new NHS Assembly, which is to be established early so as to strengthen the ability of patients, professionals and the public to contribute their views within an open consultative process.

Noted clearly as a 'key vehicle' for the achievement of both the ten-year NHS LTP and one-year operational plan is also the development of Primary Care Networks (PCNs), which are geographically based networks of approximately four to five GP Practices that collaborate, with each PCN covering 30,000–50,000 patients (Baird, 2020: 1). The aim of the 1250 PCNs is to deliver seven 'national service specifications', which are:

- structured medication reviews (e.g. stopping over-medication of people with learning disability or autism);
- enhanced health in care homes;
- anticipatory care (with community services);
- personalised care;
- supporting early cancer diagnosis;
- cardiovascular disease case-finding; and
- locally agreed action to tackle inequalities.

Baird (2020) adds that by such collaboration, GP practices can share such services as 'first contact' physiotherapists, clinical pharmacists, social prescribing link workers, etc., which is a further improvement from the development of large primary care centres of the past, and polyclinics. PCNs are funded and overseen by CCGs and, as an example, under South Warwickshire CCG, there are seven PCNs covering 32 GP surgeries for a population of 278,000 (South Warwickshire CCG, 2020).

Evolving Modes of Care Provision

Having presented an account of current healthcare strategies, policy and legislation that affect daily care, the following section on evolving modes of care provision explores the new Sustainability and Transformation Partnerships (STPs) and Integrated Care Systems (ICSs) models of care delivery, and briefly the regulation of care professions, and the roles of royal colleges and professional bodies, and the Chief Nursing Officer and Chief Professions Officers roles.

Sustainability and Transformation Partnerships, and Integrated Care Systems

To emphasise the significance of Integrated Care Systems (ICSs) (NHSE, 2020c), it is noteworthy that these are created as part of STPs' activities, and they constitute a fundamental part of NHS LTP. They are instituted to enable healthcare providers, local authorities and third sector bodies to take on collective responsibility for the resources and health of the population of a defined area, with the aim of delivering better, more health-social integrated care for patients (an example is given shortly). Collaboration between the organisations enable early intervention and prevent service users waiting an unduly long time to be seen in A&E departments. ICSs are based on alliance agreements between healthcare organisations involved in commissioning care contracts (e.g. CCGs) and providers, and thereby there is shared commitment to manage resources, to deliver services, and for governance matters.

By June 2019, 14 ICSs had been established covering a third of the English population, and 42 STPs, and it was anticipated that by April 2021 all STPs would develop to become ICSs (NHSE, 2019b: 14), covering the whole of England, which was effectively achieved on time as noted earlier (NHS News, 2021). In a critical review of progress with ICSs, however, Ruane (2019) noted there is an underlying assumption related to ICSs, the NHS LTP, as well as the HSCA, that increased care in the 'community' and service users' own homes will result in reduced hospital admissions, and consequently reduce NHS costs, which might or might not materialise. Ruane also indicates that additional use of community services has often not been accompanied by additional funding.

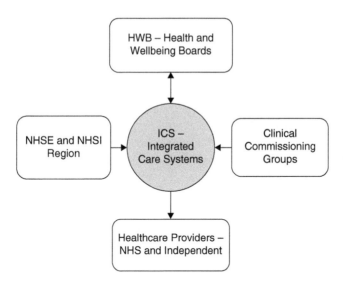

Figure 1.4   Direction of instructions involving ICSs

A significant example of ICS-type care provision is the Greater Manchester Health and Social Care Partnership (2020), whose purpose is to provide integrated health and social care for the Greater Manchester population of 2.8 million people living in its ten boroughs with a £6 billion budget, using a single strategic plan. It involves collaboration and trust between all NHS organisations and councils, primary care providers, NHS England, the voluntary community and social enterprise sector, Healthwatch, the Greater Manchester Combined Authority,

Greater Manchester Police, social care, GP services, mental health services and private sector providers.

Hospital-based services and health-social integrated care is provided through 13 NHS trusts and NHS Foundation trusts and the associated community health services. This has resulted in various benefits including reduced duplication of services across the city, the pooling of financial resources for urgent, intermediate, residential and nursing care delivery, and reduced pressures on hospital providers (Marsh, 2018).

The development of ICSs during 2019 to 2021 period was overseen by NHSE and NHSI's regional teams with delineation of various forms of guidance and support, and their 'performance' and 'support needs' were identified using 'Oversight metrics' which has 65 criteria under the five headings: service models, preventing ill health, quality outcomes, leadership and financial performance (NHSE+I, 2020a).

In the context of endeavours to integrate care systems, Anastas et al. (2019) report on their research which identified facilitators and challenges related to integration. They indicate that facilitators include clear staff roles, flexible scheduling, inter-disciplinary huddles and staff trainings. Challenges to integration include workforce, limited use of electronic health records and differing professional cultures.

At the beginning of the year 2022, a new Health and Care Bill was going through UK parliament, whose aim includes strengthening health-social care integration further. This is due to happen through the formation of Integrated Care Boards (ICBs) and Integrated Care Partnerships (DHSC, 2021). The aim is therefore for ICBs to take on the NHS commissioning functions of CCGs as well as some of NHS England's commissioning functions. ICSs will simultaneously develop into ICPs across England.

How policies are implemented into practice are examined in detail in Chapter 9 under the management of change, and also discussed in Chapter 8 in relation to ensuring quality of care.

Regulation of care professions, and the roles of Royal Colleges and professional bodies

In addition to the government's requirements of health services through its numerous policy directives, the duties of health service staff are also markedly influenced by professional regulators (e.g. NMC, HCPC, General Medical Council [GMC]) of health and social care professions. The role of professional regulators is to maintain live registers of qualified healthcare professionals who are eligible to practise in the UK, publish and regularly review the codes of practice for each healthcare profession; and also to review and periodically publish the content of pre-registration programmes.

The code of practice for nurses, midwives and nursing associates, for example, is stated in the NMC's (2018b) *The Code: Professional standards of practice and behaviour for nurses, midwives and nursing associates.* For healthcare professions regulated by the HCPC, the latest code is published in the HCPC's (2016) *Standards of Conduct, Performance and Ethics*, and all registrants on any of the fourteen professions, which include physiotherapists, clinical scientists, etc. must abide by this code.

Professional regulators also monitor the quality of health and social care delivered to service users, and when alleged malpractice has been reported to them, they conduct investigations and take action as they deem appropriate. The work of the ten regulatory bodies in the UK for health and social care is directed by various Acts of Parliament and scrutinised by the Professional Standards Authority for Health and Social Care (PSA) (2020), which was established under the HSCA 2012. Before the PSA, its roles were fulfilled by the Council for Healthcare Regulatory Excellence in the UK following discovery of malpractice in paediatric cardiac surgery at a hospital in the west of England around the year 2000.

The PSA is an independent UK health regulatory body and is funded partly by the DHSC and the UK health and social care professional regulators (e.g. NMC), and is accountable to Parliament. One of its roles is to co-ordinate standards and good practice amongst the professional regulators. On the other hand, the CQC's role is to monitor the quality of services provided to recipients of health and social care in both the NHS and the independent sector.

Professional bodies and Royal Colleges

In addition to professional regulators, healthcare and social care professionals' roles are also guided by each healthcare profession's own professional body or royal college whose key roles include developing guidelines for safe and effective practice, conducting research, and providing educational support. Healthcare profession colleges include the Royal College of General Practitioners, Royal College of Psychiatrists, Royal College of Nursing, etc.

The Royal College of Nursing, for example, is a professional college which was set up and is sustained by members' subscription, and its activities are collegial in that they build a body of knowledge for their profession through conducting research and through publishing guidelines constituted by experts on the actions to take when faced with specific issues.

The Chief Nursing Officer's and Chief Professions Officers' roles

In addition to healthcare legislation, central policies and national strategies issued by the UK government departments, England, Wales, Northern Ireland and Scotland separately, each also has an appointed Chief Nursing Officer (CNO) who provides leadership and additional key guidance for nurses on the delivery of high-quality care, and to advise on national health issues. The first Chief Midwifery

Officer (CMO) in UK was appointed in 2020, and Chief Allied Health Professions Officers as advocates for AHPs have also being appointed for the four UK countries.

To provide leadership, the CNO for England at NHS England, for example, in collaboration with the then Director of Nursing at the DHSC and Lead Nurse for PHE in 2012, published *Compassion in Practice – Nursing, Midwifery and Care Staff: Our Vision and Strategy* (DH, 2012), which was a strategy for enhancing a culture of compassionate care and treatment across the health services. The strategy set out the components of compassionate care as care, compassion, competence, communication, courage and commitment (the '6Cs'), and these were later incorporated into NHS England's (2016) strategy and framework for nursing, midwifery and care staff. The strategy also supports the work of FYFV and preventive measures to reduce the three gaps in care provision; namely, gaps in health and wellbeing, in quality of care, and in funding and efficiency (i.e. the 'triple aim'). Nurses, midwives and care staff can contribute to the 6C strategy at local levels by for example:

- working with individuals, families and communities to equip them to make informed choices and manage their own health;
- championing the use of technology and informatics to improve practice.

In 2019, the newly appointed CNO for England, while recognising the aims of the NHS LTP (NHSE, 2019a; May, 2019), also endorsed the *Pathway to Excellence* (American Nurses Credentialing Center, 2020) programme, which aligns closely with CNO's national vision to establish an England-wide collective leadership model with a focus on transformational leadership, research and innovation. Collective leadership entails empowering all nurses, midwives and care staff to be involved in shared decision-making within their organisations, and therefore focused on engaging front line staff in key decisions, and thereby also enabling them to lead change. The *Pathway to Excellence* is a 'nursing excellence' framework which is recognised globally.

Chief Professions Officers (e.g. CNOs, CMOs) are furthermore part of the National Workforce Group (NHSE, 2019a: 79, 82) that includes the Chief Allied Health Professions Officer for AHPs, along with NHSE+I, HEE and Royal Colleges, for example, to redress the supply and demand issue of staff for the health services.

Guidance for Working Effectively within Contemporary Care Provision

The following comprises guidelines for working effectively within contemporary care provision that you should find useful.

- As FHM, ensure you remain familiar with new national and local policies (e.g. the *NHS Long Term Plan*) and guidelines by being aware of them through professional journals, professional bodies and information from your senior managers.
- Attend information sessions and workshops aimed at the application of new policies and guidelines to your specialist area of practice and work setting.
- Explore ways in which new policies and all relevant current legislations affect and are being implemented in your employing organisation.
- Be knowledgeable of the clauses in your healthcare profession's code of practice that has been issued by your professional regulator.
- Keep in focus the characteristics that followers believe effective leaders should have, which were identified early in this chapter.
- Constantly reflect on your performance as a frontline manager and the effects they have on team members as well as on service user outcomes.
- Have a working understanding of the roles and interrelationships of various organisations identified in the NHS structure (Figure 1.3) and how they currently relate to your duties and your organisation.
- Be conversant with evolving modes of care provision such as Sustainability and Transformation Partnerships and Integrated Care Systems.

Chapter Summary

Frontline healthcare managers have to have good knowledge of ways in which effective leadership and management is and can be provided in contemporary healthcare. This chapter has therefore examined the broader context of care management, which included considering a range of factors related to the contemporary social context in which care is delivered, and subsequently explored the various policies that affect current care delivery, and has consequently addressed:

- The significance of effective leadership and management in healthcare, and the pre-registration education that newly qualified healthcare professionals will have received for leading and managing care delivery;
- The wide range of roles and duties undertaken by FHMs specifically in relation to their leadership and management responsibilities in practice settings;
- The contemporary demographic, social, economic, technological and political contexts in which health services are currently provided;
- The current legislation, policies and strategies that underpin care delivery and their relevance for FHMs in their leadership and management roles;
- Analysis of workforce requirements, and the issues they pose in relation to health and social care provision and delivery; and

- The role of professional regulation of care professions and codes of practice that care professionals must abide by, for compassionate, competent, safe and effective care delivery.

Further Reading

- The *NHS Constitution* documents the principles and values of the NHS in England, including the rights of patients, the public and staff, as well as the pledges that the NHS is committed to achieve. For further details, see: Department of Health and Social Care, Public Health England (2019a) *Handbook to the NHS Constitution for England*. Available at: www.gov.uk/government/publications/supplements-to-the-nhs-constitution-for-england. Accessed Date: 26 January 2020.
- For the 2019/2028, 10-Year *NHS Long Term Plan* document and details of progress with the plan, see: Department of Health and Social Care (2019b) *The NHS Long Term Plan*. Available at: www.longtermplan.nhs.uk/publication/nhs-long-term-plan/ Accessed Date: 18 December 2019.
- See NHS Providers website for the essential work that this organisation does on behalf of all its members that constitute NHS hospitals, mental health, community and ambulance services that treat patients and service users in the NHS; and that enable them to learn from each other, acting as their public voice and helping shape the system in which they operate. NHS Providers (2020) *About Us*. Available at: https://nhsproviders.org/about-us. Accessed Date: 1 May 2020.

2

Transition from Newly Qualified Registrant to Frontline Manager

---

Chapter Objectives

The chapter objectives for frontline healthcare managers in relation to transition from newly qualified registrant to frontline manager are:

- Appreciate the scope of responsibilities bestowed on newly qualified healthcare professionals and their evolving aspirations from becoming a qualified healthcare professional to becoming a team member;
- Assimilate the requirements of preceptorship programmes for newly registered healthcare professionals (NRHP), the organisational culture in care settings, and delivering and leading person-centred and evidence-informed care competently;
- Develop skills in ways of fulfilling responsibilities related to organising, and leading daily care competently, and managing communication related to delegation, record keeping, and statement writing and report writing;
- Fulfil accountability and deliver ethical practice by ensuring safe, effective and compassionate practice through ensuring adherence to the profession's code of practice, and being accountable to the employer for the achievement of agreed objectives;
- Manage teaching and supervision of team members' learning requirements, and those of students and other learners;

- Be cognisant of challenges encountered by frontline care professionals such as feeling stressed, bullied or harassed, and managing them through pointing to a wide range of formal and non-formal support mechanisms that can be accessed by healthcare professionals;
- Develop competence in personal self-management through caring for own health and wellbeing, and through developing emotional resilience and other strategies, and utilising available resources.

Introduction

Over more than three decades, research in nursing and other healthcare professions has consistently highlighted that despite the three- or four-year-long pre-registration preparation programme to become a qualified healthcare professional, at the point of registration many NRHPs experience awe, anxiety and uncertainty at the prospect of the responsibility of being a registrant, and of the expectations that accompany being employed as a qualified professional. These feelings are in addition to the anticipation and excitement of being employed, and the autonomy, wages, etc. that being a qualified healthcare professional will bring. For these reasons, the final year of the pre-registration programmes incorporates various specific preparation activities for students aimed at easing the transition from student to registrant.

However, the transition from being a novice registrant to one who feels competent and confident to assess, plan and deliver care autonomously in most specialisms takes time. The process can be eased with the appropriate supervised learning and support in situ, which is usually already available in many care settings. Nonetheless, current research still highlights deficits in the transition process, principally in terms of support (e.g. Kumaran and Carney, 2014; Wain, 2017).

Twenty-four different strategies to support graduate transition into the workplace were identified from an integrative review conducted by Rogers et al. (2021), which include preceptoring programme, supernumerary/shadowing time, structured peer-learning activities, clinical skill competency assessments and regular feedback sessions from preceptors. However, Rogers et al also conclude that the efficacy of these strategies should focus on work readiness, which in turn include personal work characteristics of the individual, their work competence, as well as 'social intelligence' and 'organisational acumen'.

While NRHPs' responsibilities, accountability and challenges are examined in detail in this chapter, other key components of NRHPs' duties are only briefly addressed here because they are explored extensively in other chapters of this book, and are signposted accordingly. Continuing learning in healthcare professionals' careers includes learning relevant specialist clinical skills, then later attending specialist or advanced practice courses (see Figure 10.1 for illustration), and components of management training.

On Becoming a Qualified Healthcare Professional

As noted in the introduction, this chapter begins by examining the expectations and experiences of NRHPs. More specifically, it explores the responsibilities of NRHPs as employees beginning to become part of a team of healthcare professionals in practice settings, awareness of the local and organisational culture, delivering and managing person-centred, evidence-based care, and developing confidence and competence after the initial induction programme.

The responsibilities of the newly qualified healthcare professional as a team member

On gaining employment and starting work as a healthcare professional, becoming part of a team is usually a very rewarding experience as NRHPs are normally welcomed by the clinical team. Nonetheless, it often becomes apparent that the responsibilities and workload of the registrant is much more wide-ranging than experienced as finalist students on management practice placements.

As noted in the introduction section of Chapter 1 of this book, healthcare professionals' duties can be grouped under the six headings: clinical role; organising care for the span of duty; managing care resources; engaging with research; educating students, service users and others; and leadership. There are several strands to the registrant's job role that the NRHP has to develop professionally, as partly illustrated in Figure 2.1, and more shortly in this chapter under roles of the FHMs.

Brief details of these job role considerations or demands on NRHPs are as follows:

Social	Work is often a social activity (in teams), belongingness, team-working.
Psychological	Adaptation to the job requirements, rewarding to see patients recover health.
Personal	More responsibility, a salary.
Autonomy	Performing clinical interventions unsupervised professionally and being accountable for each action.
Support	With developing clinical skills and knowledge.
Skill development	The felt need to learn or further develop own clinical interventions skills.
Workload	Registrants' perceptions of workload as comfortable, never-ending, or in-between.

The preparation for transition from final year student to registrant is usually comprehensive, based on the NMC's (2018a) competencies that have to be achieved

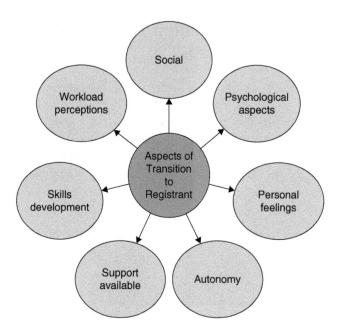

Figure 2.1 Aspects of newly qualified registrant's job role

before being allowed to join the NMC's register, and therefore should be a smooth journey. However, despite the pre-registration educational preparation, issues are likely to surface that will need to be resolved. As, for example, Wain's (2017) qualitative research found, there are situations that would prove tricky for the NRHP to resolve such as inequality in preceptorship provision, protected time with preceptors, and inadequate staffing that may be due to shortage of supply of staff to recruit from, and therefore of time and support.

ACTION POINT 2.1
Registrants' workload

A number of daily professional duties and roles of FHMs were identified in relation to Action point 1.1 in Chapter 1 of this book. Approach a recently qualified registrant and ask them if they could tell you a bit about the following.

1. Their perceptions of their workload
2. What are the effects of not having a practice supervisor to go to for advice and support as a NRHP, which finalist students have?

Several management activities were cited in response to Action point 1.1. Many of the challenges that newly registered nurses (NRN) could encounter as frontline managers will be discussed later in this chapter and throughout this book, followed by support that may be available. A general guide to the employee's responsibilities are outlined in their own job description, which in turn is based on the relevant section of the *Knowledge and Skills Framework* (NHS KSF) (DH, 2004; NHS Employers, 2019b). A number of aspects of NRHPs' responsibilities during the transitional stage are now examined.

Preceptorship programmes for NRHPs

Newly qualified care setting managers' responsibilities in relation to managing learning in the care setting include consolidation of own previous learning as well as substantial new learning, and managing learning for all team members and learners, and education for service users and their carers. It also includes accommodating learning for the wider inter-disciplinary team members. Managing learning implies much of the teaching is performed by appropriate healthcare professionals in the team, not necessarily by the FHM.

For NRHPs, starting work as a qualified professional is a prospect full of hope and anticipation, but can also be anxiety-provoking, which is the reason for the widespread availability of preceptorship programmes, which entails supervised practice for a specified length of time (with some flexibility built in). Structured preceptorship programmes contribute to making care settings more attractive for recruitment and retention purposes as well.

The aim of structured preceptorship programmes is to ease NRHPs into functioning competently as registrants, and being accountable for their practice, as well as to enable further development of their competence in the area of employment. These programmes encompass having supernumerary status and structured protected time for precepteeship, which involve enabling the preceptee to maximise learning while in this role, and maybe constituting a personal development plan. The FHM's role comprises enabling new colleagues' transition from NRHP to competent healthcare professional, and includes providing feedback when in the preceptor role.

Preceptorship constitutes a fully structured time-defined period of supervised clinical learning, and a preceptor is a registrant who has had at least 12 months' experience in the same area of practice as the NRHP, and who is willing to teach, counsel and be a role model for the professional development of NRHPs; that is, to enable them to develop clinical skills, and for socialisation and integration into the team.

While the preceptor role refers specifically to facilitation of practice-based learning for NRHPs, other such roles include 'practice supervisor' and 'clinical educator', which tend to refer to facilitation of learning for pre-registration students while on placement in care settings. The term preceptor also has different meanings in different countries, but in the UK, preceptorship refers to implementing a specified but flexible period of supervised practice for NRHPs. The Department of Health (2010b: 6) defines a preceptor as 'a registered practitioner who has been given a formal responsibility to support a newly registered practitioner through preceptorship'.

So, at care setting level, preceptorship often incorporates its induction programme, which in addition to brief orientation to the care setting includes learning many competencies that are pertinent for service user care in the specific care setting. The organisation's induction programme for all new employees generally include familiarisation with its mission statement and aims, the trust's policies on safety procedures, etc.

ACTION POINT 2.2
Anticipations of NRHPs

As a FHM, think back to the time when you were a NRHP and took your first employment as a registrant on Band 5, and think of your feelings since the point of applying for the post and a few days into the post. Consider your hopes and anxieties as a newly registered healthcare appointee, and jot down these hopes and anxieties, followed by some of the possible reasons for them as well as potential solutions.

Different hopes and apprehensions can be experienced by NRHPs about to start their first employment after gaining their professional qualification and registering it with the relevant regulatory body. Examples of hopes include being initially accepted as a person and a professional by members of the team that the NRHP is joining, and support from them in terms of being allowed to take time to become accustomed with new care interventions and activities. They might hope to be given a comprehensive orientation to the practice setting and associated areas, and systems, introduction to team members and an identified period of preceptorship, and later to be valued and supported for further professional learning.

Apprehensions expressed by NRHPs might include:

- not fitting in with the clinical team;
- isolation (lack of support) due to staff shortages;
- lack of access to preceptor;
- personal expectations of care standards not being met;
- not being valued;
- making mistakes;
- personality clashes;

- aggressive patients/staff;
- lacking in competence, and fear of litigation;
- insufficient professional development time;
- being unable to deal with complaints due to lack of experience.

As can be deduced from the responses to Action point 2.2, the NRHP requires more than orientation to the new care setting and to the healthcare organisation's policies and competencies. To manage some of the new registrants' fears or apprehensions, some of the actions that FHMs can take are as follows. For fear of feeling a lack of support, or of making mistakes, FHMs can encourage NRHPs to ensure they follow the set clinical guidelines and procedures, and learn from more experienced colleagues who they consider to be role models. They can also advise them to attend appropriate structured learning events and activities.

For fear of personality clashes, NRHPs need to learn to resolve these by using systematic problem-solving approaches (see Chapter 7) if they occur. For lack of self-confidence in dealing with complaints, the NRHP can familiarise themselves fully with appropriate policies and procedures, which include documentation. Structured preceptorship or 'facilitated transition' can incorporate discussions on ways to manage such apprehensions.

That NRHPs need support for effective transition from NRHP to confident practitioner has been documented over a number of years (e.g. Kramer, 1974; Labrague and De los Santos, 2020), and the absence of such support tends to lead to dissatisfaction at work and to attrition. Therefore, formal recognition of the role of preceptorship is required by management and a culture of support, along with preparation for preceptorship.

In their cross-sectional study of NRHPs' transition to autonomous professional, Labrague and De los Santos (2020) found that NRHPs' greatest challenges were related to their expectations in the work environment, balancing their professional and personal lives, and that higher levels of reality shock were associated with adverse patient events. They recommend provision of flexible work arrangement, reasonable workload, adequate staffing, limited mandatory overtime and self-scheduling to facilitate a reasonable work–life balance.

However, even relatively recent research has revealed that transition from student to staff nurse remains 'a difficult time for many new graduate nurses, with significant numbers of graduates being dissatisfied, ultimately considering leaving or exiting the profession' (Phillips et al., 2015: 118). To resolve such difficulties, preceptorship should include addressing autonomous working, teamworking, conflict resolution, etc., which should lead to greater levels of job satisfaction, increased commitment to an organisation and thereby staff retention. Staff retention strategies are explored in detail in Chapter 5 of this book in relation to human resources.

Preceptorship programmes tend to vary in length, mode of delivery and content. The *Flying Start* programme (NHS Education for Scotland, 2021), for example, is delivered either entirely online, or in combination with a one-day workshop and subsequent problem-solving support as deemed appropriate.

A few programmes comprise a credit-rated preceptorship module at university, with extensive work-based learning components, but remains without a formal professional preceptor qualification. In the majority of instances, however, preceptorship comprises between six- to twelve-month programmes run by the employing healthcare organisation, with some flexibility built in, depending on the NRHP's individual learning needs. The programmes can include identifying the preceptee's learning style, reflective practice, etc., and they often incorporate induction to the organisation and the practice setting.

On empirical evaluation of a mandatory preceptorship programme for Band 5 NRNs, Forde-Johnston (2017) found that the programme had positive value and improved the experience of NRNs during their first year of clinical practice, amongst several other benefits. The year-long programme content comprised components previously suggested by NRNs, and include communication, team working, documentation, clinical skills, risk assessment and clinical governance.

Furthermore, preceptorship is often also available for registrants who return to practice following a long break in employment, registered professionals joining a new part of the NMC register, individuals returning to practice after re-joining the register, and for qualified nurses coming to work in the UK from other countries (NMC, 2020a).

The FHM may have to take on the preceptor role for one of the novice registrants, with other NRHPs being allocated to other team members who have had preparation to do so. As noted earlier in this section, the ways in which front-line managers manage preceptorship in their care setting is examined further in Chapter 10 of this book.

Organisational culture

New appointees such as NRHPs generally appreciate that each organisation and care setting often have a culture and sub-culture of their own respectively, which in essence refers to the team's values, beliefs, terminologies and abbreviations used, customs, etc. that make them unique. To settle into the team and become a team member who feels they are an integral part of the team, NRHPs need to become aware of the nature of the sub-culture and endeavour to integrate some of the elements in their day-to-day work activities.

Organisational culture that supports high-quality care is explored in some depth in Chapter 8 of this book and in Chapter 10 in the context of learning culture in care organisations.

ACTION POINT 2.3
Organisational culture

Consider the following questions:

1. Does organisational culture have an effect on the level of person-centred care provided in your practice setting, or in another practice setting that you are very familiar with?
2. How does the culture in the practice setting affect how fully NRHPs settle and feel they belong to the setting's team?
3. What are the problems or issues that you have encountered in your endeavour to be fully accepted as a team member, if any? If you encountered difficulties, did you constitute a personal action plan to resolve or overcome these problems?

Delivering and leading person-centred and evidence-informed care

As a role model for learners and team members, and in the interest of highest quality of care, FHMs have to apply person-centred care in their normal day-to-day activities, and do so with confidence. The application of person-centred care is advocated in several policy documents and also explained by many, and FHMs will have examined the concept in detail during their pre-registration programmes.

Detailed explanation of the term is provided by the Skills for Health (2021), for example, which indicates that person-centred care describes care which is responsive to an individual's personal circumstances, values, needs and preferences – care which is specific to the patient's individual requirements and, therefore, focusing on caring about a patient's needs rather than the needs of the service. It is based on four principles:

- Care is personalised.
- Care is co-ordinated.
- Care is enabling.
- The person is treated with dignity, compassion, respect.

Providing person-centred care also means being aware of their spiritual wellbeing, that is person's religious beliefs, it takes into consideration relationships and family members, values and some individuals' need for self-expression, maybe their employment worries, and thereby improving the quality of healthcare provided, and a more positive patient experience while accessing health services.

Furthermore, leadership in person-centred healthcare is enhanced by 'shared values' (e.g. Kouzes and Posner, 2017), which the NHS Constitution (DHSC, 2019a) refers to as 'NHS values'. McCarthy and Rose (2010) refer to professional values as going beyond evidence-based practice (EBP), which is seen as mechanical, and then incorporating humanistic values that are inherent components of holistic care, professional judgement, intuition and considering service users' preferences. Values include care and compassion, awareness of self and of others, respect, maintaining human dignity, tolerance and being ethical, which are also integral to the profession's code of practice (e.g. NMC, 2018b).

Evidence-informed practice is discussed in fair detail in Chapter 9 of this book in relation to managing change and improvement.

Frontline Managers' Responsibilities Related to Organising Care

Frontline managers' responsibilities incorporate leadership in organising care for the shift, and communicating planned care which includes delegation, record keeping and ensuring evidence-based practice. This section explores some of the options available to FHMs for ways of organising day-to-day care.

Organising daily care

An important dimension of the management of service users' care is the day-to-day organisation of their care so that their plans of care are safely, effectively and sensitively implemented, and all objectives of the shift are achieved. Care is of course delivered collaboratively with doctors and AHPs as identified in the patient's individualised care pathway, and is also influenced by various codes of practice, policies, guidance and legislation, as well as service users' individual choice whenever feasible.

Healthcare is provided and delivered 24 hours per day, every single day of the year, and it has to be done efficiently and effectively, and therefore the modes in which care is organised is very important. These modes can affect the results of patient satisfaction surveys, level of complaints, clinical effectiveness and other quality metrics. It is also important to note that a combination of higher number of registrants and lower number of unqualified healthcare staff usually results in higher quality of care (e.g. Francis, 2013), as acknowledged in Chapter 8.

When organising care, FHMs also have to take into account the continuity of care of service users already under their care, the assessment of newly admitted service users and planning their care, individual patients' dependency level, communication with various parties, the resources that are available to them including skill mix (registered to non-registered staff ratio – discussed in Chapter 5) and the level of supervision and developmental needs of junior staff and learners.

The majority of care that FHMs are involved in is based on integrated care pathways (ICPs), which are widely used in acute care settings to manage the decision-making and care processes together with inter-disciplinary input, resulting in improved quality of care, increased patient satisfaction, reduced risk and enhanced efficiency, as noted by Oosterholt et al. (2017).

An ICP can be defined as a multidisciplinary outline of anticipated care and organisation of care processes, for a well-defined group of patients or set of symptoms for an appropriate timeframe, to help a patient progress smoothly through to positive outcomes. Consequently, care pathways comprise a standardised and effective approach that enables mutual decision-making with the service user based on multi-professional assessment of their health problems, and include specification of goals and evaluation points on the patient's journey through health and/or social care services.

Another key benefit of care pathways is that it is a one-stop shop for documentation and record-keeping with inter-disciplinary team members recording their interventions and observations in one document. ICPs can be developed through process mapping (e.g. NHSI, 2020b), which essentially constitutes full details of the service user's anticipated journey through care systems.

However, several generalised care pathways are already available on NICE (2020a), Scottish Intercollegiate Guidelines Network (SIGN) and other organisations' websites for numerous health conditions and interventions, including 'Sepsis: recognition, diagnosis and early management', 'Obsessive-compulsive disorder and body dysmorphic disorder', which tend to begin with a flowchart, and has icons for further details, resources, etc.

For implementation of care, the FHM would be aware of different modes of organisation of care. The most popular current modes of care organisation are named nurse and team nursing (with equivalent titles for other healthcare professions). Other modes that are appropriate for specific settings include key-worker method, case management, care programme approach, task allocation, etc.

The named nurse is a RN with responsibility for delivering and co-ordinating all the care interventions required for a designated service user, thereby ensuring that all required care that is due during the span of duty is delivered. It was instituted several years ago and is also one of the several recommendations of the Francis Report (2013). It has previously also been known as 'case method', 'patient allocation' and 'total patient care' and is consistent with holistic approach and person-centred care.

Team nursing usually comprises a skill mix of team members such as a Band 6 registered practitioner as team leader, a Band 5 registered practitioner and healthcare support workers (HSWs) who are allocated groups of patients for the span of duty or longer. The team leader plans, delegates, co-ordinates, supervises, monitors and evaluates the care delivered, and assigns patients based on the competencies of individual team members. It is based on collaborative teamwork and facilitates the supervision of more junior team members, but also fosters patient satisfaction as it supports the delivery of holistic care.

Many of the ways of organising care initially came into being either from research or as innovations. However, each of these methods can have weaknesses in spite of their advantages, and therefore cannot be applied universally. In particular, for task allocation, several decades ago Menzies (1960) identified problems with this method of care organisation, indicating that task-orientated nursing alienates patients from staff because of the impersonal and mechanical nature of this mode of caring for service users. It demotivates staff and is counter to the philosophy of holistic care, which is a concept and practice that uniquely distinguishes nursing from other care professions.

For the named nurse method of organising care, despite its wide implementation and advantages, it can be challenging when working 12-hour shifts or part-time short shifts. This method also requires a high level of expertise, and the named nurse is accountable for all their actions, as all registrants are of course, and therefore should assume the responsibility only when competent and confident, and under supervision for as long as required especially in more acute settings. They should, however, be able to delegate interventions to other team members including HSWs as appropriate.

From another perspective, from a systematic review of a wide range of ways of organising care compared to team nursing, Fernandez et al. (2012) concluded that with team nursing there are lower incidences of medication errors, significantly lower pain scores, less adverse events related to intravenous medication and earlier discharge from hospital, although there was no difference in incidence of falls, pressure injuries and nurses' job satisfaction.

Frontline healthcare managers would be aware that successful organisation of service users' care, which is often based on ICPs, requires collaboration and effective communication, which is explored next.

Management communication

In addition to being a crucially important element of care delivery, communication also forms a fundamental basis of teamwork. Communication is also examined in fair detail in Chapters 4 and 6 of this book in the context of principles of management in healthcare and of teamworking respectively. Only two forms of management communication – delegation and record keeping – are explored in this section of the book. Suggestions are made in relation to more details regarding statement writing and report writing.

A widely implemented model of day-to-day communication used for handover reports, etc. is the Situation-Background-Assessment-Recommendation (SBAR) framework. SBAR provides an effective means of communication of information to team members which is sufficient and succinct while also supporting a culture of patient safety as well as effectiveness and efficiency.

SBAR focuses attention on healthcare professionals' input throughout the patient journey, and across primary, secondary, community and social care, and its utilisation is acknowledged by NHSI (2018a). Using the example of patient handover (also known as 'handoff') reports, or in everyday communication situations such as telephoning a doctor to request a review of a patient, or transferring the care of a patient to a district nurse or GP, the minimum information that needs to be imparted under the four sections of SBAR are:

1. *Situation:* Your name, title and workplace; the name of the patient and reason for the communication; the issue or concern.
2. *Background:* Relevant information about the patient, e.g. reason for, and date of, admission; procedure of interventions already performed; and the last set of observations.
3. *Assessment:* Your assessment of the current situation, e.g. deteriorating vital signs, is in severe pain, showing signs of delirium.
4. *Recommendation:* What you need, e.g. doctor to assess the patient, district nurse to visit; ask if there is anything you should do while waiting for doctor to arrive; any medication change.

For example, at the handover report or when contacting a doctor regarding a patient with left hip replacement (background) and who is in pain (assessment), etc., if not all team members know each other, then 'situation' does include knowing in what capacity the person reporting is speaking (e.g. as the ward sister, or as a final year student). As for the 'Recommendation' section, more junior team members may be reluctant to make recommendations, but this could also be addressed by the communicator asking the addressee what interventions they recommend are to be performed straightway.

Other examples of when SBAR contributes to improving communication is (1) when the A&E Department or the admission ward at the acute hospital contacts a nursing home to report on a resident who was sent to the hospital; and (2) when the nurse contacts the on-call doctor regarding a patient whose condition is deteriorating.

Evidence of the effectiveness of SBAR includes a review of research by Shahid and Thomas (2018) who concluded that SBAR comprises a structured reliable and validated communication tool which has also shown a reduction in adverse events in a hospital setting, and thereby tends to contribute to patient safety.

Delegation

Recognising that delegation of healthcare duties to appropriately skilled team members is one of the primary functions of frontline managers, this management activity is discussed in detail in Chapter 4 of this book in relation to management communication, where it indicates that the principles of delegation are also identified in the NMC's (2018b) Code of practice, for example, and specific guidelines have been published by the RCN (2017a) and other organisations. It also addresses five styles of delegation identified by Magnusson et al. (2017), as well as stages of effective delegation in Figure 4.5.

Record keeping and record management

Yet another crucial component of FHMs' role is accurate documentation of all care activities. Encompassing documentation, at times referred to as record-keeping, is records management, which reflects the bigger picture of information documented. Accurate documentation as an aspect of the FHM's daily management activity is also analysed in fair detail in Chapter 4 of this book.

Interestingly, the concept has also been analysed in the context of the phrase, 'If it's not written down; it didn't happen ....'. Andrews and St Aubyn (2015) investigated this well-publicised statement made previously in a court of law, and re-emphasise the significance of accurate record keeping of patient-related activities. Consequently, they suggest 6Cs of good record keeping as follows, but it is advisable to read the whole article (details in Further Reading section) and with the NMC's (2018b) code of practice. The characteristic 6Cs of skilled record-keeping are:

1. *Contemporaneous* – complete the documentation as soon after the event as is possible.
2. *Continuity* – date and time all entries chronologically, with the patient's name on each page.
3. *Correct* – clear writing; clear message; clear communication; clear conscience. Write legibly and with clarity, accurately, and without expressing opinions, and without abbreviations if possible.
4. *Claim* – include your name on your records, and your designation, and sign your entries.
5. *Candour* – the quality of being frank and honest about events in the care setting in the interest of maintaining patient safety.
6. *Contain* – maintain confidentiality and store all records according to local policies/procedures.

Statement writing and report writing

Other areas of management communication including statement writing and report writing, which are integral to healthcare professionals' and FHMs' duties. A written statement may be required in relation to an incident in the practice setting. In *Statements: how to write them*, the RCN (2021) indicates that healthcare professionals could be asked to write a statement on an incident as an involved person; or as a witness; or for an inquest or criminal court. The NMC (2018b) code of practice indicates that nurses and midwives have a duty to assist in investigations, which also implies statement writing.

Detailed recommendations on statement writing is also offered by the RCN (2021a), which include ensuring the request to write a statement is itself in writing; not to sign if someone else has prepared a statement for you; and keeping a copy of your written statement. More statement writing guidelines are available over the internet, but the above-mentioned RCN's recommendations constitute comprehensive advice on how to do so safely.

Report writing is often based on a project that you may have led, or an educational visit to explore how an innovation is being applied elsewhere in your specialism. Reports usually start with either 'Terms of Reference' or 'Aims' of the report directly following the title page. You may consider writing an executive summary, but before this, including a contents list with page numbers adds substantial clarity related to what the report is about. Thereafter, it has to have an introduction, and later a conclusion and recommendations. In the body of the report there will be a number of themes, or main areas. Detailed guidelines for writing reports are also generously available on the internet, for example University of Leicester (2018).

Accountability and Ethical Practice

'Registered nurses play a vital role in providing, leading and co-ordinating care that is compassionate, evidence-based and person-centred', states the NMC's (2018b: 3) code of practice, and are accountable for their practice and fitness to practise. As is well documented, healthcare professionals are accountable to various parties. We are accountable to our respective regulatory bodies (e.g. NMC, HCPC), to the patient, the public, our employer, etc. The NRHP is accountable for their practice both as an individual and as part of a team of healthcare professionals.

Accountability and ethical practice can be achieved by ensuring adherence to the profession's code of practice, and accountability to the employer through individual development and performance review (IDPR) meetings, for example.

ACTION POINT 2.4
Your accountability

Remind yourself all parties you are accountable to in the course of your work duties, and for which actions/interventions, and list them.

Healthcare professionals' accountability is clearly identified in their professional regulatory body's code of practice, for example HCPC's (2016) *Standards of Conduct, Performance and Ethics*, and, as the title indicates, codes are based on principles of ethical practice.

Ensuring adherence to the profession's code of practice and duty of candour

The importance of healthcare professionals' code of practice was highlighted in Chapter 1 of this book and, as expected, all healthcare professionals have a duty to comply with all the clauses of the respective professional regulators' code of practice.

Ethical practice constitutes professionalism, which in turn incorporates duty of candour when patient safety incidents occur. In the context of healthcare professionals encountering mistakes, failures and patient incidents, the NMC and GMC (2019: 1) jointly indicate that registrants have to 'be open and honest in reporting adverse incidents or near misses that may have led to harm', which is also a way of achieving and maintaining a culture of quality. Openness, honesty, frankness and truthfulness are states that are consistent with the concept 'duty of candour'.

The CQC (2015) also indicates that it expects all healthcare providers to meet duty of candour requirements, which was also one of the many recommendations in the Francis Report (2013), which asserted the need for transparency, which in turn signifies allowing information about patient incidents, performance and outcomes to be shared with staff, service users and the public. The Report indicated that fulfilling the duty of candour means that any service user harmed through the provision of healthcare is informed of the incident and an appropriate remedy offered, regardless of whether the service user or their family or carer have questioned or raised a complaint about the incident.

The British Association for Counselling and Psychotherapy (BACP) (2018) also suggests that healthcare professionals demonstrate accountability and candour by: (a) being willing to discuss with clients openly and honestly any known risks involved in the work and how best to work towards our clients' desired outcomes by communicating any benefits, costs and commitments that clients may reasonably expect.

Accountability to employer and performance appraisal

Staff performance appraisal and their training needs have been a feature of human resource management for several years. It gathered impetus with the introduction of management by objectives (MBO) (e.g. Drucker, 2007: 11), a style of management that is discussed further in Chapter 4 of this book. As the term implies, the manager has to agree the team member's professional objectives, typically for one year at a time. MBO is the opposite of more autocratic management styles whereupon the manager determines all the employee's work-related activities.

MBO features in the organisation's business plan in the form of operational and strategic objectives, which the organisation's employees have to achieve on behalf of the organisation. Consequently, individual employees' work objectives for the year contributes to the organisation's objectives; the specific objectives will have been negotiated and agreed between the team member and their line manager during IDPR. At IDPR meetings between manager and employee, the focus is on individual employees' strengths and achievements at work as well as their further development and training needs.

Guidance on annual IDPRs for care professionals working in health services is indicated in the NHS KSF (DH, 2004). The framework provides a structure that directly links the care organisation's skill needs for the achievement of its corporate objectives with the individual employee's clinical skills and responsibilities, and their professional development needs. These skills and responsibilities are identified as competence items under six core dimensions (see Figure 2.2).

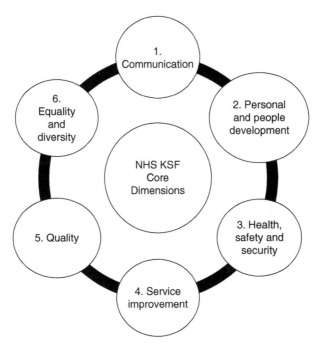

Figure 2.2   Dimensions of NHS Knowledge and Skills Framework

Later versions of the NHS KSF (NHS Employers, 2019b) include the optional leadership and management dimension aimed at more senior roles in response to feedback from employers. Furthermore, to complement the NHS

KSF skills, other frameworks are published by professional organisations. For social work, for example, the 'Professional Capabilities Framework' published by British Association of Social Workers (2020) identifies professional capabilities that can be achieved at different stages during career progression. The capabilities are identified under nine domains which are grouped under the three super-domains purpose, practice and impact that, on qualifying, social workers should be capable of performing competently, before moving on with their careers.

One of the nine domains is professional leadership, under which one of the capabilities is 'contribute to collective/collaborative professional leadership through participating in or initiating purposeful peer support, social work forums and meetings within and/or outside my organisation' (p. 1). The regulator of social workers is Social Work England (2020), which has also published the professional standards that all social workers in England must be competent in, along with other necessary guidance publication on, for example, their education and training, CPD, etc.

More broadly, eight 'job performance factors' have been identified by Arnold et al. (2020), which are:

1. Job-specific core task proficiency
2. Non-job-specific proficiency
3. Written and oral communication
4. Demonstrating effort
5. Maintaining discipline
6. Facilitating team/peer performance
7. Supervision/leadership
8. Management/administration

When preparing for an IDPR or appraisal meeting, the registrant needs to be aware of such job performance factors, but more directly, they should revisit their job description to reacquaint themselves with the components of their job role to self-ascertain their performance over the past year, and identify training needs for either the same post or for career progression, from Band 5 for example to Band 6. This includes constituting a personal development plan (PDP), which is also included in the NHS KSF.

The personal development objectives in PDPs should also meet the criteria for SMART objectives, with the acronym signifying specific, measurable, achievable, realistic (or relevant) and time-bound. These criteria can be applied to all objectives, be they annual objectives or shorter-term ones. However, some of the objectives are less measurable, for example, building working relationship with team members, delivering excellent service, respect and compassion.

ACTION POINT 2.5
Personal Development Plans

The aim of this Action point is to prompt you to create a PDP for yourself to ensure first-hand experience at compiling PDPs, in readiness for enabling more junior registrants to do so.

Based on the six components of healthcare professional roles identified in Figure 1.2, and the seven dimensions of the NHS KSF (those presented on Figures 2.2 as well as the leadership dimension), create a PDP where you identify how you are going to enhance your competence and self-confidence in either of the component areas with a view to enhancing both your own development and service user care.

Teaching and learning supervision

The NRHP role as frontline manager encompasses teaching and practice supervision, which includes supervising students and having current knowledge of students' curricula. It is also FHMs' job requirement to teach all team members as well as service users and their relatives as required. Of course, a vast number of teaching duties are delegated implicitly or explicitly to other appropriately competent registrants. Teaching and supervision of learning duties of frontline healthcare managers is explored in some detail in Chapter 10 of this book.

Challenges for Frontline Care Professionals

Frontline healthcare managers have continuing demands made of them by various parties, who seek further information related to service users, or have queries related to any other aspect of the service being provided, both during any single span of duty and over longer periods of time. This is in addition to their service user care obligations. A number of these demands on FHMs are due to insufficient time being available, including:

- queries from patients' relatives that need to be responded to sensitively and with time;
- evidence base of care interventions;
- monitoring competence of novice registrants and responding to their queries;
- care co-ordination with MDT members;
- attending to students' education needs;
- quality monitoring metrics;
- queries related to bed availability;

- staff transfers;
- report of staff bullying or harassment incidents.

A range of demands on FHMs will have been identified in response to Action points 2.1 and 2.2, which can be added to those identified above. Another challenge is the constantly repeated requirement in health service policy for the need for efficiency savings while still ensuring best outcomes for service users. Furthermore, an unexpected patient death in the care setting, or an unanticipated physically aggressive episode by a service user, for instance, could prove emotionally demanding, and mechanisms and time for a debrief following such incidents often prove most valuable when feeling stressed from such demands.

Managing stress, bullying, etc. and their aftermaths

Health and care professions have often been recognised as some of the most demanding and potentially stressful occupations (e.g. Dean, 2012; RCN, 2015a), and frontline managers have a duty to prevent staff feeling stressed in their care settings. They also have to manage their own feelings of stress.

Several factors could cause stress in care professions such as interruptions when attending to a patient, working with inexperienced staff, insufficient resources, competing demands on your time, sickness and vacancies, unannounced changes in off-duty roster, lack of career opportunities, managing under-achieving students and multitasking. Sources of stress for community care professionals can include having to learn to use new medical and digital devices, increased caseloads, etc.

Stress tends to manifest itself with such symptoms as fatigue, physical unwellness, distress and feeling emotionally overwhelmed, according to Hawkins and McMahon (2020), as well as loss of appetite, insomnia, headaches or migraine, indigestion, inability to concentrate, paranoid thoughts, avoiding friends/colleagues, increased alcohol intake and even overeating. Over time, unrelieved stress results in 'burnout', which Hawkins and McMahon (2020) suggest is a state of emotional and physical exhaustion accompanied by a lack of interest in one's job, low trust in others, a loss of caring, cynicism towards others, self-deprecation, low morale and a sense of failure. This is because burnout can also have negative effects on quality of care, it can lower patient satisfaction and increase medical errors.

Similar problems are encountered by UK GPs, according to Lacobucci (2020), in that a substantial number of GPs feel stressed and overburdened because of short patient appointment times, increasing number of patients, etc. Research by Jones-Berry (2016) revealed that almost a third of intensive care nurses experience severe burnout, which puts them at risk of post-traumatic stress disorder, possibly alcohol abuse and even suicidal thoughts.

A study conducted by the *British Medical Journal* less than a decade ago revealed that 42% of nurses in England stated that they felt they were experiencing burnout (Dean, 2012). In a more recent survey of nurses, midwives and nursing associates entering and leaving its register, the NMC (2019) reports that almost a third of those who left cited stress and/or their mental health as the reason for leaving.

Healthcare employers therefore should monitor job dissatisfaction and burn-out rates among employees regularly and manage them promptly when they occur. Such consequences could be avoided, or their effects reduced markedly, if appropriate support mechanisms or structures are instituted and utilised.

Support mechanisms, which can be mutual, that can be instituted by employing organisations include buddying, clinical supervision and socialisation opportunities, that in turn can facilitate prevention or reduction of stress and enable care professionals to manage challenging situations more objectively. Instituting such mechanisms is also consistent with the human relations theory of management, which is explored in Chapter 4.

ACTION POINT 2.6
Support available for staff
experiencing excessive stress

Access the document 'Stress and You: A Short Guide to Coping with Pressure and Stress' (RCN, 2015a) (available at: www.rcn.org.uk/professional-development/publications/pub-004966), and view page 6 which identifies a number of the symptoms of stress experienced by nurses.

Then, consider whether you personally experience any of these symptoms. If you do, think of those who you turn to for support either in your personal life or at the workplace when feeling stressed. Consider also which other forms of support might be available at the employment base, and even regional or national support mechanisms for healthcare professionals.

The RCN (2015a) document mentioned in Action point 2.6 also provides a short 'Top Tips' tick box list of ways of managing stress, which includes ways of improving our mental wellbeing and resilience. Further positive ways of preventing or managing stress that can be adopted by healthcare staff include moderate physical exercise, eating healthily and general personal care, as opposed to giving in to negative strategies such as ruminating on the day's issues. Potential ways of resolving those challenging situations also include broaching difficult situations at team meetings, or using group reflection-on-practice or debriefing mechanisms.

NHS.uk (2018) suggests various 'stress busting' actions that healthcare staff can purposefully engage in for their own psychological health, which include being active, connecting with friendly people, having some 'me time', avoiding unhealthy habits and accepting the things that are outside our control. Such actions can also promote staff resilience, and endeavours to become resilient are worth investing efforts into to manage disproportionate amount of work stress.

Furthermore, in a systematic review of randomised controlled trials (RCTs) exploring the effects of the use of stress reduction techniques such as mindfulness-based stress reduction programme, yoga, cognitive behavioural therapy, massage therapy and relaxation techniques, Alkhawaldeh et al. (2020) found that overall such programmes are effective in reducing occupational stress levels.

On the other hand, the results of the *International Standard for Organisations (ISO)* accredited 2019 NHS England Survey Co-ordination Centre [NHSESCC] (2020) revealed that in addition to over 40% of NHS staff in England reporting having felt unwell as a result of work-related stress, 29% experienced at least one incident of harassment, bullying or abuse at work from patients/service users, their relatives or other members of the public, and even violence.

Earlier research by NHS Employers (2013) also found that 20% of staff in the NHS reported having been bullied by other staff, of whom 51% indicated that the most common source of bullying was supervisors/managers themselves, which caused them psychological distress and affected patient care. Prevention or management of bullying by managers is one of the NHSE+I's (2020a) criteria (metrics) for ICSs, representing standards that they (which includes all healthcare providers) have to meet to be deemed 'autonomous'.

Bullying can be verbal or physical, explicit or covert, and is characterised by offensive, insulting or intimidating behaviour, and an abuse or misuse of power that undermines, humiliates or emotionally injures the recipient. In their online cross-sectional survey of experience of workplace bullying among nurses, Brewer et al. (2020) found that repeated occurrence of being bullied results in burnout, job dissatisfaction and absenteeism.

Based on the various guidelines on the actions that organisations, employers, managers and individuals should take in relation to bullying or harassment at work, the following comprise the main actions that should be taken:

- Ask the person to stop the behaviour.
- Explain to the person bullying how their behaviour makes you feel.
- Explain to the person how it is interfering with your work.
- Maintain a written log or diary of bullying incidents.
- Keep a note of everything that is said.
- Update your knowledge of workplace policy, and discuss with a trade union representative.
- Inform your manager or senior colleague if the person continues to bully you.

Such practical steps to prevent and manage bullying or harassment usually feature in health service organisations' own local policies, guidelines and procedures as well.

Support Mechanisms for Healthcare Staff

The provision of support mechanisms that have been instituted for healthcare practitioners is consistent with the human relations theory of management, which takes into account the social aspects of work, together with employees' personal aspirations at work, as discussed in Chapter 4 of this book. It can be provided as formal facilities, non-formal and informal. Support mechanisms that are usually available for care practitioners to draw on comprise a number of formal mechanisms, for example the Occupational Health Department of the organisation.

Additionally, there are non-formal mechanisms, which are those that staff self-negotiate amongst their peers and colleagues, which they initiate themselves with people of their choice, on topics of their choice, at places of their mutual choosing and in their own time, and include, for example, staff socialisation encouraged by managers.

It is useful for frontline managers to have knowledge of the organisational, personal and professional support mechanisms that are available so that they can direct team members to them if required.

Formal support mechanisms

The support mechanisms that have been formally instituted to support staff manage the challenges that they encounter (noted earlier in this chapter) can be available at individual level, organisational level and supra-organisational level. Table 2.1 identifies some of the most common formal support mechanisms.

Line managers, for example, comprise an important and easily accessed source of formal support that NRNs can access, and which FHMs should provide to those who they manage. Being genuinely interested in the welfare of staff that care managers manage and providing them with an appropriate level of support are components of the human relations theory of management. This includes considering the social aspects of work, together with employees' personal circumstance, beside ensuring that the day's work is completed to a high standard.

Additionally, healthcare professionals might have access to counselling, cognitive behavioural therapy (CBT), meditation and hypnotherapy (Dean, 2012: 18). Another mechanism is clinical supervision (e.g. Driscoll et al., 2019), which comprises emotional support from non-managerial sources. Clinical supervision entails clinical supervisor and supervisee holding regular pre-arranged support meetings to facilitate the supervisee to reflect on their work and areas of their development for both self-improvement and enhancement of patient care.

Also referred to as 'clinical support' or 'peer supervision', clinical supervision should occur throughout healthcare professionals' careers as a mechanism for continuing professional development. It can be conducted at one-to-one level

Table 2.1 Formal support mechanisms for health and social care practitioners

Support mechanism	Details
Own line manager	FHMs can provide a fair level of support to their colleagues and team members in the form of empathetic listening and guidance; and they can access support for themselves from their own line managers when required.
Action learning sets	Comprise small discussion groups, with pre-agreed membership, who meet regularly to discuss proposed service improvement, issues, new policies or guidelines and professional development needs.
The occupational health department	For *ad hoc* advice and for counselling on work-related issues; for 'return to work' programmes, for early retirement on grounds of poor health, etc., which are provided via telephone or on a 'drop-in' basis.
Flexible shifts and agile working	Work scheduling to accommodate family commitments where feasible, and agile working facilities to accommodate employees' other commitments aimed at enabling staff to lead more balanced working lives and thereby improve their mental wellbeing and resilience, and motivation to work.
Reflection-on-action mechanisms and huddles	Structured reflection can be undertaken by individuals through writing up on incidents, or through mentor/supervisor facilitation. Huddles are short meetings directly addressing patient safety risks, which can be reflected upon afterwards.
Clinical supervision	Structured sessions for professional peer support (more details below).
Preceptorship	Structured learning programmes to facilitate smooth transition from finalist student to competent practitioner (discussed earlier in this chapter).
Peer learning	Recognition and support for colleagues learning from each other, which includes colleagues bringing new knowledge and skills acquired from conferences and workshops, and sharing with the team.
Professional forums	Comprise special interest groups that have been formed by clinical specialists locally or nationally for peer guidance and organising formal conferences. The RCN has approximately 85 professional forums, including forums for critical care nurses, mental health nurses, etc.
Personal life coach	Personal fee-based coaching addressing career and personal aspirations.

with a more experienced care practitioner supervising someone less experienced, or as small group supervision. However, the supervisor–supervisee relationship needs to be non-competitive, clear and objectives-focused.

It also needs to be supported by the conditions of therapeutic relationships, which according to Rogers and Freiberg (1994) include unconditional 'acceptance' of the supervisee for who they are and the situation that they find themselves in;

genuineness (i.e. being honest about oneself as a person); and empathy. A thorough analysis of the ways in which effective working relationships are formed is presented in Chapter 2 of Gopee's (2010) book entitled *Practice Teaching in Healthcare.*

A possible weakness of clinical supervision is that care practitioners might be apprehensive about this provision, fearing that it could be associated with individuals' weaknesses being identified by management. Another is the erratic implementation of clinical supervision, and yet others include insufficient adequately trained supervisors, and the cost associated with time taken for clinical supervision. If the supervisor–supervisee relationship breaks down, this can be problematic as well. Consequently, career-long mentorship-type programmes have been mooted to extend clinical supervision-type support beyond episodic events to a more continuous activity.

The practice of clinical supervision can be strengthened by a systematic approach through the use of a framework or model of clinical supervision. Two popular models of clinical supervision are: (1) Proctor's (2001) three-function interactive approach – normative, formative and restorative; and (2) Heron's (1989) six-category intervention analysis framework comprising prescriptive, informative, confronting, cathartic, catalytic and supportive interventions.

Non-formal support mechanisms

The various non-formal (and informal) support mechanisms that healthcare staff can utilise as and when they need them include peer support, peer-mentoring and buddying systems amongst peers, and peer review; professional forums; and social and peer learning mechanisms. Non-formal support mechanisms are those that are available either within the institutional setting or outside that individuals can access by virtue of being healthcare professionals.

The term peer basically signifies other registrants who are approximately or very slightly ahead in their careers as healthcare professionals. The concept of 'support' can entail someone of appropriate status giving the FHM time, and actively listening to an issue or problem that the FHM is involved in. Peer support can be obtained informally from colleagues, and in a more structured way through clinical supervision.

For peer-mentoring, Johnston et al. (2020) report on the successful implementation of a peer-mentoring programme for Marie Curie nurses whose role tends to entail working remotely and in isolation, whereupon named peer-mentors respond to the needs of newly appointed RNs and provide support and guidance as required.

Yet another form of peer support ensues from peer reviews, which refer to knowledgeable professionals in the same clinical specialism and similar professional status from a different care organisation providing feedback to individuals on proposed new ways of working. Thus, when the healthcare professional or team is allocated a new clinical activity or project, then after planning the activity (e.g. a new procedure) in detail, they forward it to peers in the same specialism for critical review and comments, and maybe pose questions on any key component that is not stated sufficiently clearly.

Work associated with peer review can also be useful for senior healthcare professionals (e.g. clinical nurse specialists, lead nurses) who, as they become more autonomous in their practices and decision-making, feel they could benefit from periodic feedback on their practices. It is also implemented in medicine in relation to performance assessment of doctors when concerns have been expressed in relation to their competence.

Personal Resources and Self-Management

In addition to the wide variety of potential staff support avenues just discussed, the NRHP also needs to draw on personal resources through self-care and self-management of one's own health and wellbeing as a basis for developing essential personal skills and coping strategies such as emotional resilience which includes emotional intelligence and self-awareness.

Caring for own health and wellbeing

Increasingly, healthcare professionals are being made aware that it is important to care for their own health and wellbeing, which is also referred to as self-management or managing oneself, which constitutes intentional and planned efforts made by individuals to develop their physical, mental, social and economic resources. These personal resources can form a sound platform for developing such coping strategies as resilience and mindfulness, which are concepts and skills that registrants will normally have encountered during undergraduate programmes.

ACTION POINT 2.7
Your own health and wellbeing

Having realised the extent of the range of FHMs' duties soon after acceding to the role, consider and identify a full range of strategies and sources of support that you can draw on to maintain your own emotional resilience.

Consider and identify also all the strategies that you use, and those that you could also use, to ensure your own health and wellbeing. Allow 10 minutes for this Action point and write down some details.

Experience of stress is one of various psychological imbalances felt by individuals and, therefore, individuals' mental health and wellbeing have gradually become more prominent in the thinking of health and policy makers, along with funding to provide support for dealing with ensuing mental health issues, as also identified in NHS LTP (NHSE, 2019a: 117). Psychological health and wellbeing impact directly on physical and social wellbeing, and vice versa, which is why FHMs need to be cognisant of the organisational, personal and professional support mechanisms that are available to access and to direct staff to for help.

Additionally, NHSE+I and NHS Employers (2018) have collaboratively published the NHS *Workforce Health and Wellbeing Framework*, along with a 'Diagnostic tool', which is an interactive document that provides guidance on how organisations can plan and deliver a staff health and wellbeing strategy. The document also presents 'actionable steps' under 14 headings.

The authors argue that investing in staff health and wellbeing delivers benefits for employees, the employing organisation and ultimately the service users in the healthcare professional's care. The 14 component areas that should be considered by employers include effective line management, engaging with staff, psychological interventions for mental health of staff, lifestyle change interventions, etc.

Attributes of resilience include being emotionally intelligent, which in turn incorporates utilising self-awareness skills, and being capable of exercising mindfulness and empathy.

Developing emotional resilience and other strategies

A range of strategies can be harnessed by healthcare professionals for managing challenging situations. Resilience is one of them, which is a personal quality that can be developed by FHMs and team members, which refers to people's ability to recover quickly (or to 'bounce back') from problematic or adverse situations that has caused stress and possibly burnout. With reference to non-humans, in metallurgy for example, it refers to the ability of metal to absorb stress but return to normal shape straight afterwards.

Resilience is thus 'the ability to adapt to adverse conditions while maintaining a sense of purpose, balance and positive mental and physical well-being', indicate Hatler and Sturgeon (2013: 33). The characteristics of resilience include optimism, having courage, toughness, compassion, humility, willingness to take risks, altruism, tolerance and accepting differences, etc., and learning from mistakes. Resilience can be developed by healthcare professionals at individual level, at team level and organisational level.

Integral to resilience are also emotional intelligence (EI) and mindfulness. The emotionally intelligent person is someone who has wide-ranging interpersonal skills, including empathy, self-awareness and self-management. Emotional intelligence is the ability to identify, assess, manage and control one's own emotions and to react to other people's (e.g. service users') emotions, the emotions being felt 'here and now', instead of suppressing them, according to Karimi et al. (2014: 178). Furthermore, from their research on EI among nurses, Raeissi et al. (2019) conclude that well-developed EI enhances communication skills among nurses.

Consequently, emotionally intelligent people know what to say during interactions in emotional situations, and when and how not to engage with others. Healthcare professionals can develop EI through mindfulness and higher self-awareness of their own feelings (e.g. of frustration, anger, excitement, etc.) in any given situation, their preferences, values and biases. Mindfulness can be developed through, for example, enhancing attention and concentration, by increasing flexibility and creativity, and acting with compassion and kindness, indicates NHS. UK (2019).

In a systematic review of mindfulness related to the effects of mindfulness-based interventions for informal palliative care givers, Jaffray et al. (2016) found that such interventions are beneficial, feasible and acceptable to care givers. However, rarer mindful interventions, such as possibly meditation classes, yoga and tai chi which are not widely available under the NHS, should only be offered with the service user's informed consent. Furthermore, mindfulness enables individuals to develop the attributes of compassionate leadership, which in turn contributes to the provision of safe and high-quality care, asserts NHSE (2014a).

Guidance for Managing Transition to Competent Autonomous Healthcare Professional

The following comprise guidance for NRHPs to manage frontline healthcare responsibilities and duties competently.

- Continually ascertain all your responsibilities, for which you are accountable, as a NRHP and a frontline manager.
- Harness opportunities to further develop and advance your competence related to safe, effective and compassionate clinical practice that is also person-centred and evidence-informed.
- Continually develop your competence related to your responsibility for leading daily care, and organise daily care delivery based on service users' care needs, and allocate named service users to staff with the relevant competence.
- Ensure you always adhere to your profession's code of practice and to legislation related to healthcare provision and delivery, and that all team members also do.
- Ensure time is put aside to ensure new employees joining your team including NRHPs are welcomed to the care setting and sufficient time is given to them to acquaint themselves with the setting, and their questions attended to.

- Constantly check that the organisational culture in the care setting supports delivery of competent person-centred and evidence-informed care under your leadership.
- Reflect on your management communication such as in delegation and documentation to ensure they are effective.
- Develop your skills at conducting individual development and performance reviews (IDPR) for junior team members, which include ensuring that the agreed objectives meet SMART criteria.
- Be cognisant of your responsibilities towards education and practice supervision of students on placement in your care setting, and at managing all other team members' learning needs, including learning related to IDPR objectives.
- Accept that challenging situations could be encountered by frontline care professionals such as when team members feel stressed, and bullied or harassed, and manage them yourself or through directing them to available support mechanisms.
- Develop competence in personal resources and self-management through caring for own health and wellbeing, and through developing emotional resilience and other coping strategies.

Chapter Summary

The transition from newly qualified registrant to frontline manager is a substantial leap in activity and responsibilities in the delivery and management of care, and in the various inherent components within them. Consequently, this chapter has focused on:

- The scope of responsibilities bestowed on newly qualified healthcare professionals and their own evolving aspirations from becoming a qualified healthcare professional to becoming a team member, preceptorship programmes for NRHPs, the organisational culture in care settings, and on delivering and leading person-centred and evidence-informed care competently;
- Ways of fulfilling responsibilities related to organising, and leading daily care competently, and management communication related to delegation, record keeping, and statement writing and report writing;
- Accountability and ethical practice by engaging in safe, effective and compassionate practice through ensuring adherence to the profession's code of practice and being accountable to employer for the achievement of agreed objectives;
- Managing teaching and practice supervision of students on placement and attending to team members' and other learners' learning needs;

- Challenges encountered by FHMs which include stress, and bullying or harassment, and managing them through formal and non-formal support mechanisms that can be accessed by healthcare professionals; and
- Developing personal resources and self-management through caring for own health and wellbeing, and through developing emotional resilience and other coping strategies.

Further Reading

- For a comprehensive analysis of record-keeping, see: Andrews A, St Aubyn B (2015) 'If it's not written down; it didn't happen...'. *Journal of Clinical Nursing,* 29 (5): 20–22.
- For a comprehensive discussion on the what, why and how of preceptorship, see: Capital Nurse (2017) *Preceptorship Framework.* Available at: www.hee. nhs.uk/sites/default/files/documents/CapitalNurse%20Preceptorship%20 Framework.pdf. Accessed Date: 25 March 2021.
- For guidance on ways to improve staff experience of working in the healthcare organisation though direct and sincere consideration of each employee's wellbeing, see: NHS Improvement and NHS Employers (June 2018) *Start Well: Stay Well – a model to support new starter.* Available at: file:///C:/Users/lgope/ AppData/Local/Packages/Microsoft.MicrosoftEdge_8wekyb3d8bbwe/TempState/ Downloads/CUH-case-study-Final—June-2018%20(1).pdf. Accessed Date: 22 March 2020.

3

Competent Leadership in Healthcare Settings

Chapter Objectives

The chapter objectives for frontline healthcare managers in relation to competent healthcare leadership are:

- Gain understanding of what leadership is and what leadership in care settings entails, which also includes distinguishing between leadership and management;
- Ascertain the reasons for leadership in health services and its benefits, and precisely who are the healthcare professionals who provide it;
- Discuss the different styles of leadership and their impact in care settings;
- Identify several earlier theories of leadership along with the more informed current approaches to leadership provision to team members;
- Explore leadership development programmes that are based on models and frameworks of leadership that reflect comprehensive skill-set for this function;
- Perform self-assessment of leadership skills to identify strengths and areas for further development.

Introduction

As noted in Chapter 1 of this book, the widely recommended NHS Leadership Academy's (2020) *Healthcare Leadership Model*, which comprises a nine-dimensioned framework of the key characteristics, attitudes and behaviours of effective healthcare leaders, represents one of the main contemporary guidance on ways in which leadership should feature in health services. Effective leadership by all healthcare professionals is the lynchpin of safe, effective and compassionate care delivery in clinical settings, and as the NMC (2018b: 22) recognises, 'Throughout their career, all our registrants will have opportunities to demonstrate leadership qualities, regardless of whether or not they occupy formal leadership positions'.

Figure 1.1 in Chapter 1 provided succinctly the four most significant characteristics that followers believe each leader should have, and now this chapter provides an in-depth examination of the extensive knowledge base on leadership that currently prevails, such as research on leadership, and leadership skills for healthcare. This is based on the rationale that FHMs are required to exercise leadership skills in the course of their daily duties.

The chapter approaches leadership in healthcare in distinct components, which are: what is leadership; why is it important to have competent leadership in healthcare; who provides leadership; and then how to provide leadership. The last component on how to provide leadership is divided into four sections, which are: (1) styles of leadership; (2) enduring earlier theories of leadership; (3) current more-informed leadership theories; and (4) skills and frameworks of leadership (this fourth section includes guidance on self-assessment of leadership skills, and an action plan for further development of these skills as deemed relevant in health or social care situations).

Understanding the Nature of Leadership – Defining an Elusive Concept

The effectiveness of leadership in healthcare, or the need for it, features regularly in healthcare journals. At times they document ways in which it has been implemented successfully, at other times they argue that leadership needs to be strengthened. Yet leadership is not a new concept in healthcare as it was, for example, highly recommended by Fretwell (1980) several decades ago, and today national health organisations provide recommendations and detailed ways in which leadership can be implemented systematically and, therefore, more effectively.

The concept 'leadership', however, is a noun that can have four possible meanings: (1) the activity of leading; (2) the body of people who lead a group; (3) the status of the leader; and (4) the ability to lead. In all forms, leaders influence the behaviour of those they lead. The word 'influence' appears frequently in the definitions of the term leadership. Buchanan and Huczynski (2019), for example, indicate that leadership is the process of *influencing* the activities of an organised group in its efforts towards goal-setting and goal achievement.

Similarly, leadership is a relationship through which one person *influences* the behaviour or actions of other people, according to Mullins (2019). From his comprehensive review of literature on leadership, Dinibutun (2020: 46) deduces that leadership is 'the ability to involve others in the process of accomplishing a goal within some larger system or environment'.

These standard definitions of leadership usually incorporate or imply *influence*, or some degree of authority, over people, and in the context of the FHM's role, leadership entails involving or influencing the behaviour of team members at inter-disciplinary level. Thus, leadership is a two-way process based on a leader–follower type relationship. FHMs thereby involve, inspire and energise team members towards the achievement of the organisation's or the care setting's goals while performing both manager and leader duties.

Furthermore, leadership can be distinguished between vertical leadership and horizontal leadership (e.g. Chin, 2015) (see also Table 3.1) – vertical referring to top-down approach, while horizontal refers to a much more equality of status between leader and team members, and between team members. Furthermore, the form of leadership is affected by the personal characteristics of the leader, and by the attitude and needs of the followers, to some extent by the structure and purpose of the organisation, as well as by the tasks that have to be performed.

The current *Healthcare Leadership Model* (NHS Leadership Academy, 2021) identifies nine leadership behaviours that include inspiring shared purpose, engaging the team, etc. Brief details of effective healthcare leadership related to the components identified in Figure 1.1 (in Chapter 1 of this book) are as follows:

- *Honest* – Exercises full honesty in all clinical matters at all times, and genuineness; 'acceptance' of every team member, for their strengths and improvement areas.
- *Forward-looking* – Is visionary, and proactive in anticipating ways in which clinical matters are likely to evolve in future.
- *Competent* – Knowledgeable and competent as an evidence-informed practitioner, organiser of care and in leadership; willing to learn and improve; sees issues or problems as opportunities.
- *Inspiring* – Takes responsibility, and is a role model of highest standard of clinical practice.

So, in what ways are leaders different from managers, or more usefully, in what ways are leaders' functions different from those of managers'?

ACTION POINT 3.1
Distinguishing between leaders' and managers' functions

Reflect on your personal experiences of managers and leaders in care settings as well as more broadly, and think of the similarities and differences between these functions. Then identify what the distinct differences between these two functions are.

Following a comprehensive literature review of leadership and management, Jennings et al. (2007) identified almost 900 competencies related to leadership and management, of which 862 competencies are exercised by both leaders and managers, despite the two concepts being very different. Jennings et al. identify 'human resource management' and 'information management' more as management competencies, whereas leadership competencies include 'setting the vision' and 'developing people'. They suggest that those who run management and leadership courses should be aware of these differences in competencies and incorporate them in their courses appropriately.

In the context of healthcare, the two activities management and leadership can be distinguished as illustrated in Figure 3.1.

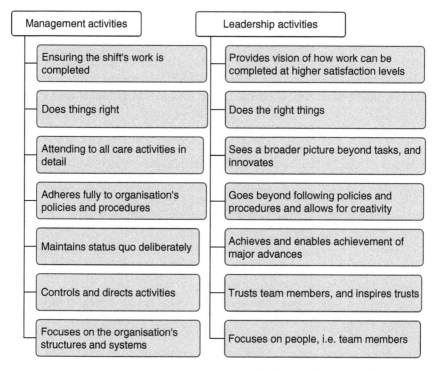

Figure 3.1   Distinguishing between management and leadership activities

Leadership competencies and capabilities form part of the skill-set of FHMs, which they exercise through ensuring that the care settings' obligations are fulfilled dutifully and to very high standards, and thereby in the achievement of departmental and organisational goals. Frontline healthcare managers will have learned leadership competence and capabilities during their pre-registration education, by both observing successful leaders, and through any leadership development programmes subsequently attended.

Leadership competencies are specified in the SOPs that healthcare profession students have to achieve by, for example, the NMC (2018a) who indicates that the outcomes that RNs will have achieved in the course of their pre-registration programme to prepare them for their post-qualifying duties. Particularly under Platform 5 'Leading and managing nursing care and working in teams', leadership outcomes include (p. 20):

> 5.5 safely and effectively lead and manage the nursing care of a group of people, demonstrating appropriate prioritisation, delegation and assignment of care responsibilities to others involved in providing care.

> 5.6 exhibit leadership potential by demonstrating an ability to guide, support and motivate individuals and interact confidently with other members of the care team.

Clearly, the NMC is stating that leading care involves appropriate prioritisation, delegation, supporting and motivating team members, etc., which FHMs have to perform competently. As for management, this refers to ensuring day-to-day duties are completed in good time, it is about adherence to policies and procedures, maximising outputs and productivity while working within allocated resources, monitoring performance against pre-determined outcomes, etc. These are examined in comprehensive detail in Chapter 4 of this book, where it is also noted that leadership is often a subset of management in healthcare. Alternatively, leadership and management can be seen as two distinctive but complementary activities, according to Kotter (2009).

Why Is Leadership Required in Health Services?

There are several reasons for the application of effective leadership in healthcare. For example, based on his extensive research over several years, Mintzberg (2011) identifies effective leadership as one of the key roles of all managers, which is consistent with suggestions made by current healthcare practitioners as deliberated in detail in Chapter 4 under the heading 'Roles and Styles of Frontline Managers'.

As an example of the benefits of effective leadership in healthcare, in a systematic review exploring the relationship between transformational (relational) (defined shortly) leadership and patient outcomes, Wong et al. (2013) concluded that this form of leadership, which is based on strong positive relationships (referred to as positive relational leadership styles) between colleagues, tends to result in increased patient satisfaction and decreased patient mortality, decreased patient falls, less medication errors, less restraint use and less hospital-acquired infection.

However, Francis (2013) stipulated that the scandalous malpractice and patient neglect that prevailed at a UK hospital around a decade ago was the consequence of 'dysfunctional leadership' in all parts of the organisation, from top level managers/administrators to ancillary staff, including senior medical, nursing and allied health profession staff. This had become ingrained in a culture that was focused on the trust's business (purchaser-provider model) instead of on service users, with a great degree of tolerance of poor standards and of risk to patients, and an assumption that monitoring standards and performance management was the responsibility of someone else, etc.

In a more recent systematic review of healthcare organisations that are repeatedly unable to improve quality, Vaughn et al. (2019) found various areas of concern, which they group under: poor organisation culture, inadequate infrastructure, lack of cohesive vision and mission, and dysfunctional external relations. Often, the reason for these weaknesses are poor, or lack of, leadership, which prevailed in the form of:

- unsupportive leadership,
- under-developed leaders; and
- lack of transparency.

Thus, it is clear that the sustainability of the organisation and the quality of care received by service users are both dependent upon the competence of its leaders. It is for this reason that leadership competence development by all healthcare professionals is considered not only a necessity, but also a requirement and an imperative.

Ultimately, the suggestion that there should be leadership at all levels in health services (e.g. May, 2019) is supported by the realisation that all healthcare professionals can take leadership roles after receiving leadership training, because there does not seem to be any evidence that leadership qualities are inherited, or belong to one particular type of person. Furthermore, research (e.g. Jennings et al., 2007; Kouzes and Posner, 2017) has often signposted that leadership comprises competencies that can be learned through appropriate development programmes. Therefore, FHMs should assure themselves of their own leadership competence against the content of such programmes, and subsequently support and facilitate the potential for team members to be effective leaders themselves.

Furthermore, in the context of the clinical governance framework of quality enhancement, the RCN (2020b) asserts that appropriate leadership, such as collective leadership, contributes to team cohesion, lower stress levels, higher empowerment, more potent self-efficacy and quality outcomes in care settings, which in turn 'provide motivation and stimulate creativity and innovation'.

Consequently, leadership development programmes for healthcare professionals has been urged for at least two decades in various policy publications including *The NHS Plan* (DH, 2000b), the *NHS Change Model* (NHS England, 2020c) and the NHS LTP (NHSE, 2019b: 23). A number of leadership development programmes are available for health and social care professionals from various organisations (e.g. RCN, 2020a), which are examined later in this chapter.

Who Provides Leadership in Health Services?

Having clarified that leadership entails influencing the actions and behaviour of team members, and having differentiated between leaders' and managers' roles, this section explores the different forms of leadership that prevail in healthcare and the different postholders who provide those forms of leadership in addition to FHMs. As noted above, there can be leadership at all levels in the hierarchy, and therefore leadership is also a component of more senior managers' roles. Closely related is the type of formal power that is inherent within leadership (addressed later in this section).

ACTION POINT 3.2
Leaders in care settings

In the context of the healthcare organisation and the care setting where you work, thinking of the diverse aspects of your work, ascertain the ways in which you approach your work differently based on whether you are led and supervised, to when you lead.

Other than the leadership roles of managers, often in care settings leadership is associated with the healthcare professional's particular interest in certain specific aspects of care, such as in tissue viability, or being the key worker for 'moving and handling' or patient safety, and so on. Leadership is also provided by colleagues in specialist practice or advanced clinical practice (ACP) positions. In both instances, leadership is not provided from someone in a managerial post, but someone who is 'an authority' in the specific area of clinical practice. As Anderson (2018) notes, ACPs provide leadership by empowering colleagues with specific knowledge and skills.

Healthcare leaders are usually appointed to the position by the organisation, or they emerge through leadership qualities, or through their specialist clinical expertise. There are various diverse forms or types of leadership, and Table 3.1. lists and briefly explains a number of key forms of leadership, which is different from leadership theories which are discussed shortly in this chapter.

On and off, some of the different forms of leadership identified on Table 3.1 tend to prevail in different care settings. With regards to formal leadership, it is

Table 3.1   Diverse forms of leadership

Attempted leadership	An individual attempts to take the leadership role for a specific group, by implication unsuccessfully
Authentic leadership/ Values-based leadership	A model of leadership, which is also known as 'values-based leadership', whereupon authentic leaders are guided by their own and their team members' values and beliefs, whereby the leader's behaviour encourages openness in sharing information needed to make decisions, resulting in enhanced professional collaboration
Charismatic leadership	A leader who emerges naturally based on their personal attraction
Elected leadership	Achieved leadership through democratic election
Formal leadership	Leadership granted to an appointee, who therefore has *legitimate authority* and status to lead a team, e.g. a formally appointed care manager or a project leader; is also referred to as legal/rational leader
Imposed leadership	Leadership based on the role being given to an individual, who accepts it willingly or reluctantly. It also refers to someone who declares themselves the leader but wasn't appointed or invited to the role
Informal leadership	A form of leadership based on personal knowledge and skills and on ability to influence and guide others on specific activities related to the organisation, not necessarily based on appointment to a post
Political leadership	Is based on the person taking the lead through favouring specific policies that are supported by other people who take the same stance
Relational leadership	Is based on strong positive relationships between colleagues, and is often a feature of transformational leadership
Shared leadership	When two or more Band 5 or 6 registrants share leadership in a practice setting for different aspects of care or based on different areas of knowledge or skill
Successful leadership	A leader who is effective in achieving pre-determined goals
Traditional leadership	Leadership achieved through forefathers having traditionally and historically been leaders, or through social norms, and which comes with very strong authority or power

reflected in job titles such as 'clinical leader' and 'team leader', which represent formal leadership duties at the practice edge of care provision. Shared leadership, which is also referred to as collective leadership, prevails in teams in which different teams' members of similar job status have leadership duties, as found in community care teams, or in intensive care units.

Additionally, the idea of self-leadership and self-management are also mooted in healthcare. Self-management is often associated with service users managing their health condition when the individual is coping with chronic health conditions or multi-morbidity, whereupon with the relevant education and support the individual takes responsibility for managing their illness and healthcare regime. Self-leadership, on the other hand, is more about all individuals taking responsibility for influencing their life holistically; the term holistic implying physical health, psychological, inter-personal, financial and spiritual health.

Taking responsibility for physical health incorporates ensuring appropriate nutrition, hydration, rest, exercise, etc. For financial health, this includes getting relevant education or training and consequently an employment with financial rewards. It also involves identifying one's strengths, and building on them, especially through knowledge acquisition, emotional intelligence and feedback from trusted individuals. Balancing one's plans and priorities, actively managing own time and workload more effectively without compromising one's own health are other features of self-leadership.

In *Going Nowhere? Lead Yourself,* Gopee (2018) analyses in extensive detail numerous ways of engaging in self-leadership, which starts with deliberately taking charge of all aspects of one's life and career, regular self-appraisal, deciding on directions to take and choosing opportunities to pursue. Self-inspiration, self-influencing and self-change are further components of self-leadership, which consequently constitutes a platform for more effective leadership in people organisations, such as healthcare organisations.

ACTION POINT 3.3
Attributes of effective leaders

What are the personal qualities of 'good' or effective leaders? Thinking about this question from a broader perspective, e.g. a popular prime minister, captain of your favourite sports team, the chief nurse at your workplace, or the leader of a special interest society that you subscribe to, consider and identify their personal attributes that make them good leaders from the point of view of the people they lead. Make a list of some of their personal attributes.

This Action point might well have seemed easy to undertake, as you may have thought of leaders who influence you personally in some way, or of health or care leaders who lead by example, and who inspire others in the workplace. They might be Band 5 staff nurses at the frontline of healthcare, or more senior managers, clinical nurse specialists, nurse (or AHP) consultants, etc.

Being role models of practice is a characteristic that healthcare professionals start to develop early in their vocation. The NMC's (2018a) SOP for pre-registration courses for nurses, for example, indicates that being a good role model is a component of registrants' leadership in healthcare settings. Having good role models in practice settings has a direct beneficial impact on learning, as found by Baldwin et al. (2014) in their integrative literature review, as such role models have qualities that include being approachable, having a clear set of values, selflessness and acceptance of others, commitment, being passionate and always being positive and calm, and who support learning and are usually available to listen to suggestions for more effective ways of working.

Furthermore, role models either instigate the process of socialisation in practice settings or they continue with socialisation that learners initiate, in order to foster a sense of belonging to the team. Conversely, in a study of the influence of senior healthcare professionals as role models, Felstead and Springett (2016) also observed poor and undesirable behaviours, and they conclude that healthcare professionals in management and leadership positions should be mindful of the impact of their job roles in shaping the outlook of the future workforce by being more self-aware and leading by example.

As for individuals who are not as effective, those who are poor leaders, that could be so because they have unwillingly accepted the leadership role, or because they lack appropriate resources to be effective. Different leaders view their roles from different perspectives, which those who have studied leadership in depth refer to as theories or models of leadership. The attributes of effective leaders are discussed later in this chapter under trait theory and characteristics of 'admired' leaders. However, there is no doubt that being in the leader role carries extra specific responsibility and, therefore, also requires preparatory work before meeting team members to discuss aspects of care.

Leadership Influence and Power

As noted earlier, the definitions of leadership often include the word 'influence'; that is, influence of the leader over the people or team members who they lead. The word influence signifies having an effect or affecting the behaviour of other people, which in turn denotes a sense of authority or power over them. Consequently, leadership tends to be associated with power, which signifies the capacity to produce or prevent a specific change in people. Thus, power can be associated with control, which has negative connotations, but shouldn't, dependent upon the type of power exercised by the leader. Table 3.2 identifies and provides brief details of the types of power that leaders can exercise over those they lead.

In general, healthcare leaders wouldn't want to be associated with the notions control and authority in aspects of healthcare that they endeavour to lead and influence. For instance, being associated with expert power, or referent power or reward power (see Table 3.2) are positive forms of power that are more acceptable, but authority power and information power need to be managed more carefully.

Frontline managers can apply their leadership influence and power for the mutual benefit of leader and led in the following ways: For reward power, for example, FHMs could:

- offer the type of rewards that people desire;
- ensure that rewards are fair and ethical;

Table 3.2 Types of power that leaders can exercise

Organisational power

Authority power *(or legitimate power)*	Based on the position (or job and rank) that the individual holds within the hierarchy of the organisation, and therefore the leader's right to 'command and control' because of their position in the organisation.
Coercive power *(or punishment power)*	Based on threats of penalties that the leader is in a position to impose on an individual or a group such as withdrawal of support, invoking disciplinary procedures, etc.
Information power	Based on possession of and access to useful information.
Reward power	Based on inducements such as pay, promotion, praise and recognition that the leader can offer group members in exchange for co-operation and contributions towards the achievement of the group's objectives.

Personal power

Connection power	Based on the individual's formal and informal links with influential individuals within and outside an area or organisation.
Expert power *(or profession power)*	Based on very high level of knowledge and competence associated with their role; often limited to narrow, well-defined specialism.
Referent power *(or ascribed or status power)*	Based on admiration and respect for the leader by others for their charisma, attractiveness, wealth, etc. and high position in society, and on identification with the leader.

- not make promises of more than can be delivered;
- identify and publish simple criteria for giving rewards;
- provide rewards as promised when requirements have been met;
- use rewards symbolically (not in a manipulative way).

On the other hand, when using legitimate power or authority, FHMs could:

- use politeness and clarity when making requests;
- explain the reasons for requests;
- not exceed their scope of authority;
- verify authority if necessary;
- follow agreed organisational channels;
- follow up to ascertain compliance;
- insist on compliance if necessary.

So far, this chapter has approached leadership in healthcare in distinct components, which are: what is leadership; why is it important to have competent leadership in healthcare; who provides leadership; and then how to provide leadership. The next section covers further theoretical and practical aspects of how to provide leadership, which it does in four sections, which are: (1) styles of leadership;

(2) earlier theories of leadership; (3) current more-informed leadership theories; and (4) skills and frameworks of leadership.

Multifarious theories of leadership have been suggested, which are summarised in Figure 3.2, and then analysed in some detail subsequently. It is noteworthy that a number of these theories are still suggestions or exhortations, others are at experimental stages, but others are empirically generated, that is research-based.

Styles of Leadership

The kind of leadership that frontline managers can provide is partly dependent upon how they view their leadership role, on their own personality and the leadership training that they may have attended. This mode of self-determined leadership activity tends to be referred to as styles of leadership. Leadership style refers to the ways in which the leader conducts their leadership role on a day-to-day basis, together with the way in which the leader is perceived as typically behaving towards their followers. Such styles or patterns of behaviour are developed through their own life experiences, their personal perceptions of the role and experiences of being led by seniors at work in the past.

The most widely known styles of leadership are democratic style, autocratic, permissive, bureaucratic and the people versus product-oriented style (see Table 3.3). Note also the different types of leadership identified on Table 3.1, some of which, such as political leadership, may be perceived as styles of leadership.

These different styles of leadership are easy to detect amongst those in leadership roles, each having either helpful or unhelpful (or positive or negative) overtones and consequences. As briefly noted on Table 3.3, the democratic or participative style, for example, might be the most widely accepted style as it takes each follower's views into account before deciding on courses of action. There might also be scope for the autocratic or authoritarian style, exercised by, say, a senior consultant physician towards their team, it is a style that is unlikely to thrive for long in the NHS.

For permissive or laissez-faire style of leadership, it obviously depends on interpretation and application of the style by the individual leader. Parish (2006) reports on a study of a range of different leadership styles applied in acute hospital wards; namely, directive, visionary, affiliative, participative, pace-setting and coaching leadership. The study concluded that high-performing ward managers are able to choose from and use a wide range of leadership styles, while lower-performing managers choose from a limited range of styles.

Additionally, each leadership style is likely to have advantages and disadvantages associated with it. As to which leadership styles you may wish to adopt as a FHM, this can vary according to the requirements of particular situations, e.g. an emergency versus a team-building day – the style in the former is likely to be directive, and in the latter laissez-faire.

Table 3.3   Styles of leadership

Democratic or participative	• Leader formally seeks input from all relevant team members • Achieves consensus in the team through their involvement • Consults and works with individuals and teams • Engages in open two-way communication • Encourages collaborative teamwork
Authoritative or autocratic	• Portrays and exercises position power • Feels the need to exercise authority and approval of status by those they lead • Exercises control and directive behaviour • Makes decisions alone and expects obedience of instructions • Is decisive when changes or clear direction are required
Bureaucratic	• Complies in full with established policies and rules and expects all staff to do so as well • Exercises power by inflexible adherence to rules • Communication is impersonal
Affiliative	• Promotes harmony and emotional bond in the work environment • Motivates people even during difficult times
Coercive	• Requires immediate compliance all the time • Provides directives in crisis situations and is decisive with problem employees
Coaching	• Nurtures team members with the future in mind • Helps employees improve their performance
Pacesetting	• Sets high standards and expects excellence from the team • Is most effective when there is a need to receive quick results • Expects team to be highly motivated
Permissive or laissez-faire	• Allows team members extensive freedom of choice • Intervenes only when approaching or reached crisis point • Appears relaxed about rules and policies • Monitors performance from a distance, and therefore appears detached

Enduring Earlier Theories of Leadership

Several theories of leadership have been developed over the years that seek to explain how best to apply leadership in organisations in order to ensure that they are effective in the services they provide or their products, as well as for improvement of these. The wide variety of theories can make it problematic to decide which one(s) can be most usefully applied to one's own care setting. In this section on how FHMs can provide leadership, the theories are divided into three main categories (see Figure 3.2), which are: (1) the earlier but enduring theories, some of which are based on research, others on speculations but are still applied effectively in some areas; (2) theories that are currently applied in healthcare with good levels of success; and (3) leadership frameworks and models that are applied by organisations, and are often used for leadership training.

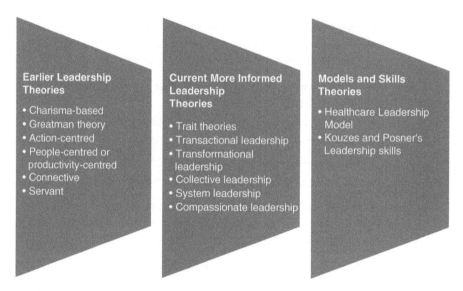

Figure 3.2 Three main groups of leadership theories

Based on the classification of leadership theories presented in Figure 3.2, a number of the most commonly encountered theories are now explored in some detail. They are charismatic and greatman theories of leadership, action-centred leadership, connective leadership and servant leadership. People-centred or productivity-centred leadership, which is also perceived as a management theory, is discussed in Chapter 4 of this book. Covey (2006) provides details of further leadership theories including psychoanalytical and personal-situational leadership theories.

Charisma-based and greatman theories

Being a charismatic leader entails being popular with people generally because of one's natural self-confidence, pleasantness, exceptional ability to persuade people, and novel ideas and strong convictions. The leader's personality arouses affection and emotional commitment to both the leader and to their beliefs and their views about the organisation.

Similarly, greatman theory of leadership comprises the leader's persuasiveness that inspires or motivates followers to readily endorse the leader's ideas. The theory refers to those with ability to lead at national level which very few people possess.

On their own, neither charismatic leadership nor greatman theory of leadership are applicable to healthcare settings and care delivery. This is principally because their scientific basis is non-existent, and both concepts are difficult to define and therefore cannot be acquired through training or education, while in healthcare, leadership skills are developed and exercised by the majority of healthcare professionals though appropriate education and exposure.

Action-centred leadership

Another theory of leadership that has been widely debated and that features in leadership development workshops periodically is action-centred leadership (ACL). The principal advocate of this form of leadership is Adair (2005), according to whom the leader operates by ensuring three sets of needs of the organisation are met, which are: task needs, individual needs and team maintenance needs.

Effective action-centred leadership is dependent upon these three areas of needs being adequately met within each department, unit or care setting. Therefore, in healthcare organisations, care leaders such as FHMs have to pay full attention to these sets of needs for the care setting to function effectively. This is because too much concern to any one of these three areas, say too much attention to individual or task needs at the expense of team maintenance needs, can cause imbalance and obstruct effective teamworking, which, in turn, could negatively affect the quality of care outcomes, and the morale and motivation in the care setting.

Frontline healthcare managers can apply Adair's (2005) ACL in a number of ways. For example, briefly, for meeting task needs, they can ensure that the objectives of the work group are achieved, resources are allocated as appropriate and they delegate according to individuals' capabilities. For meeting team or group needs, FHMs can hold regular team meetings, ensure full and timely communication, make themselves approachable and available, and provide feedback. For meeting individual needs, FHMs can ensure that IDPRs are conducted on time, be available for one-to-one meetings, and manage any conflict and potential problem areas in interpersonal relationships within the team.

Connective leadership

With a major emphasis on markedly wide-ranging collaborative working within the health and social care organisations, as well as building inter-organisational working relationships with the focus staying on achievement of organisational goals, connective leadership accordingly involves leading by fostering extensive networks of connections. Thus, the ability and activities of leaders that create inter-connections within and across practice settings, intra-organisationally and inter-organisationally, is valued; the result from which is better co-ordination and integration of service user care services in a caring, non-competitive, mutually beneficial way.

To achieve this form of results, the leader takes concerted actions to create connections and to foster integration by valuing and working with actual and potential collaborators in varied settings, and facilitating interdependent interactions, and sharing information and vision with each collaborator.

Research by Yan et al. (2016) into connective leadership concluded that it is positively related to employee goal commitment and for conflict management. However, this theory seems limited as a complete leadership theory because being appropriately connected with similar other experts through networking and so on is already a recognised essential attribute that effective leaders must possess.

Servant leadership

Also identified as a distinct theory of leadership is servant leadership which belongs to instances when leaders are elected democratically to leadership positions, an example being elected politicians and trade union leaders who tend to claim that they are in a leadership position through their desire to serve the public who elected them. Serving incorporates stewardship, and the characteristics of servant leaders include personal integrity, courage to speak up and advocate, altruism and empowerment of team members, according to Best (2020).

However, in healthcare all these components of servant leadership mustn't detract from the organisation's purpose and goals to provide care and treatment to service users as and when required. Furthermore, Waterman (2011) suggests that the term 'servant' is ancient and has religious connotations and might not be acceptable to current-day nurses who endeavour to ensure that their practice is evidence-informed.

Current More Informed Healthcare Leadership Theories

Either building on, or despite earlier theories of leadership just discussed such as charismatic and greatman theory, action-centred leadership, etc. (each of which still have their proponents), the most prominent and widely applied contemporary leadership theories are: traits theory, transactional leadership and transformational leadership, collective leadership, system leadership and compassionate leadership.

Trait theories

Numerous research has been conducted since the 1950s on the specific character-istics of effective leaders (e.g. Handy, 1993). Initially, it was known as 'great man' or 'great woman' theories of leadership, which attempted to identify innate traits of successful leaders, so that potential leaders could be supported to develop these qualities and become effective leaders. These characteristics were also referred to as 'traits' or qualities, and the traits of successful leaders have been identified as including self-confidence, motivation, intelligence, using own initiative, visionary, and so on.

After examining several studies on traits of successful leaders, Bass (1990) categorised their traits into three areas: (1) *intelligence,* including judgement, deci-siveness, knowledge, fluency; (2) *personality* traits such as adaptability, alertness, integrity, nonconformity; and (3) *ability* such as co-operativeness, popularity, tact.

However, the trait theory has not been universally accepted based on the reasoning that no one person could have or develop all the traits identified by researchers. Furthermore, the traits (e.g. decisiveness, popularity) themselves are abstract, subjective and difficult to define into a common understanding; and also there are a number of exceptional leaders who do not possess all the traits that research has identified. There are also many who believe that 'leaders are born, not made', which is contrary to and not applicable to healthcare where leadership is exercised by most healthcare professionals.

Nonetheless, researchers have continued to explore the qualities or charac-teristics of successful or effective leaders, but without using the term 'trait'. For example, Kouzes and Posner (2017) have been conducting extensive worldwide ongoing research over several years to identify the specific characteristics of 'Admired Leaders', and from one of their most recent surveys they identified the following characteristics:

Honest (approximately 89% of participants)
Forward looking (approximately 71%)
Competent (approximately 69%)
Inspiring (approximately 65%).

Kouzes and Posner (2017) also report that other important leadership charac-teristics include being intelligent, broad-minded, fair-minded, dependable, sup-portive, straightforward, co-operative and determined; and less frequently cited characteristics of effective leaders include being courageous, ambitious, caring, loyal, imaginative, mature, self-controlled and independent. However, there isn't a complete set of qualities, traits or characteristics that everyone agrees on as those required by healthcare professionals to ensure they are effective leaders.

Nonetheless, in the context of personal qualities required for effective nurse leadership Lucas (2019) asserts that the list of qualities (similar to traits) can be categorised into four 'intelligences', namely spiritual, emotional, business or practice, and political. While lists of leadership qualities or traits can be grouped under any set of headings researchers choose, it is useful to see political intelligences identified by Lucas, which in essence entails networking widely (internally and externally), being involved in professional forums or groups, and developing report-writing and presentation skills that are audience-friendly and persuasive.

Transactional leadership and transformational leadership

As noted earlier in this chapter, some leaders lead by virtue of being appointed to their posts with leadership activities, while other leaders emerge. The FHM is appointed to a management position within the healthcare provider's management hierarchy, which is one that includes substantial leadership functions. With the FHM's priority being to ensure all the day's service user tasks are completed to the required standard, which is in the context of the achievement of organisational goals, this form of leadership is referred to as transactional leadership.

Successful or effective transactional healthcare leaders first of all ensure all duties are completed in full accordance with the organisation's policies and procedures, and thereby maintain equilibrium and harmony. They motivate and reward staff by open recognition of their contribution and other incentives to enhance employee loyalty and performance, according to Bass and Riggio (2006). This approach supports and maintains the status quo, and has firm elements of predictability of the manager-leader's behaviour and actions. However, its weakness is that it is markedly short-term focused, without longer-term vision or strategy for the enhancement of the service.

Moreover, currently one of the most widely advocated forms of leadership for healthcare professionals is transformational leadership, which entails merging the goals, desires and values of leaders with those of their followers into a common set of goals (Kouzes and Posner, 2017). The aim of the transformation is to generate employees' commitment to the organisation's vision and mission, in conjunction with their own and team members' individual aspirations and aims as employees of the organisation.

Deducing from the extensive literature on transformational leadership in healthcare, the following key points tend to reflect the general behaviour of transformational leaders (i.e. what they do, as different from their personal qualities or characteristics):

- Merges the organisation's, own and followers' goals, aspirations and values into a common goal.
- Enables individuals to consider their personal beliefs about healthcare, their attitudes and behaviours, and to pursue higher values (i.e. transforming).
- Communicates in persuasive and appealing ways.

- Acquires employee commitment to organisational goals and radical changes.
- Encourages team members to exercise leadership and inspire them to achieve organisational and personal goals.
- Stimulates growth and development, and discourages dependence.
- Acts as a catalyst for creativity and innovation in daily duties.
- Focuses on transforming the outlook and behaviour of team members by facilitating significant change within themselves, which, in turn, has effect on the employing organisation.
- Transforms team members' behaviour without exercising authority or coercion.
- Challenges and rewards informally and formally where possible.

Consequently, it can be concluded that transformational leadership is one of the most appropriate form of leadership for health and social care, which can form the basis for facilitating the prevailing endeavours in continuous service improvement and service transformation. Based on her concept analysis of transformational leadership in nursing, Fischer (2016) also concluded that although transformational leadership is associated with high-performing teams and improved patient care, the concept and its elements remains ambiguous and lacks an operational definition.

Nonetheless, according to Kouzes and Posner (2017), transformational leadership constitutes keeping a strategic or 'helicopter view' of the whole, and entails aspiring to effect radical changes in work practices. Transformational leaders, however, also tend to display substantially more energy and enthusiasm than other categories of leaders, and consequently may sometimes appear pushy.

Moreover, transformational leadership can be portrayed as comprising four elements (referred to as 4 Is) (Arnold et al., 2020; Collins et al., 2020), which when applied to healthcare means:

- *Individualised consideration* – Leader respects each team member for their individual merits and supports their development through delegation and supervision of their learning.
- *Idealised influence* – Leader is a role model, shows determination and high standards, and shares success with team members.
- *Inspirational motivation* – Leader demonstrates clear vision of team objectives and creates optimism towards its attainability.
- *Intellectual stimulation* – Leader encourages individuals to think for themselves, encourages creativity and innovation, and to apply their individual capabilities.

On summarising the extensive publications of transformational leadership, the following specific characteristics and common elements of the transformational leaders stand out, in addition to what transformational leaders do:

- Is visionary in the ways in which organisational goals can be achieved to a high degree of excellence.

- Is self-aware, balanced and confident within inter-disciplinary team-working.
- Displays honesty, integrity, commitment and credibility.
- Portrays self-belief in followers, and thereby inspires them.
- Is comfortable with team members' independent, responsible and autonomous decision-making.
- Shows high self-esteem, self-regard and self-awareness.
- Is passionate about the organisation's existing and new ventures.
- Treats home life and work life as a continuum, not as separate entities.
- Is a role model of interpersonal relationships, teamwork and care delivery.

ACTION POINT 3.4
What is transformed through
transformational leadership?

As indicated already, in the term 'transformational' the word transform implies fundamental change; that is, change to the vision, and the subsequent ideas for improvement, and then implementing them.

What might be your vision of how care can be transformed for the better in your own care setting, or in your organisation?

The above list of characteristics clearly suggests that transformational leaders need to have the capability to merge the organisation's, own and followers' goals, aspirations and values into a common entity. Consequently, they transform team members' views and approach, and enable them to understand and engage with the leader's vision of the work setting's or organisation's goals.

From a systematic review of transformational leadership, Holly and Igwee (2011) concluded that this form of leadership comprises intellectual stimulation by encouraging new ideas through individual consideration of followers' capabilities. It inspires motivation in team members, stimulates creativity, transmits optimism, and thereby provides a sense of direction while simultaneously instilling pride in their work.

Transactional leadership, on the other hand, is predominantly about managerial 'transactions' between the manager and the managed, and leaders are directive in their approach to team members' work, and also keep their home life completely separate from work. However, despite the slightly negative tone reflected in transactional leadership, this form of leadership has a definite place in healthcare, as it enables short-term goals to be achieved and all tasks to be completed, as also argued by Richards (2020) for example, although it needs to be combined with other forms of leadership for optimum effectiveness in care settings.

In their analysis of the relevance of transformational leadership for nursing, Collins et al. (2020) conclude that this form of leadership is highly motivational and empowering, and results in better staff engagement and, therefore, more effective and creative team members. However, the downside of transformational leadership, they argue, could be that the requirement to adhere to very high levels of engagement and creativity can be felt as pressure that can lead to 'burnout in some employees, and might also be emotionally draining for the leader' (Collins et al., 2020: 62) (staff motivation is discussed later in Chapter 6).

Collective leadership

Currently, leadership is valued as a function that can be exercised by all healthcare professionals, that is at all levels, and not as the exclusive role of postholders with supervisory and management duties, and is known as collective leadership. Also known as distributive or shared leadership, collective leadership involves shared responsibility and decision-making with regards to care delivery, accountability, and creativity and genuine engagement – as different from looking up to the skills of just one leader.

The well-recommended collective leadership theory is implemented sporadically in healthcare settings, and where it is applied systematically, it is one of the most suitable leadership approaches for achieving the goals of the health service. Previously in the form of the 'keyworker' model, the theory and concept indicate that it entails several members of the clinical team taking leadership roles for different aspects of practice in care settings (e.g. for infection prevention and control, auditing NEWS2, etc.), formally or informally.

ACTION POINT 3.5
Shared leadership

Pause for a moment and consider whether leadership at all levels and collective leadership prevails in your practice setting. For example, do staff members feel they are able to be creative and specialise in certain aspects of care in the practice setting? Then, is specialist expertise disseminated to team members?

Collective leadership involves developing a leadership culture in care settings whereupon leadership responsibilities are endowed on individual team members based on their expertise in specific areas of practice, and formal and informal leaders work collaboratively. Thus, the FHM may be the Band 5 or Band 6 front line manager for the care setting, who under collective leadership is able to share leadership with appropriate members of the team. The FHM would be the formal leader, by virtue of their appointment to the post, and various inter-disciplinary team members are delegated to lead in specific aspects of care and are generally seen as 'informal' leaders as they usually lead by virtue of their knowledge base and special expertise.

The benefit of collective leadership is that by empowering team members to take the lead, it also enhances staff engagement, promotes patient safety, clinical effectiveness and therefore high-quality care, and more likelihood of raising and documenting concerns when poor practice is suspected or detected. Staff members respect each other's and informal leaders' roles, responsibilities and their areas of expertise.

Collective leadership is also highly recommended in the NHS LTP (NHSE, 2019a) in the context of creating a culture of 'leadership at all levels'. It was earlier advocated by West et al. (2014), based at the King's Fund Centre, who also identify the specific capabilities of collective leaders, including:

- readily able to adapt to change in a coherent and collective manner;
- being responsive to patients and carers in a manner that demonstrates shared responsibility;
- proactively solving system issues and making improvement that require collaboration across internal or external departments or organisational boundaries, such as acute hospitals and community care.

However, collective leaders naturally must self-evaluate their effectiveness in the leadership role, in addition to updating their area of expertise and, as Nightingale (2020) notes, informal leaders also need to make plans to handover to other team members when the time comes to move on from their post due to promotion or otherwise.

Ultimately, as noted in Chapter 1 of this book, collective leadership is firmly endorsed by England's Chief Nursing Officer who asserts that this form of leadership involves empowering all healthcare professionals through shared decision-making which, in turn, enables them to lead change.

System leadership

Inherent within the structure of Integrated Care Systems (ICSs) that has been developed under the aegis of the NHS LTP (NHSE, 2019a), is the systems approach to management in health services. In relation to service users with complex and long-term conditions in particular, systems management incorporates working across different health and social care systems and organisational boundaries, as suggested by Timmins (2015) at the King's Fund for example. It also requires system leadership, which entails actively involving staff and their expertise from different departments of the organisation, for example radiology, social services, clinical psychology, etc., as well as those from other organisations.

Thus, through system leadership, health and care is co-ordinated and collaboratively supported by various service agencies (systems) in order to achieve care goals, or to enhance patient outcomes, which novel models of care such as ICSs and 'out-of-hospital care' aim to achieve. System leadership is consequently characterised by wide-ranging teamwork, and at all levels.

The difference between these two forms of leadership is that while collective leadership refers to a 'collection' of staff, i.e. team members in one care setting, system leadership incorporates an extensive range of people including service users and carers, social services, voluntary organisations, etc. that contribute to the wellbeing of the service user. Both concepts were referred to in Chapter 1 of this book, and collective leadership will be encountered again in the context of team-working in Chapter 6.

Compassionate leadership

Another widely advocated current avenue of providing leadership, especially since the recommendation made by Francis (2013) to provide compassionate care, is compassionate leadership. Compassionate care involves attending to service users' health problems by demonstrating understanding and by empathising with them, an approach that needs to be instituted as the core cultural value of healthcare (West et al., 2017). Furthermore, research on key stakeholders' perspectives on compassionate practice conducted by Kneafsey et al. (2016) suggests that such practice is more effective through applying active and effective communication and interpersonal skills, and by personal engagement and sustaining relationships.

Going beyond compassionate care, compassionate leadership extends to valuing people, and to the action they take to listen to the views of those they lead, empathising with them, and creating co-operation within the team. Compassionate leadership entails understanding the factors that motivate staff at work, acknowledging their aspirations and problems, and creating support mechanisms for people to achieve self-actualisation in their workplace.

Based on research exploring the impact of compassionate leadership on organisations, Boedker (2012) found that this form of leadership has substantial influence on organisational performance and productivity, partly by leaders being receptive and responsive to people's suggestions. It therefore also entails being a trustworthy person, who creates and maintains a compassionate and happier workplace that fosters engagement, an approach that is to some extent consistent with the people-centred (as opposed to productivity-centred) style of management, which is discussed in Chapter 4.

Furthermore, for compassionate leadership to be effective in healthcare settings, it needs to be implemented after careful planning at five levels according to West et al. (2017): (1) individual level but self-driven; (2) team and frontline manager level; (3) inter-disciplinary team level; (4) organisation level; and (5) system-wide. Compassionate leadership thereby becomes fully embedded in the organisational culture, resulting in positive outcomes, as it motivates team members to find new and improved ways of working because they feel they are listened to, valued and supported.

The six currently applied theories of leadership relate to the prevailing knowledge of leadership, some of which are based on extensive research studies (e.g. Holly and Igwee, 2011 – on transformational leadership; Boedker 2012 – compassionate leadership), and are useful theories that healthcare professionals (e.g. FHMs) can apply to leading care in practice settings. Further research should in future enhance our knowledge base of which theories apply most to different care settings. Table 3.4 provides a brief summary of the six widely applied current leadership approaches.

Table 3.4   Brief summary and differentiating between current leadership approaches

Traits theory	Refers to leaders' personal qualities
Transactional leadership	Management-focused leadership
Transformational leadership	Forward-looking, visionary and inspiring
Collective leadership	Components of healthcare led by different team members
System leadership	Leadership based on harnessing different systems in health and care provision
Compassionate leadership	Leading through respect for service users, maintaining dignity, listening

However, based on workshops using an action learning approach, Bonner and McLaughlin (2014) identify that ward managers struggle to participate in and demonstrate their clinical leadership role, and thereby also struggle to act as role models of practice for their juniors. This is because of the amount of administrative duties that they have to perform, for which they are inadequately trained, and Bonner and McLaughlin suggest that some of the administrative duties such as audits can be delegated back to their senior managers. Such action could free ward managers to engage in more effective clinical leadership, including participation in change management (covered in Chapter 9 of this book).

Leadership Skills and Frameworks Theories

Moving on from, first, the earlier theories of leadership such as charismatic and greatman theories, action-centred leadership, etc. and, second, the widely implemented current more-informed approaches that include transformational leadership, collective leadership and system leadership, this third section on how to lead is on models and frameworks of leadership, whose added purpose is to form the basis for leadership skills development programmes.

Models and frameworks of leadership that focus on the skills of effective leaders include the following (two of which were mentioned earlier in Figure 3.2):

- The nine-dimension *Healthcare Leadership Model* published by the NHS Leadership Academy (2021)
- Leadership Practices Inventory (LPI) and development programme by Kouzes and Posner (2017)
- The RCN Clinical Leadership Programme and the RCN System Leadership Programme (RCN, 2020a)
- The Clinical Leadership Competency Framework by NHS Leadership Academy (2012)

In healthcare, one of the most widely adopted frameworks in the nine-dimension *Healthcare Leadership Model* (NHS Leadership Academy, 2021), which comprises key behaviours that are inherent components of effective leadership. Each component of the model consists of a range of sub-concepts that need to be mastered to be successful as a leader, which are also influenced by the culture and climate of the work setting, and specific personal qualities such as self-awareness, resilience and flexibility.

These nine dimensions of the NHS Leadership Academy's (2021) *Healthcare Leadership Model* are:

1. Inspiring shared purpose.
2. Leading with care.
3. Evaluating information.
4. Connecting our service.
5. Sharing the vision.
6. Engaging the team.
7. Holding to account.
8. Developing capability.
9. Influencing for results.

Each dimension in the model comprises questions, against which FHMs or individual practitioners can rate themselves using a scale from 'strong' or 'exemplary' level to development required. An alternative to the nine-dimension leadership model is the more universal 'Five key practices and commitments' of leaders model that is deduced from worldwide original research by Kouzes and Posner's (2017), which constitute:

1. Modelling the way (i.e. leading by example, etc.).
2. Inspiring a shared vision.

3. Challenging the process.
4. Enabling others to act.
5. Encouraging the heart.

These five practices are developed into the Leadership Practices Inventory (LPI) by Kouzes and Posner, and each practice has two commitments (total ten commitments), which can be utilised for leadership self-assessment and development purposes. The NHS Leadership Academy's (2012) framework will also be elaborated on shortly, but the RCN's (2020a) frameworks can normally only be accessed after registering on its development programmes.

Developing Leadership Skills

Recognition of the need for effective clinical leadership in the frontline has been gaining prominence for more than two decades (e.g. DH, 2000b; NHS Leadership Academy, 2021). As is noted in Chapter 1 of this book, all health and care professionals should be equipped with the capability to take the lead in different components of care delivery and certain aspects of healthcare, which is rapidly becoming a reality NHS-wide.

An evaluation of the impact of a transformational leadership training programme based on Kouzes and Posner's synthesis of effective leaders for charge nurses in Turkey concluded that leadership practices 'increased statistically significantly with the implementation of the programme' (Duygulu and Kublay, 2011: 633). On the other hand, three perspectives on clinical leadership were identified from a qualitative study of leadership on healthcare by Generation Y (people born between 1980 to 1995) nurses (Dyess et al., 2016):

- Idealistic expectations of leaders – i.e. expectations of top-level leaders are too high, unrealistic, etc.;
- Leading in a challenging practice environment – e.g. staffing levels, national and local targets, availability of equipment;
- Cautious but optimistic outlook about their own leadership and future, as nurses are willing to adopt leadership roles so that they can influence the work environment, teamwork, etc.

Issues with leadership development programmes have been raised previously in that they are sometimes seen by nurses as not directly relevant to the real world of practice (e.g. Byrne, 2007). Consequently, recipients of leadership programmes should be provided with supported or supervised continuing opportunities for the application of theories within care delivery settings.

It has often been stated that organisations should not wait for frontline leaders to be appointed, but to identify existing employees with leadership potential and enable them to develop or improve their leadership skills and performance through training (e.g. Kotter, 2009). Such is the significance of leadership skill development that increasingly there has been the recommendation to include leadership awareness from the very first year of healthcare professionals' pre-registration programmes (e.g. Francis, 2013; Vaughn et al., 2019). This is now incorporated in pre-registration curricula.

Crucially, however, students should be exposed to leadership competence not only in theory sessions at university, but also to positive leadership role modelling in practice settings and be provided supervised opportunity to develop their leadership competence along with feedback from supervisors.

For registrants, on the other hand, they can develop leadership competence through practice-based structured learning, or a balanced combination of theory and practice opportunities, usually as part of a master's level course. Learning is often based on one of the published frameworks of leadership, such as the nine-dimension leadership framework offered by the NHS Leadership Academy (2021).

Leadership self-assessment tools are also available in textbooks (e.g. Kouzes and Posner, 2017), and via the internet (e.g. NHS Leadership Academy, 2012), which is normally followed by identifying areas for personal development. Many development programmes aim to enable attendees to develop transformational leadership skills, because this form of leadership has been widely researched and because transformation signifies making changes and implementing innovations in order to ultimately ensure that service users' experience of healthcare remain positive. Components of other leadership theories and approaches can be incorporated as deemed appropriate, especially as healthcare leadership models and frameworks are not meant to be rigid and complete, but adaptable instead.

Frontline healthcare managers can also further develop their own leadership skills by attending leadership skill development workshops or courses. There has been a cumulative proliferation of leadership skill development programmes over the last decade or two, ranging from master's courses to much shorter ones, from interactive face-to-face workshops to online learning facilities, some of which are self-funded while others may be supported financially by employers. Ongoing self-development in leadership as well as other components such as management, clinical competence and research skills is consistent with the notion of lifelong learning by healthcare professionals (Gopee, 2001; Davis et al., 2014).

Some of the longer and more prominent leadership development programmes that are based on the five models are mentioned at the beginning of this section. The NHS Leadership Academy (2012: 2) programme, for example, comprises five domains: (1) demonstrating personal qualities; (2) working with others; (3) managing services; (4) improving services; and (5) setting direction. Each domain consists of four elements with associated 'competence statements', and as an example, the four elements under 'Demonstrating personal qualities' are:

- Developing self-awareness by being aware of their own values, principles and assumptions, and by being able to learn from experiences;
- Managing yourself by organising and managing oneself while taking account of the needs and priorities of others;
- Continuing personal development by learning through participating in continuing professional development and from experience and feedback;
- Acting with integrity by behaving in an open, honest and ethical manner.

Therefore, the above four bullet points are specific examples of leadership competence against which healthcare professionals can self-assess themselves, and maybe identify professional development areas. The specific competencies in the nine-dimension *Healthcare Leadership Model* published by the NHS Leadership Academy (2021) can also be accessed on the internet, but the reader might need to register (which is free) with the organisation to do so.

ACTION POINT 3.6
Self-assessment of leadership competencies

Access the NHS Leadership Academy's (2012) Clinical Leadership Competency Framework Self-assessment tool on its website at: CLCF Self-Assessment Layout 1 (leadershipacademy.nhs.uk).

The whole twelve-page document is very easy to follow and interesting to look through and reflect on. As noted above, it includes competence statements related to 'Demonstrating personal qualities'; for example, under the sub-headings 'Developing self-awareness' 'Managing yourself, 'Continuing professional development' and 'Acting with integrity'.

Perform a self-assessment on the competence statements, and the comprehensive 'Personal Action Plan' in the latter part of the document which includes development need, resources required, obstacles and how they can be overcome, etc.

Sometime after completing the self-assessment and action plan, you might decide to discuss them with a colleague of senior or equal status to obtain external views of your development plans, a concept and exercise referred to as '360-degree feedback' (e.g. Kouzes and Posner, 2017) when feedback is sought from a variety of professionals. With 360-degree feedback it is essential that a supportive medium is created, possibly by using an external facilitator so that the receiver of the feedback does not feel over-criticised. Furthermore, you might decide to broach specific components to discuss with your line manager at your next IDPR.

Guidance for Effective Leadership by Frontline Care Managers

The following comprises guidance for effective leadership by frontline healthcare managers.

- As an effective leader, genuinely respect individual team members, be considerate, empathise and facilitate an open working relationship within the team.
- Endorse and assimilate forms of leadership that are currently most appropriate for healthcare, such as collective leadership, compassionate leadership, transformational leadership.
- Always keep in mind the benefits of functional (opposite of dysfunctional) leadership in terms of benefits to service users as well as to staff and in the achievement of organisational goals.
- Heed the qualities of leadership such as honesty, forward-looking, competence and inspiring that followers believe each leader should have (noted in Chapter 1 of this book), and those discussed extensively in this chapter.
- Be fully aware of the styles of leadership that you adopt, both routinely and as situations deem right.
- Have a working knowledge of all leadership theories, and their application and suitability for different care settings and circumstances.
- Although leaders may be in a position to exercise different forms of power, remember leadership is about empowering team members (as opposed to wielding coercive power).
- Enable and support team members to develop their own leadership skills in aspects of the organisation's goals, remembering that as the leader you are also the role model who leads by example.
- In appropriate circumstances, obtain feedback periodically on your leadership activities and take self-development action to enhance your leadership skills and styles as appropriate.

Chapter Summary

As elaborated in ample detail in this chapter, the FHM's leadership role is pivotal for ensuring that service users receive person-centred, safe and effective healthcare when needed. Extensive literature on healthcare leadership can be found easily in health profession journals and in policy and guidance documents. Furthermore, various leadership development programmes can be accessed by healthcare professionals to further their own leadership competence with the prime purpose being the provision of highest quality of care. This chapter has endeavoured to explain the evolution of leadership over recent years, and provided detailed analysis and application of the more current and better informed leadership approaches, which provide comprehensive guidance on leadership to frontline healthcare managers. It has, therefore, focused on:

- understanding of what leadership is and what leadership in care settings entail, which also involves distinguishing between leadership and management; and examining research on leadership;
- ascertaining the reasons for leadership in health services and its benefits, and precisely who are the healthcare professionals who provide it;
- the different styles of leadership and their impact in care settings, as well as different types of power associated with leadership;
- earlier theories of leadership along with the more informed current approaches to healthcare leadership provision to team members;
- leadership development programmes that are based on models and frameworks of leadership that reflect a comprehensive skill-set for this function; and
- undertaking self-assessment of leadership skills to identify strengths and areas for further development.

Further Reading

- For some basic reflective exercises for developing self-awareness as a leader, and on positive role modelling, see Major D (2019) Developing effective nurse leadership skills. *Nursing Standard,* 34(6): 61–66.
- For research findings based on data from generation Y nurses' perspectives on leadership in healthcare, see: Dyess S M, Sherman R O, Pratt B A, Chiang-Hanisko L (2016) Growing nurse leaders: Their perspectives on nursing leadership and today's practice environment. *Online Journal of Issues in Nursing,* 21(1): 1–7.
- For NHS Leadership Academy's healthcare leadership self-assessment tool, see: NHS Leadership Academy (2021) *Healthcare Leadership Model – The nine dimensions of leadership behaviour.* Available at: www.leadershipacademy. nhs.uk/resources/healthcare-leadership-model/nine-leadership-dimensions/. Accessed Date: 4 April 2021.

4

Effective Management in Healthcare Settings

Chapter Objectives

The chapter objectives for frontline healthcare managers in relation to effective management in healthcare are:

- Articulate the specific day-to-day managerial duties that frontline health-care managers tend to engage in.
- Show substantial insight into how organisations in general and healthcare organisations specifically function, and recognise the structures and staff hierarchies within them.
- Show clear knowledge of what managers and management signify, where management fits into the organisation and where FHMs fit into healthcare management structures.
- Demonstrate knowledge and comprehension of different well-established research-driven theories of management, and of their application to care settings.
- Identify established styles of management that FHMs can apply in the course of their day-to-day duties.
- Establish the various ways in which the FHM communicates daily care effectively in collaboration with relevant services, along with more specific management communication such as delegation of duties and accurate documentation.

Introduction

The majority of organisations that employ approximately one hundred or more workers have four basic levels of management: top level managers, middle managers, first-line managers and team leaders, with managers at times being referred to as leaders, supervisors or administrators. This textbook focuses on first-line managers and team leaders in healthcare, and they are referred to as frontline healthcare managers (FHMs).

Health services are provided in numerous service-user facing settings, ranging from acute emergency settings to longer-term care within the community, caring for mothers and babies and to end-of-life care. Healthcare may be accessed by individuals at any point during their lifespan. FHMs are tasked with managing care effectively and efficiently in their designated areas of responsibility, while ensuring that the care provided is 'safe, effective and focused on patient experience', as noted in the *NHS Constitution* (DHSC, 2019a: 2).

Having ascertained the social and financial context in which healthcare is delivered in the UK in Chapter 1 of this book, various facets of NRHPs' roles in Chapter 2 and competent leadership in Chapter 3, this chapter converges on ways of managing care effectively and, therefore, examines the various known underpinning principles, conceptions, theories, styles and features that determine the manner in which care managers manage the human and non-human resources made available for their care settings.

The chapter begins by delving into day-to-day management duties and roles of FHMs, which is followed by discussion on service provider organisations, and then by well-established and widely advocated theories and styles of management, and related research, and their application to healthcare management. It concludes by examining multiple types of management-specific communication, such as delegation and documentation, and then the interpersonal skills and personal qualities of FHMs.

Determining Frontline Managers' Duties in Service Provider Organisations

Numerous activities that FHMs engage in were identified in response to Action point 1.1, Chapter 1. However, for some decades now, concerns have remained high about the financial challenges being encountered by the NHS, about the adequacy of the workforce and about the need for improvement in the quality of care. Yet, scientific advances continually discover new and more effective ways of treating human illnesses, which, with changes in demographic and environmental factors, tend to cumulatively increase the costs of health and care provisions. Both effective and efficient management of care delivery is therefore an imperative through careful utilisation of resources, while also maintaining high-quality evidence-informed care.

On and off, frontline managers such as FHMs might seem to spend a substantial amount of their day engaged in administrative duties (at times referred to as 'doing the paperwork') or participating in formal meetings within or outside the department. At other times, they may appear to do no more than ensure that healthcare professionals in their team are conducting their roles correctly, intervening only when problems are anticipated or arise. However, as noted above in relation to Action point 1.1, all activities that frontline managers engage in are centred around the health recovery and wellbeing of service users.

Your list of managerial duties in response to Action point 1.1 may have included many of those identified in the list presented after the Action point. They are management duties or activities identified by RNs taking management courses or modules at university, and by finalist pre-registration student nurses, separately. For ease of understanding, these day-to-day activities/duties are here grouped under ten categories or roles, as illustrated in Figure 4.1.

All the regular daily activities and roles that FHMs perform can also be grouped under the five main areas identified in the introduction to Chapter 1, but grouping them under the ten categories or roles in Figure 4.1 shows a more comprehensive picture of roles that form the basis for safe and effective care management in clinical settings.

In their qualitative study of the roles of first-line healthcare managers, Cziraki et al. (2014) re-affirm that healthcare professionals in frontline healthcare management positions facilitate the attainment of organisational goals, which, in turn, has positive effects on patient safety and job satisfaction; and that their role includes being skilled and visionary leaders, advocates, communicators, educators and change agents. They engage in decision-making, to ensure a safe environment for all in the clinical setting, and in risk management.

However, when Carlin and Duffy (2013) researched practitioners' perceptions of the management and leadership responsibilities, and the qualities of senior charge nurses in acute hospital settings, they found that research participants had difficulty articulating clearly the leadership aspects of charge nurses' roles. With regard to management, they concluded that increased workload related to quality improvement, such as infection control precautions, reduced managerial staff's visibility in clinical settings, which, in turn, led to reduced feedback to practitioners, diminished presence of charge nurses as role models and lessened approachability. Lack of visibility of healthcare leaders in practice settings is antithetical to the concept of 'clinical leadership' (see Chapter 3).

Following his study of management activities, Fayol (2012) placed these activities (or functions) in five groups as planning, organising, commanding, co-ordinating and controlling (feedback), which has been widely adopted across organisations. Further details related to the managerial role components derived from Action point 1.1 are presented in Table 4.1.

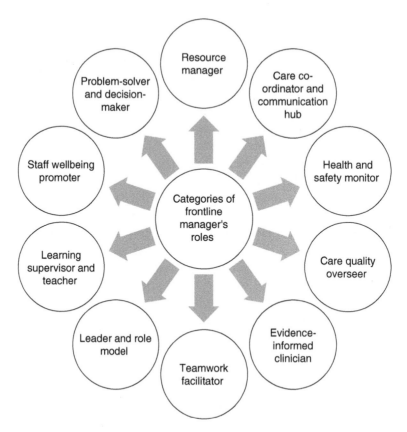

Figure 4.1   Categories of frontline managers' roles

The managerial components in Table 4.1 are presented as discrete elements in the endeavour to group them as themes. However, more than one component is often accomplished simultaneously while engaged in work-based activities, such as being a resource manager, decision-maker and problem-solver at the same time. The table represents quite an accurate overall picture of contemporary managerial role components of FHMs' healthcare organisational activities undertaken across various hospital wards, clinics, departments, etc in the organisation.

Alternatively, Mintzberg (2011: 45) clusters management activities as ten groups of 'the manager's working roles' (as discussed later in this chapter). However, Drucker (2007: 14, 11) categorises management activities at organisational level under only four categories, which are managing the business, managing managers, managing workers and managing work. The work of frontline managers (as different from management) are grouped under five 'basic operations', which are setting objectives, organising, motivating and communicating, measuring, and developing people.

Fayol (2012) and others also group the very wide range of managers' activities into just a few categories of more generalised terms, although this can result in loss

Table 4.1 Components of the FHM's management roles – in no particular order (see also Table 10.1)

Managerial role component	Brief details
Resource manager	Manage human resources – recruiting, retaining, motivating, developing staff Manage non-human resources, e.g. equipment, consumables, etc. Manage budget, promote efficiency Plan, prioritise and manage workload; supervise
Care co-ordinator and communication hub	Communicate care requirements, delegate, record-keeping, facilitate meetings Collaborate across disciplines
Health and safety monitor	Ensure health and safety of all; policy adherence Adhere to professional codes Devise/adapt clinical guidelines
Care quality overseer	Promote highest standards of care; service improvement; audits, evaluation of care Monitor quality of patient care informally and formally Manage change and innovation
Evidence-informed clinician	Knowledgeable, competent and up-to-date practitioner Knowledge of relevant policies and procedures Patient/service user advocate
Teamwork facilitator	Inter-disciplinary team-worker, team advocate, team builder Maintain inter-disciplinary team cohesiveness Exercise social skills and capabilities
Leader and role model	Role model, team leader, provide leadership, pro-active, creative, devolve leadership Ensure and support equality and diversity Link and network with other organisations
Learning supervisor and teacher	Educate students from different disciplines, teach apprentices Identify, contribute to and monitor team members' professional development Support continuing learning for all
Staff wellbeing promoter	Knowledge of facilities and support that staff can draw on Advise on staff wellbeing Support colleagues experiencing stress/burnout Emotionally resilient and self-aware
Problem-solver and decision-maker	Prevent/manage disruptions in the care setting Make decisions at operational level; conflict resolution Manage poor performance

of detail of the multiple and complex activities that especially FHMs engage in during every span of duty.

Furthermore, in healthcare, although FHMs' roles and activities focus attention on the practical aspects of their role during a typical span of duty, FHMs' own line managers, as middle managers, are also likely to have a good degree of responsibility and accountability for the functioning of care settings.

Defining Manager and Management

Moving on from the duties and roles of FHMs, this section explores the terms manager and management in the context of healthcare provision, and the general structure and functions of organisations like hospitals and other providers.

The terms 'manager' and 'management' have been studied and analysed for several years, mostly since the nineteenth-century industrial revolution in Britain and other countries. Terms like industrial revolution and modernism are characterised by mass production of goods such as cars, light bulbs, television sets, etc. in large factories employing hundreds or thousands of employees. The employees had to be managed to ensure expected productivity, and the resources for production needed to be managed.

There have been various definitions of the terms 'manager' and 'management' over the years. Drucker (2007: 6), for example, identifies a manager simply as 'someone who directs the work of others and who does his work by getting other people to do theirs'. Such definitions clearly suggest that a manager is a person who has the responsibility to oversee and ensure that employees perform their allocated duties which thereby enable specific objectives set by the organisation or a department to be met.

Furthermore, in her study of the key characteristics and the necessary personal skills of effective nurse managers, Calpin-Davies (2000) identified the key characteristics as including being service oriented, radiating positive energy, being synergistic, regular professional updating and believing in other people. The personal skills of effective nurse managers according to Calpin-Davies' research include having good communication skills, the ability to motivate people, the ability to influence others, adaptability and ability to respond positively to change.

Subsequent research by Cziraki et al. (2014) concluded that the characteristics of first-line healthcare managers include being passionate and proud about their work (i.e. about their specialism, their colleagues, etc.), being accountable for their responsibilities and appropriate use of resources, being committed to professional development, being reflective and self-directed, and tenacious and resilient.

As a health service frontline manager, the FHM is an employee who has been appointed by the management of the organisation specifically to ensure that the objectives of their area of responsibility are achieved in full with the knowledge and expertise that they hold. They, therefore, decide and prioritise the specific tasks or activities that need to be performed, and ensure that the activities that they have delegated to appropriately skilled team members are performed according to the organisation's policies and guidelines.

Considering the management of the healthcare organisation, this is often made up of a group of managers who are senior to the FHM, and includes relevant post-holders such as finance officer, senior doctor, Chief Executive Officer, etc. Drucker (2007: 15) defines management as 'a multi-purpose organ that manages a business, manages managers, and manages worker and work', and asserts that if any of these components is missing then the business will not thrive. The term 'organ' is deliberately included to emphasise the live and dynamic nature of businesses and organisations, in their quest for the achievement of their objectives.

To achieve specific objectives, however, the right resources are required, and if problems do arise, they need to be resolved instantly to bring it back to normal functioning again. At the frontline FHM level, Drucker's definition also applies to service user facing level, and comprises a team of appropriately qualified individuals who engage in multiple activities aimed at effective and efficient delivery of care.

As for the terms effective and efficient, 'effective' is an adjective which refers to being able to achieve or accomplish results. To 'effect' is to 'accomplish', and the noun 'effect' refers to 'something attained or acquired as the result of an action'. The closely related term 'efficient' also refers to being effective, but with the use of the least amount of effort and resources. Therefore, the effective and efficient FHM is one who achieves results at a pre-determined standard and does so without wastage of available human and non-human resources.

Healthcare Providers as Organisations

Over and above managers and management of the healthcare organisation is the organisation itself as an entity in its own right in that managers as employees of the organisation can leave at any time, definitely in their lifetime, but the organisation outlives each employee and endures over a number of generations, centuries sometimes, to ensure the healthcare needs of the local population is met. At times they merge with other local healthcare organisation into more efficient larger ones, and occasionally they are disbanded as one was in the West Midlands in the UK following the Francis (2013) Report.

Organisations are generally viewed as belonging to one of two generic groups: first, the public sector organisations and, second, those in the private sector. The distinction between the two is that public sector organisations are non-profit-making organisations (although they may end the financial year in surplus or in deficit), they are 'owned' by taxpayers, and their main aim is to provide a service that is concerned with the wellbeing of the people who live in a defined geographical area. Private sector organisations are usually of a commercial nature and put together by groups of individuals with the aim of making profit from its business and growing bigger for even more profit. Care organisations are public sector non-profit-making service organisations.

Organisations consequently vary according to the nature of the work they have been created to undertake. For example, contrasting a school with a car manufacturer, or a hospital with a public library, shows that each has distinct functions. These functions determine the specific people skills they require, how simple or complex those skills need to be, the number of people they need to employ, and their overall size which is determined by the volume of their output.

How Organisations Function

Organisations are often led by a Chief Executive Officer (CEO), who, in turn, is accountable to the chairperson of the Board of the organisation, with the Board comprising unpaid members whose aim is to ensure the viability and the longevity of the organisation. For healthcare in England, it's at the NHS trust Board level, with the CEO or equivalent being accountable to NHS England, and to the Secretary of State for Health.

At Trust level, the care organisation is housed in a complex of buildings, has different departments and the staffing structure incorporates all individuals employed by the organisation, with the precise division of responsibilities and individual tasks for each employee. Responsibilities and tasks of senior and junior staff are clearly demarcated and hierarchical. The hierarchy, therefore, manifests the reporting relationships within the organisation, but there are also parallel relationships between equivalent posts, as well as the co-ordination of their activities, the purpose being to achieve the aims and objectives of the organisation.

Hierarchical structure of staff responsibilities represents the line management through which the activities of the organisation are established, communicated and monitored, using different mechanisms such as individual and groups emails, face-to-face communication, team briefs, staff meetings, bulletins and staff training notifications on notice boards, etc.

Each department's work is normally clearly defined, and duties divided among employees based on their skill and knowledge, but with teamwork, and with appropriate level of supervision. The posts that individuals are appointed to have identified job descriptions, whether they are at registrant level or specialist level, and are accompanied by their areas of accountability. The degree of specialisation required to achieve the objectives of the organisation are usually clearly delineated.

Nonetheless, a good structure of the organisation does not singularly guarantee success, which is because each individual employee's input impacts on the organisation's outcomes and objectives, and therefore staff morale, motivation and job satisfaction are important elements. Consequently, appropriate leadership and management styles are also significant elements, and systems for monitoring effectiveness.

The formal structure of the organisation is precisely designed to fulfil a purpose and deliver a service, but another unplanned dimension always exists, which is referred to as an 'informal organisation'. This comprises informal small groups of employees, but serves as a tentative unofficial voice of employees whereby personal complaints are shared with peers, or group suggestions for improvement of the service can be suggested to the organisation.

Informal organisations, therefore, essentially constitute a sub-culture that has undefined lines of communication, at times led by personalities, and may be in conflict with the formal organisation, and even constitute political motives. Nonetheless, informal organisations make an important contribution to the organisation's wellbeing through the peer support that employees can derive from them. They satisfy the social needs of employees to communicate their thoughts and feelings about their posts and the organisation.

Informal organisations also comprise a medium for social interaction with its additional channels of communication, e.g. the 'grapevine' and social media, through which thoughts and ideas get communicated quickly. It can also be a medium for gaining a sense of personal identity, belongingness, feeling of stability and security, and even social status.

Informal organisations can have significant influence on the job satisfaction and performance of staff, their morale and motivation, and the prevailing beliefs, assumptions and values of the organisation (i.e. organisational culture – see Chapters 2, 8 and 9 of this book for more analysis of organisational culture), but may also be a route for voicing ways in which improvements can be made in the formal organisation for staff and the clientele.

The formal staff management structure of organisations just discussed can be represented diagrammatically as a hierarchy or in the shape of a pyramid (see Figure 4.2 as an example of a range of titles for nursing staff), and much debate has taken place about how flat or steep the hierarchy should be.

Where there are steep structures, there are several levels of management, each upper level being more senior and the bottom-most level being the frontline

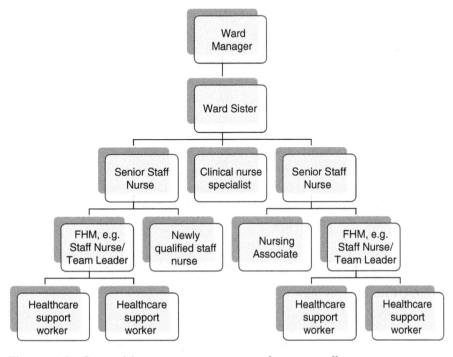

Figure 4.2 Pyramidal management structure of nursing staff

workers. With flatter structures, there are fewer levels of management to answer to, with more management responsibilities given to those who are in lower management positions.

Note the boundaries between these roles are not always clear and distinct, as they vary according to the salary band the manager is on, progress with their own continuing learning, and their specific scope of responsibilities within the specialism. Thus, ward manager equivalent roles could include charge nurse, senior sister, clinical manager, clinical sister, etc.

ACTION POINT 4.1
Staff hierarchy in your own workplace

Think about the management structure in your work setting, and then draw a diagram as in Figure 4.2 showing the actual staffing hierarchy and lines of responsibilities in the team, department or organisation.

Check how many levels of management there are, and consider if the management structure and levels within your care setting are appropriate. What management structure do you consider to be ideal?

Drucker's (2007) suggestion that management is an organ implies that the structure within the overall parameter can change to add more or fewer levels, or more or fewer posts at each level, along with changing individual responsibilities. Management structures can be affected by continual changes, or influenced by internal and external factors, problematic matters could surface, which means that the existing structure may need to be reviewed and changed to strengthen its impact.

One potential problem with steep pyramidal structures is that they can be the cause of ineffective communication because of too many go-between levels of managers, which, in turn, could lead to misrepresentations and misunderstandings. Flatter management structures could resolve some of the issues related to pyramidal structures and enable smoother communication and be more rewarding for employees through more responsibilities.

Research-Driven Evolution of Management Theories

Moving on from the nature of organisations and how managers function within them, the next section endeavours to focus on the evidence base underlying management. The reason for exploring the evidence base is to ascertain the research that is available for frontline managers to draw on in addition to the management skills that they have learnt through experience, through management workshops, and through guidance from their own senior managers.

On examination of evidence-based management, Pfeffer and Sutton (2006) observe that many managers engage in management of their resources, and in decision-making, etc. based on management practices from their own past experiences, or they endeavour to practise it in the way that high-performing managers (or experts) in their field are perceived as doing. This mode of learning management skills from experts is referred to as 'experiential evidence', which Walshe (2016) asserts is widely accepted as evidence base, particularly because of the dearth of well-designed research on management.

With the prevailing ethos of evidence-based practice, the question can rightly be asked as to what is 'evidence-based management'. For example, is there any research or systematic reviews of research whose findings guide the way we manage? Well, the answer is yes, there are some. Let's, however, first establish what is evidence-based management. According to Briner et al. (2009: 19), evidence-based management (usually abbreviated as EBMgt) is about making decisions through the conscientious, explicit and judicious use of four sources of evidence:

1. practitioner expertise and judgment;
2. evidence from the local context;
3. critical evaluation of the best available research evidence; and
4. the perspectives of those people who might be affected by the decision made.

The above explanation of EBMgt is adapted from one of the definitions of evidence-based medicine, mainly because it appears that the concept of EBMgt has not been widely empirically investigated (i.e. researched). In the hierarchy of evidence in healthcare, normally the best evidence is those from meta-analyses, systematic reviews and randomised controlled trials, albeit expert knowledge is also seen as evidence, but a weak one.

Therefore, EBMgt refers to any evidence from any level in the above-mentioned hierarchy, be it research or expert knowledge, that justifies the ways in which managers manage the human and non-human resources at their disposal during the course of their duties. However, Stewart (2018) argues that EBMgt is primarily an attitude of mind, and although it is feasible to compare two managers' productivity to ascertain whose activities achieve set outcomes more efficiently, managers are well known for their reluctance to share information despite their networking activities. This could be because when wrong decisions are made with uncomfortable consequences, then it is the individual manager whose position in the organisation is jeopardised.

ACTION POINT 4.2

Evidence-based management by care setting managers

Thinking about the managerial activities identified by RNs and finalist pre-registration student nurses presented earlier in this chapter in Table 4.1 (as well as published ones such as those by Fayol and by Mintzberg), and considering the actions that FHMs take to perform these activities and fulfil these roles, what is the 'best available evidence' base that determine them taking these actions the way they do?

Evidence-based management remains an evolving concept, as it is affected by organisations and businesses being of very different sizes (based on their income and number of employees), being a non-profit-making public sector organisation or private sector profit-making organisation, the age of the organisation and its infrastructure, their implementation of novel technology and their sustainability, etc. An overview of some of the key research on management practices conducted over the years, and their conclusions, are summarised at the end of the next section that examines established management theories.

Well-Established Theories of Management

As noted above, many managers learn to manage through experiences of management situations and perhaps from the knowledge and advice of their own previous managers. Then, Walshe (2016) suggests, as managers progress through their managerial careers, they reflect on their ways of managing and how their ways compare with the actions indicated by established management theories, models and concepts. They will usually have gained some knowledge of management theories and principles during their pre-registration programme.

In relation to theories, it is worthwhile pausing momentarily to consider what a theory is. A theory is exactly what the word implies, which means it is a hypothesis, a generalisation or an assumption of a 'cause and effect' relationship. Our theories are based on our prediction that if we do x (cause), then y (effect) will happen. An assumption signifies that if we take a certain action, then that should lead to a specific result. A theory is constructed from ideas and concepts that emerge from experience, which then seeks to explain an ambiguous situation or a phenomenon, or is developed into ways of working, or research, that seems to resolve the issue or prevent it occurring in the first instance.

Accordingly, with management theories (discussed next), they are also based partly on general assumptions and generalisations, and partly on research. They endeavour to predict or justify management activities. In the following section, four prominent theories that apply to FHMs and healthcare are discussed: scientific management theory, human relations theory, systems theory and post-modern theories.

Scientific management theory

The scientific management theory (also known as 'Taylorism', or the classical approach) is one of the earliest management theories, but one that can also be easily observed in bureaucratic organisations today. According to this theory, managers guide the organisation to improve productivity and efficiency, the latter being a concept that has been at the top of NHS priorities and under subsequent governments' spotlight for the last two decades. The notions productivity and efficiency assume that if an organisation's formal structure is aligned so that it clearly identifies exactly which tasks for the organisation are covered by which posts, that is, the exact technical skills that each post-holder needs to have to fulfil the job requirements, and a comprehensive set of detailed rules and procedures that need to be followed for various activities are firmly established, then the organisation should be able to deliver the service it has been set up for smoothly and fully.

The organisation's formal structure includes a clear hierarchy of workforce, with clear division of work and definition of duties and responsibilities, with formal intra-organisational relationships. The scientific management theory was originally based on very detailed job analysis performed by Frederick Taylor in the nineteenth and twentieth centuries. Taylor successfully endeavoured to change managers' attitude towards work for the benefit of both the employer and employees, through analysis of each job, and asking employees for suggestions for improvement in exchange for monetary incentives, and through:

- increasing the amount of work done during a particular shift, and thereby improve productivity;
- breaking jobs into discrete tasks and 'one best way' to perform each task;
- co-operation with workers to ensure work is carried out in the prescribed way; and
- systematic selection, training and development of employees.

Other strengths include better quality of management decisions, fewer accidents and less sickness and absenteeism. Taylor's scientific method of management has, however, been criticised for being too 'bureaucratic', with too rigidly structured rules and regulations, and with employment being based predominantly on technical qualifications and skills. Other weaknesses are that:

- excessive emphasis on rules and regulations can stifle growth and initiative, and lead to failure, frustration and conflict and stereotyped behaviours;
- there is neglect of the employees' aspirations, and consequently feels impersonal.

Scientific management methods have been applied to care management more recently whereupon, for example, questions have been asked about how many minutes a GP should take to attend to each patient, and therefore how many they can see in one day's work; how long a district nurse takes to perform a dressing in a patient's home, etc. Such methods tend to overlook the post-holder's interpersonal needs for interaction between employees, and post-holders' individual views on the functioning of the organisation, compassionate person-centred care, etc.

Consequently, the scientific method of management is relatively unpopular amongst both employees and managers. Subsequent theories of management, such as the human relations approach, incorporate consideration of the personal and social experiences of individual workers, and thereby overcome this major weakness of the scientific theory.

However, another feature of the scientific management theory is efficiency in the management of healthcare. The Chartered Global Management Accountant (2015) indicates, for example, that one of the best ways to increase efficiency as well as effectiveness is to adopt 'lean management techniques', which can be applied beneficially to for-profit, as well as to not-for-profit organisations, such as education and healthcare. Lean thinking refers to the least wasteful way of providing care, which also maximises the use of resources and reduces delays. Lean management entails devolving responsibilities to teams of employees, which also enables organisations to identify and reduce waste in their processes and procedures.

Human relations theory of management

Based primarily on the highly regarded and well-documented Hawthorne experiments at the Western Electric Company in the United States between 1924 and 1932, the human relations management theory has evolved consistently over the years and prevails extensively across management today. In the experiment, it emerged that managers' focus on increasing productivity was further enabled when some of the employees' social and psychological needs were met. These needs were met when the employees were asked to change from working individually to working in small groups or teams, members of which were self-selected; and they also had short breaks during work that afforded opportunity for further informal social interaction between members.

The human relations management theory, which is also referred to as the 'behavioural' or 'informal approach', resulted in teamwork (instead of just individual work) taking root and gradually being widely established in work settings. Later developments of this approach include neo-human relations theories, as the theory and the concept teamwork were synthesised by Maslow (1987), Herzberg (2003), McGregor (1987) and others. These authors asserted that when organisations established mechanisms that enabled some of the workers' psycho-social needs to be met, that also resulted in higher staff motivation and higher productivity. Human needs and staff motivation are further discussed in the context of teamwork in Chapter 6.

Working in teams is visibly applied in the majority of healthcare settings, short refreshment breaks are structured into the day's work, and some interest in each other's personal and social life are accepted as a healthy norm. Human relations theory is clearly the most appropriate approach for managing health and social care staff, as the whole ethos of health and social care organisations is based primarily on caring and promoting the holistic wellbeing of people. Additionally, the theory enables employees to feel a sense of belonging to the organisation and to the team, and of being valued and respected, as also noted by Peek (2020).

Some of the ways in which the FHM could effectively implement the human relations approach are by:

- supporting fulfilment of social needs by encouraging staff to socialise during their breaks, recognising a team member's birthday, etc.;
- considering each individual staff member's personal aspirations from the post they are employed in, such as professional development, and prospects of promotion at some point;
- promoting teamwork ethos, rather than working as individual employees;
- ensuring new members of staff are supported individually to enable them to be assimilated into the existing team;
- asking employees individually how they are getting on, and thereby showing an appropriate level of interest in the employee's family, holidays, new baby, etc.;
- providing general peer-support through making clinical supervision and other such mechanisms available.

The human relations management approach thus facilitates an atmosphere of openness, flexibility, trust, loyalty, cohesion, belongingness to the workplace and high morale prevails in the work setting (Johansson et al., 2014: 156–7). Furthermore, certain human relations skills between manager-employee and peers are also required for this approach to be successful, which include:

- good level of empathy needs to be exercised;
- ability to multitask and prioritise, but also to complete all duties;
- flexibility in being able to adapt to workplace changes and new policies that affect daily work;
- communication using similar type of English whenever appropriate, instead of official formal language;
- when disagreement or conflict occurs, conflict resolution has to be managed sensitively.

ACTION POINT 4.3
The human relations approach in your workplace

Reflecting on the above-mentioned examples of the application of the human relations theory, think of instances that you have noticed when managers who you know have actively utilised the human relations approach in the practice setting.

While engaging in the above Action point, you will have thought of 'good' managers that you have encountered already. However, how far frontline managers can apply the features of human relations theory is also dependent upon such factors as adequate resources, levels of employees' motivation and their knowledge and competence. It could also be said, however, that it is difficult to please all staff, all of the time; and also, excessive focus on staff's human needs at the expense of scientific methods could affect productivity negatively.

Systems management theory

The evolution of multifarious technological devices for healthcare, and the departmentalisation and specialisation of healthcare provision and delivery, are two components that form the basis for the systems management theory. This theory, therefore, extends preceding theories, and top-level management sees the organisation as comprising a number of systems and sub-systems, akin to the systems of the human body, each functioning as a distinct entity, but has communication lines with all other systems so that the aim of the organisation as a whole is achieved.

Systems in organisation can feature as departments in hospitals (e.g. radiology, operating theatres, dietetics for nutrition for patients), sections, university faculties, etc; and subsystems can include units, teams, work groups, but they interrelate and work in collaboration with the other systems (i.e. not as isolated units) and collectively with the whole organisation. Working in collaboration and collectively was also noted under system leadership in Chapter 3 in this book, a current example of which is integrated care systems (ICSs).

Systems approach, therefore, incorporates aspects of both classical and human relations approaches. This approach sees organisations as either: (1) open systems with multiple channels of interaction internally and with the broader external environment; or (2) socio-technical systems, with staff continually acquainting themselves with novel technologies, with the aim of enhancing organisational outcomes as well as improving the quality of services.

Both open and socio-technical systems can be identified in healthcare organisations in the form of increased use of computers and digitalisation to increase the speed of communication, and with continuing renewal of medical equipment and devices used for a wide range of interventions and diagnostic investigations respectively. Moreover, more universal use of computers and hand-held devices facilitate speedier interventions through, for example, tele-health, telephone consultations with GPs, etc.

Open systems signify taking into consideration public involvement in decision-making where appropriate, and input from instituted organisations such as JSNA, Health and Wellbeing Boards. Both systems are incorporated in the organisation's business plans and policies.

Post-modern management theory

Research-based management theories such as scientific (Taylorism) theory and human relations theory have been linked to the industrial revolution and seen as modern methods of management, based on them being a trigger for massively increasing productivity. Post-modern management, on the other hand, refers to management thinking that evolved from the mid- to late twentieth century, and which extends the human relations approach substantially to reflect current thinking about people's work and employing organisations.

Post-modern management approach is based on post-modern philosophies and beliefs about society (e.g. Petersen and Bunton, 1997) whereby managing goes beyond the rigidity and bureaucracy of 'modern' methods in workplaces (e.g. Clegg and Kornberger, 2003), and suggests that managers think more flexibly and creatively about managing work and people. This implies that managers should listen to employees' suggestions related to management of care, their expectations from the employment, etc.

Post-modern management theory, therefore, entails managers always considering alternative but better ways of managing situations and people – alternatives that might well be unprecedented and untested – and retain sceptical and critical thinking even after the most appropriate and acceptable management decision has been made. It is about managers having the ability to change and adapt quickly, and at the same time effectively.

For example, if an incident occurs in the work setting, there is often a set procedure to follow that is legal, ethical and effective. However, the manager may well consider alternative ways of dealing with the situation, before deciding on a course of action devised by them. Another example is in relation to efficiency, sustainability, ongoing improvement in quality of care and cost-effectiveness, as overarching requirements, for which employees and employers have to work collaboratively, which also allows every employee to be creative and harness networking. The post-modern management approach can thus bring out 'the best in people, organisations and communities', through taking a 'possibility centric' approach, according to Brookes (2011: 16), with the aim of improving care and team performance.

The four management theories explored above are distinctly different from each other, except individually they each have strengths and weaknesses, and therefore might not be applicable to all management situations. Furthermore, there isn't a standard 'one-size-fits-all' management theory, argues Olden (2016). Fiedler (1967) realised this dilemma a while ago and argued that there is no one best way to manage all organisations, all of the time, and suggested the 'contingency management theory' which entails adapting to the requirements of different situations at different times such as when the organisation is affected by poor economic climate. This implies that the FHM can adjust their style or approach, say from democratic to autocratic (or vice versa), depending on (or contingent upon) the demands of the situation (and therefore at times referred to as 'situational management').

Consequently, there are multiple ways of managing and leading, and therefore FHMs need to be flexible and adaptable when they experience novel or unprecedented situations or issues. The management approach is thus dependent upon the urgency of the task in hand, the capability and receptiveness of the followers (or team members), and the nature of the resources that are available. It changed, for example, to the contingent approach during the coronavirus pandemic in 2020/2021 when a marked increase in workforce became immediately necessary, and therefore finalist healthcare students, retired professionals and others were invited to join the workforce.

Table 4.2 shows some of the empirical basis for main well-known management research on which prevailing management theories are based.

Table 4.2   Examples of landmark research that generated management theories – evidence-based management

Researcher(s)	Findings
Fayol's (2012) studies	Researched management activities, and grouped them as: forecasting, planning, organising, commanding, co-ordinating and controlling
Mintzberg's (2011) research	Researched management activities since 1973, and identified ten roles of the manager
Herzberg's (2003) research	Researched what motivates employees at work, and identified a number of 'motivators' and motivation maintenance factors
McGregor's (1987) research	Researched human motivation at work, and concluded with Theory X and Theory Y assumptions, and consequent management practices
Taylor's 'scientific management' theory (Encyclopaedia Britannica, 2020)	Scientific management (also known as Taylorism) was advocated by F. W. Taylor (1856–1915), who studied productivity and efficiency in factories by observing how long it takes to perform each task; concluded that to enhance these outcomes, workers need to be provided with appropriate tools and training, incentives related to performance
Hawthorne experiments – conducted between 1924 and 1932 by Elton Mayo	Researched productivity at work, but discovered the importance of teamwork and human relations management theory

Table 4.2 shows only the main well-known management research and, of course, there have been several research studies on management since, but they haven't been as ground-breaking as those shown in the table. Note, for example, Calpin-Davies's (2000) research which identified key characteristics and personal skills of nurse managers; and Kouzes and Posner's (2017) longitudinal international research on leadership in organisations that identified the 'practices and commitments' of effective leaders.

Styles and Roles of Frontline Managers

In addition to the four management theories discussed above, two other approaches to understanding management in healthcare organisations stand out, which are managerial role theory and styles of management. Managerial role theory is another approach to understanding management, and one of the best-known role theories is propounded by Mintzberg (2011), whose research identified ten key role areas for 'working' managers:

1. Figurehead – usually the public-facing most senior person in the area or organisation.
2. Liaison – communicates with peers and outsiders in order to exchange work-related information.
3. Leader – role model and visionary whose examples almost all follow.
4. Monitor – gauges the quality of care, often based on metrics information.
5. Disseminator – communicates information to subordinates, some of which might not otherwise be available to them.
6. Spokesperson – responds to external need for information.
7. Entrepreneur – initiates and facilitates new ways of working and use of innovation.
8. Disturbance handler – intervenes to prevent or resolve disruptions.
9. Resource allocator – determines and plans where and how resources will be deployed.
10. Negotiator – communicates with agencies and individuals when conflict occurs or seems imminent; or when consent and co-operation are required in care provision and delivery.

The first three roles are grouped as interpersonal roles, the next three as informational roles, and the final four as decisional roles. Mintzberg's ten-role theory is therefore an alternative framework that encompasses all the duties that frontline managers engage in, and that apply to FHMs as well.

Styles of Management

Another perspective on management, in addition to management theories, is styles of management, which despite being less researched, still comprises a useful complementary way of appreciating the ways in which managers manage. The term style tends to represent the manager's usual or habitual ways of interacting with those they manage; that is, the behaviour or manner in which the manager expresses themselves towards team members. Management styles are thus applied by FHMs through the ways in which they usually conduct themselves towards staff in care settings.

Although the autocratic, democratic (or participative) and laissez-faire styles of management can all be detected in organisations, the two better-informed and more useful ones that deserve attention are the '*Management by objectives*' style, and the '*People-centred versus productivity-centred*' style.

Management by objectives

One well-documented and applied style of management that is supported by Drucker (2007: 103) and was earlier promoted by Odiorne (1979) is 'management by objectives' (MBO), which constitutes recognising the organisation's short- and long-term (operational and strategic respectively) objectives. The MBO style of management focuses on these objectives, and as often occurs at IDPRs, the employee is asked to define their major areas of responsibility and clinical activities, identify their personal and professional objectives, and is subsequently asked how their objectives match the organisation's operational objectives for the financial year. The individual employee's professional development needs are then identified jointly, along with the ways in which they can be met.

According to Odiorne (1979), MBO is based on: (1) defining specific areas of responsibility, setting objectives and targets, and criteria of performance, and the continual review and appraisal of results; and (2) the professional development needs of the employee. The MBO style is widely and effectively applied in both public and private sector organisations, mainly in the form of IDPR (or staff appraisal), with the focus being on the individual employee's strengths and achievements, instead of on their weak point(s).

The organisation's employees receive financial rewards or bonuses in the private sector if annual corporate objectives in terms of goals or targets are achieved or surpassed. Conversely, not achieving corporate objectives can result in staff numbers being reduced if it occurs year after year as the company records losses rather than financial profits or surpluses. Some level of bonus payment occurs in the service sector as well for selected posts. Achievement of IDPR objectives thereby becomes a high priority for the employee, and therefore their point of focus.

During IDPR conversations, the manager concentrates on achievement of objectives, but doesn't link achievement or non-achievement to the employee's character or personality. One possible weakness of the MBO style is that it can focus too much on tasks and reflect the scientific management approach, which can feel too bureaucratic and impersonal. Another is that it also assumes that there will be complete alignment between individuals' and the organisation's annual objectives. IDPRs are also discussed in some detail in Chapter 2 of this book.

People-centred versus productivity-centred style

Another style of management is referred to as the 'concern for productivity versus concern for people' style, which has been advocated mainly by Blake and McCanse (1991). Based largely on their earlier research that explored a management style that is focused completely on productivity against a style that is focused on the people who work in the organisation, the people-centredness versus productivity-centred approaches are presented on a grid that compares the effects of each approach on their employees and on the organisation's productivity (the amount of work completed) in their area of work (see Figure 4.3). Productivity-centred style of management is also consistent with transactional mode of leadership, while people-centredness is more in tune with transformational leaders, and with the human relations theory of management.

Consequently, when applying the productivity-centred style, which is also referred to as 'high concern for productivity', the manager's principal focus is on ensuring that all the day's tasks are completed, and in full. Opposite to this is the manager who exercises a more people- or worker-centred style of management.

As also concluded from a recent literature review by Dinibutun (2020), there can be five likely outcomes for the organisation based on whether the manager's

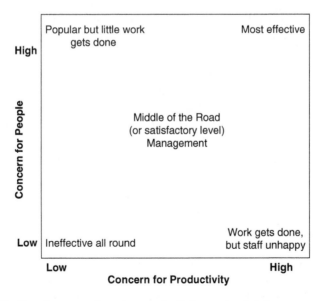

Figure 4.3 People-centred versus productivity-centred style

style is more people-centred or more productivity-centred in their area of responsibility. These outcomes are that:

High people-centred and high productivity-centred style is the most effective as it reflects 'team management' whereupon team members work together to accomplish tasks, and are content because their views are heeded by the manager.

High people-centredness and low productivity-centredness results in the leader being popular, but less work gets done, i.e. low productivity.

Low people-centredness and high productivity-centredness results in substantial work getting done, but the staff do not feel valued, nor their contribution recognised.

Low people-centredness and low productivity-centredness results in 'impoverished management' as it reflects a disinterested or incapable and ineffective manager.

Medium people-centredness and medium productivity-centredness results in mediocre performance by both leader and led, and mediocre satisfaction.

These management styles are the results of self-learned behaviours that the manager will have developed from previous experiences of management either as a manager or managed. When reflecting on the effect of each of these styles of management, you are rightly likely to deduce that the manager who demonstrates both high people-centredness and high productivity-centredness would be the most effective.

Ensuring Effective Communication in Care Settings

Communicating care intervention activities is essential for ensuring comprehensive patient assessment and effective clinical practice. By virtue of being in the frontline of clinical practice, FHMs simply have to be fully competent communicators. The NHS KSF (NHS Employers, 2019b) identifies communication as one of only six 'core dimensions' of competent healthcare employees, and earlier in this chapter Table 4.1 identified *communication hub* as being one of ten essential components of managerial duties that FHMs engage in.

All care activities that health and social care practitioners undertake require effective communication, with team members, which includes continuously recording patient information, and deciding on actions, communicating them through various means to others as and when necessary. Communication can be defined as verbal or non-verbal interchange between individuals and groups to impart and receive information. It is a process in which two or more parties endeavour to impart and comprehend messages to and from each other.

Communication therefore is a two-way process, the success of which is dependent upon the receiver interpreting the information in the way that the sender had intended. Messages sent electronically, that is without the two parties actually talking to each other, carry the risk of being misinterpreted by the receiver as they are unable to establish the associated non-verbal tone of the message.

Three sets of modes of communication can be identified, namely:

- Written: typed on a laptop and printed, handwritten, emailed, posted, texted on mobile phone, etc.
- Oral: speaking with an individual or small group face-to-face, speaking by telephone, video conferencing, lecturing, etc.
- Non-verbal: listening, gestures, posture, tone of voice, etc.

The first two modes may occur by physical interaction or by use of electronic devices. Video-conferencing, video-consultation by GPs and e-teaching are examples of virtual communication that were widely utilised during the 2020/2021 coronavirus pandemic, including via:

- Zoom
- Microsoft Teams
- Google Meet
- Skype for Business
- Cisco WebEx Meetings
- GoTo Meetings
- Slack
- WhatsApp Business
- BBB Big blue button

A closer examination of the reasons for management communication intimates that effective and efficient communication by health and social care managers is performed to:

- retain focus on the aims and specific objectives (or goals) of the care organisation;
- delineate specific ways in which the objectives can be achieved;
- organise human and other resources efficiently;
- recruit, develop and appraise employees in the organisation;
- motivate, lead and guide junior colleagues in the workplace; and
- monitor the effectiveness of care interventions.

At times, communication takes place in challenging circumstances, such as when an adverse event occurs, or a complaint has been received. It also needs to be acknowledged that all management components that managers have to engage with are underpinned by the necessary communication skills, with specific communication skills warranted by different situations, clinical specialisms and purposes. Examples of specific management communication activities are identified in Figure 4.4.

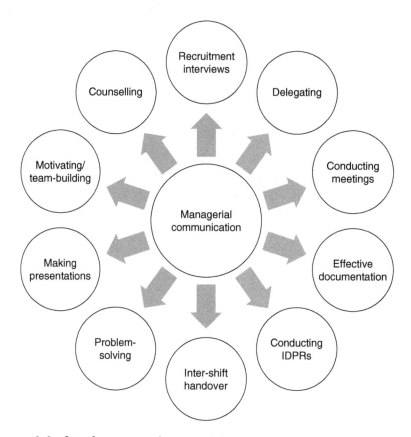

Figure 4.4 Specific managerial communication activities

Such a varied range of communication activities, in addition to the FHM's various managerial duties identified earlier in this chapter, highlights the breadth of specialist communication that FHMs have to be proficient in. Two examples of managerial communication activities identified in Figure 4.4 will now be explored in some detail to illustrate the various facets that each comprises. These are delegation of duties, and documentation and record-keeping.

Delegating the day's duties

Healthcare comprises teamwork by members of one's own profession as well as input from multiple other healthcare disciplines, and as a manager and leader, the

FHM's role includes delegating the work that needs to be carried out to appropriate members of the team on duty (as also noted in Chapter 2 of this book). In particular, this is because the FHM has full oversight of the group of service users' healthcare needs in their particular practice setting, but cannot physically perform all care interventions by themselves. Moreover, careful delegation of duties and responsibilities has become increasingly important because of issues around skill mix, unfilled vacancies and additional expanded roles becoming part of healthcare professionals' skill-set.

The NMC's (2018b) Code of Practice recognises delegation of nursing and midwifery work as an integral component of daily duties, and states further in clause 11 that nurses and midwives must: 'Be accountable for your decisions to delegate tasks and duties to other people'. It goes on to specify that the RN or RM must only delegate tasks and duties that are within the delegatee's scope of competence and that they are adequately supervised and supported, because the responsibility for delegated tasks remains with the delegator.

Professional associations such as the RCN (2017a) also indicate that tasks have to be delegated appropriately, that is within the team member's scope of competence and associated accountability, be they other registrants, HSWs, assistant practitioners, trainee nursing associates, or nursing apprentices. Furthermore, in their qualitative study of ways in which NRNs learn to organise, delegate and supervise care in practice settings, Magnusson et al. (2017) identified five styles of delegation, which are:

- Do-it-all style – completes most of the work themselves;
- Justifier style – over-explains the reasons for decisions and is sometimes defensive;
- Buddy style – endeavours to be everybody's friend and avoids assuming authority;
- Role model style – anticipates others will copy their best practice; and
- Inspector style – constantly checks the work of others, based on their awareness of their accountability.

Magnusson et al. (2017: 46) concluded that educational and organisational support is required for NRNs 'to develop safe and effective delegation skills, because suboptimal or no delegation can have negative effects on patient safety and care'. Nonetheless, delegation of care must always be in the best interests of the service user, and any clinical risk involved in delegating must have been thoroughly considered beforehand. There are various stages of effective delegation, as illustrated in Figure 4.5.

Although each stage of the process is distinctly separated out, at times two of the steps may be undertaken simultaneously, e.g. steps 5 and 6. Other points that have to be considered in effective delegation include:

- Staff morale can improve through the responsibility that delegation confers.

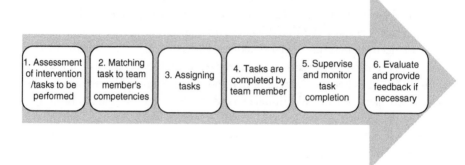

Figure 4.5   Stages of effective delegation

- Awareness that delegation can provide subordinates with opportunities to learn, and can support their career development.
- All delegation involves some risk, but can be minimised by measured coaching and effective supervision.
- Despite careful preparation mistakes could still occur, and FHMs should learn from them and not avoid delegating.

At times, however, some managers tend to be reluctant to delegate care tasks, believing that juniors are unlikely to perform them as thoroughly as them. However, this is unlikely to present as an issue because pre-registration programmes now include clinical experience in leadership and organisation of care; and also due to the staffing shortages issue in health services noted by NHSE (2019a). Frontline managers can also use certain strategies with regards to delegation, such as coaching, and having a contingency plan should any issue arise.

Accurate documentation and record-keeping

One of the most essential modes of communication is keeping accurate and up-to-date records (often referred to as 'documentation') of care interventions provided to every service user, be it in paper form or electronically. Doing this is an important activity undertaken by healthcare professionals, although on-and-off in the past, poor healthcare records have been under the spotlight when complaints or failures in care have surfaced, or even made the national news.

Effective record-keeping is therefore a very important means of communicating patient care activities, and it represents evidence of care delivered. The International Organization for Standardization (abbreviated ISO) (National Archives, 2010: 3) defines records as, 'Information created, received and maintained as evidence and information by an organization or person, in pursuance of legal obligations or in the transaction of business'. Heriot Watt University (2020: 5) indicates that, 'A record is any piece of information created or received and maintained by an organisation or person in the course of their business or conduct of affairs and kept as evidence of such activity'.

Both definitions also indicate that the main purposes of records are that they comprise evidence of care interventions, and their quality to some extent, especially in the event of a dispute, and can act as information that is used in the decision-making process. Both definitions apply to healthcare interventions.

ACTION POINT 4.4
Documenting care activities in your workplace

Make a list of specific care activities that are documented in your workplace. Consider this in relation to both routine activities and unexpected events.

There are, of course, several different ways and modes of keeping health records, such as hand-written patient records, records stored in a computer (including copies of emails), hand-held records, letters written to patients, investigation reports, x-ray photographs, print-outs, scanned documents, video recordings (of e.g. a chronic wound or rash), photographs, etc. Further examples of service user care activities that are documented and kept include assessment of service users' health problem, care delivery (including medication administration), informed written or verbal consent, CPR decisions, risk assessment, audit forms, refusal of care, incidents of aggressive or violent behaviour in care settings.

Poor record-keeping is one of the reasons for registered practitioners having to appear before their professional regulator. Detailed guidance on the benefits of good record-keeping, the dos and don'ts of effective record-keeping, and the consequences of poor record-keeping have been published by various organisations. The Royal College of Nursing's (2017b) *Record keeping – The Facts* is one example, and the NMC (2018b, clause 10) is another, which under the theme 'Practise effectively' identifies the requirements with regard to effective record-keeping by nurses and midwives, including patient records, and states for example that registrants must:

- Complete records at the time or as soon as possible after an event, but clearly stating if they were documented sometime after the event.
- Complete records accurately and without any falsification, taking immediate and appropriate action if you become aware that someone has not kept to these requirements.
- Take all steps to make sure that records are kept securely.
- Attribute any entries you make in any paper or electronic records to yourself, making sure they are clearly written, dated and timed, and do not include unnecessary abbreviations, jargon or speculation.

Additionally, service user records have to meet confidentiality requirements, but service users can apply to see the records kept about them, as is also noted in the *NHS Constitution* (DHSC, 2019a: 8), indicating that service users have the right to access their health records and to request any factual inaccuracies to be rectified. One way in which FHMs can monitor or ensure accurate record-keeping (for risk assessment – see Chapter 8) is to conduct audits of these in their workplace, and take appropriate action if inadequacies are identified.

Record-keeping is, however, sometimes referred to as 'doing the paperwork', and that is treating it as of secondary importance. Furthermore, a RCN survey found that nursing staff spend 'more than a million hours a week on paperwork' (Lomas, 2012), and questions are asked about whether some of this time should be spent in direct patient care activities instead, and suggests that it could be reduced through a lean approach (see Chapter 8), or if more administrative support was available to staff. However, Lomas also draws attention to the finding that ward manager and charge nurse administrative support (such as ward clerks) have gradually diminished, and in many instances ceased completely.

Communicating patient progress at inter-shift handover is discussed to some extent in Chapter 6 under team communication, which includes the application of the situation-background-assessment-recommendation (SBAR) tool.

Furthermore, the NHS LTP (NHSE, 2019a) provides details of 'digital road maps', which involves maintaining electronic health records (EHR) for patients whereby local health and care systems can use digital technology to keep paperless records. Guidance on records management is also provided by NHSX (2021a), which addresses components including legal, professional, organisational and individual responsibilities when managing records, as well as a retention schedule, i.e. for how long each type of record should be kept.

This section on management communication has addressed mainly delegation and documentation and record-keeping, as fundamental managerial duties, and as the analysis of these components shows, each management communication component comprises a whole range of activities that might not be immediately apparent.

Guidance for Managing Effectively and Efficiently

Effective management of care is the central function of frontline care managers, and the following constitutes good practice guidelines for doing so.

- Develop a clear sense of what management is about (covered in the chapters of this book), which includes leadership manifested by frontline healthcare managers.

- Ensure acquisition of comprehensive knowledge of published theories and research of management of staff and all other resources, based on which you develop your management skills and behaviour.
- Develop insights into the mechanics of the ways in which healthcare organisations function, and awareness of the role of informal organisations.
- Ensure full and effective top-down and bottom-up communication of all plans and actions related to day-to-day care in care settings, and effective management-specific communication such as in delegating duties and accurate documentation.
- Delegate duties appropriately and with professional accountability, and supervise work to ensure that they are completed to the required standard.
- Overtly see team members as your most valuable resource and ensure they know that their expertise and contribution to care and team objectives are appreciated.
- Apply appropriate mechanisms that enable employees to meet their work-related social and psychological growth needs.
- Be aware that team members and the healthcare organisation have certain expectations from the employment, and work collaboratively to meet these expectations as much as feasible.
- Distribute workload, responsibilities and new opportunities equitably and be accessible and approachable to each team member.
- Develop an understanding of relevant legislation and national policies, and how they relate to your practice.

Chapter Summary

Effective management of care is the prime role of FHMs and they have to draw on a range of knowledge base and competence to do so. This chapter has focused on effective management in healthcare settings, and to do this, it has explored the prevailing and enduring approaches to management that FHMs can apply to their day-to-day management duties, in order to ensure achievement of care organisations' aims and objectives through the human and non-human resources at their disposal. It has therefore addressed:

- the wide range of day-to-day managerial duties that FHMs engage in to ensure effective management of care;
- detailed insights into how organisations in general and healthcare organisations specifically function, and recognised the structures and staff hierarchies within them;
- knowledge of what managers and management signify, and where management fits into the organisation and where FHMs fit into healthcare management structures;

- knowledge and comprehension of different well-established research-driven existing knowledge of theories or principles of management, such as the human relations approach and post-modern approaches, as well as managerial role theory;
- frontline healthcare managers' styles of management, that FHMs can draw on to apply to their daily duties; and
- the various ways in which FHMs communicate day-to-day care in collaboration with inter-disciplinary services, and types of management communication such as delegation of duties and accurate documentation.

Further Reading

- For a systematic review of the evolution of management theories, see: Kwok A C F (2014) *The Evolution of Management Theories: A Literature Review.* Available at: www.researchgate.net/publication/307760441_The_Evolution_of_Management_ Theories_A_Literature_Review. Accessed Date: 2 May 2020
- For detailed guidance regarding responsibility and accountability related to delegating nursing interventions, see: Royal College of Nursing (2017a) Accountability and Delegation – A Guide for the Nursing Team. Available at: www.rcn.org.uk/professional-development/publications/pub-006465 Accessed Date: 24 April 2020. Scrutinise the content of journals *Nursing Management* or *British Journal of Healthcare Management* for research articles on various components of management identified in this chapter.

5

Managing Healthcare Resources (and Human Relations)

Chapter Objectives

The chapter objectives for frontline healthcare managers in relation to managing healthcare resources are:

- Specify the necessary human and non-human resources required by service providers for effective care delivery in practice settings, and why resources have to be managed;
- Demonstrate knowledge of sources of funds required for health services, with fair knowledge of what budgets are, why budgeting is important in health services, how budgets are set and ways of maximising their use;
- Stipulate the wide range of other non-human resources that are required such as hospital buildings and other facilities, equipment, clinical guidelines and consumables that need to be managed for effective care delivery;
- Demonstrate knowledge of multiple components of human resource management, including human relations in the workplace, the recruitment and retention of staff, safe staffing and skill-mix; and
- Show awareness of the significance of staff surveys in the context of employers' and employees' expectations of each other.

Introduction

Essential resources such as appropriately skilled staff plus designated funding for paying their wages, dedicated buildings, the necessary equipment, disposable materials (for example dressings), etc. are naturally all required for the provision and delivery of healthcare. At the same time, however, only a certain proportion of national income can be allocated for health services, the remainder being allocated for other public provision such as education, public protection, etc. Thus, the effective and efficient management of available resources is fundamental to ensure that healthcare is available to everyone who needs it. Each of the wide range of resources required for the operational management of healthcare has costs associated with it, and FHMs' duties include responsible and efficient management of the resources made available to them.

This chapter examines the management of healthcare resources, covering effective and efficient utilisation of funding, human (staffing) resources, the infrastructure comprising building, departmentalisation, etc., and consumable materials.

Beyond the knowledge and competence of staff, human resources also take into consideration the human relations theory (noted in Chapter 4), and the challenges encountered by healthcare professionals. Also examined are the challenges that FHMs and team members encounter while also ensuring high-quality care delivery; the tensions in day-to-day work-life, along with the provision of organisational mechanisms and strategies; and the personal and peer resources that are available to prevent or deal with problematic situations. The chapter addresses these aspects of the FHM's role, along with some of the support facilities that could be harnessed in the endeavour to maintain a healthy work–life balance.

Which Resources Are Required for Effective Care Delivery?

An endeavour to identify all items of resources that are required for health and care in all settings, from acute (secondary) to community (primary care) settings in the UK can feel like a mammoth task. They are certainly provided in a wide range of settings, and for a wide range of health issues. As noted in Chapter 1, the NHS delivers healthcare to a total population of approximately 66.4 million people (mid-2018 figures) (ONS, 2020).

The total expenditure on health in the UK for the year 2020/2021 was approximately £178 billion, out of a total public spending of approximately £928 billion (*The Times*, 2020: 16; HM Treasury, 2020). Money for public spending comes from income tax and various other forms of tax such as business rates, value added tax, as well as from National Insurance contributions and charges to patients (e.g. dental treatment, prescription charges) (King's Fund, 2019b).

In addition to the £178 billion allocated for the year 2020/21, the then Prime Minister also announced in 2019 that the NHS will receive an average increase of 3.4% each year until 2023 (Nuffield Trust, 2020), predominantly to fund the continuing implementation of the NHS's *Five Year Forward View* new models of health-social care (NHSE, 2014a) and the NHS LTP (NHSE, 2019a). Figure 5.1 identifies the overall sums designated for this for the year 2020/2021, which includes £8.2 billion of capital budget.

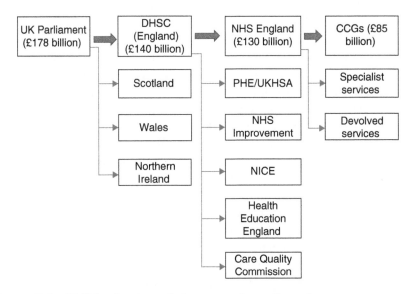

Figure 5.1   NHS funding (rounded up approximate figures)

The £178 billion allocated for the NHS is then distributed to the four UK countries, of which £140 billion is allocated to the DHSC in England, from which £130 billion is given to NHSE, 75% of which is given to the CCGs and Regional Teams in England (see Figure 5.1). The remaining £38 billion is distributed to the other three countries, based mainly on each country's total population (HM Treasury, 2020; NHSE, 2014b: 24).

Thus, in 2020, healthcare expenditure was approximately 19% of the total annual expenditure for the UK, which represents a spending of approximately £2600 per person on healthcare each year. The NHS is also the biggest employer in Europe, with 1.3 million employees across the health service just in England (an estimated 1.4 million employees in the whole of UK NHS) (NHSE, 2019a).

The government is also the main source of funding for personal social services, which are managed by local authorities along with the necessary local structures and a 2020/21 budget of £36 billion (HM Treasury, 2020: 16). The allocated funds include personal health budgets, and the Care Act 2014 (Legislation.gov. uk, 2014; DHSC, 2016, 2020) provides precise details of ways of providing integrated care and support for adults and for carers.

Before delving into details of allocation of funds, it is worthwhile seeing them in perspective by taking a look at the structure of the NHS identified in Figure 1.3 in Chapter 1, which acknowledges NHSE and CCGs as having the pivotal role of identifying and resourcing care needs and as the principal commissioners of health services. Thus, in England, NHSE apportions the financial resources for care and treatment, and CCGs then allocate money to healthcare providers (e.g. NHS trusts, and the independent sector) for spending on healthcare professionals' salaries, equipment, medication and all other materials that are required for treatment and care delivery.

Decisions on how much money is spent on each required resource are usually made by a committee chaired by the Chief Executive of the healthcare provider (e.g. a NHS trust) with the support of finance officers and healthcare professionals. Therefore, the Chief Executive (at times known as Chief Executive Officer) has to ensure that appropriate officials have been appointed in each system (discussed in Chapters 1 and 4) in the trust including Estates so that clinical activities achieve operational aims of the trust. The Chief Executive of the trust is answerable and accountable to the chairman and the trust's Board, and is responsible for ensuring appropriate structures are in place and mobilised appropriately.

The healthcare provider's aims, along with its mission statement and objectives, are stated in the operational (usually annual) or business plan, and strategic longer-term (usually five to ten years) plan. All service providers have operational and strategic plans identified in advance, including care providers in primary care, mental health services, GP practices, services for learning disabilities and autism, commissioned services in the independent sector, etc. Being in the frontline of care requires FHMs to be familiar with the aims of their department and the trust, which, in turn, usually form part of their own work objectives that have been agreed at their IDPRs.

Ultimately, the aims of service providers are underpinned by core aims of the NHS, which for England are declared in the *NHS Constitution* (DHSC, 2019a – last updated 2015), indicating that healthcare is free at the point of delivery for all British citizens who are residents of the UK, and in the DHSC's mandate to NHS England. Details of the resources that are required for achievement of the NHS's aims are examined next.

Resources Required by Service Providers

The term 'resource' tends to denote a supply of designated assets such as staff, money and policies that are calculated and allocated to an organisation (or individual) in order to achieve the aims of the organisation, which in healthcare is to provide care and treatment to the population in its area.

> ## ACTION POINT 5.1
> ## Which resources are required for your care setting?
>
> Thinking of your own workplace, with the usual expected number of service users to attend to, think of all the resources that are required to provide safe, effective and high standard of care. Spend no more than three minutes on this exercise, but do include the whole range of human resources required as well, professional and ancillary.

Two broad categories of resources required for healthcare are human resources and non-human resources. An alternative classification groups resources under human and hardware resources; examples of human resources being the staff and their clinical knowledge, skills, time, etc., and those of hardware resources include hospital buildings, beds, equipment and medical devices.

In response to Action point 5.1 you may have mentioned that the resources required for your care areas include staff with appropriate skills, their salaries, equipment, equipment maintenance, consumables such as wound suturing materials, etc. The full range of human and non-human resources that are needed to ensure safe, effective and compassionate care delivery is categorised by Gopee and Galloway (2017) under the acronym BEICHMM (though the order is not significant), which stands for:

- Buildings
- Equipment
- Information technology
- Consumables
- Human resources
- Methods
- Money.

The acronym BEICHMM therefore represents a checklist of all groups of resources required by healthcare organisations and their care settings to achieve their operational objectives. The need for *buildings* of appropriate capacity is obviously a requirement to accommodate the designated care delivery facilities. *Equipment* includes a variety of implements such as X-ray machines, telephones, manual handling aids, patient-attached equipment such as cardiac monitors or syringe drivers, and various forms of vehicles for transportation.

Information technology is of course now all-pervasive as a resource, which in healthcare often enables instant communication of service user information between the care setting and many other departments. However, a more appropriate and current heading is *Information* – in the form of data and metrics as resources, which are processed and stored in computers. For *consumables*, examples of resources comprise disposable single-use items such as syringes, catheters, endo-tracheal tubes, some medical devices, etc.

When referring to health services workforce (that is *human resources*), this denotes staff of a wide range of professions and occupations, each with their own specific skill-sets (e.g. nurses, AHPs, medical staff, HSWs, ancillary staff, managers and administrators, social care professionals, etc.). It also refers to the skill mix of staff (proportion of qualified and unqualified staff, specialists, etc.), as well as to formal communication within the workforce, and recruitment and retention of staff.

Additionally, human resources also incorporate consideration of staff sickness, pending maternity leave, retirement, etc., which, in turn, create temporary or longer-term vacancies; and also time for continuing education of staff, and time spent motivating them in their work and maintaining their morale.

As for *methods* as a resource, they include procedures, clinical guidelines and policies, together with the training and assessment of competence to utilise them competently. It includes the step-by-step procedure for meeting professional updating requirements, for instance, and for making referrals to medical staff, specialist nurses and therapists. For *money*, the resources include the cost of employing staff, maintaining the building(s), purchasing equipment, and so on. All resources cost money.

While recognising these developments, the NHS LTP has set up mechanisms such as 'Getting It Right First Time (GIRFT)' and 'NHS RightCare' to provide the evidence base for best practice, optimum care pathways and more efficient working (NHSE, 2019a). It identifies ten priority areas for strengthening efficiency, including centralisation ('aggregation' – p. 105 of NHS LTP) of purchase of consumables, clinical pharmacists to work more closely with GPs to reduce waste of prescribed medicines, and improving patient safety to reduce costs and litigation. Both GIRFT and RightCare have recently been required components of annual NHS operational plans, as stated in *NHS Operational Planning and Contracting Guidance 2020/21* (NHSE+I, 2020a).

Why Resources Have to be Managed

Healthcare managers are accountable for the efficient use of the resources allocated to their part of the organisation, and they have to use them responsibly. Management of resources designated for care and treatment can be challenging, as innovations, novel treatment methods and new medications for conditions that have thus far proved difficult to treat become available, unless extra money and manpower is made available centrally, i.e. by the government.

Efficiency in the use of resources has been a central theme exhorted by the government for a number of years. Efficiency refers to the achievement of expected outcomes at minimum financial cost, in the minimum amount of time, but to the required standard. It refers to achieving the maximum effect from available resources, to 'make the most of the NHS pound' (NHS, 2019a: 110). The associated term 'effectiveness' refers to the extent to which care is being delivered as intended, and benefits service users in terms of benefits to their health.

The UK government keeps reminding the public that the NHS is funded primarily from taxpayers' money and, therefore, those who the money is allocated to are accountable for spending it responsibly; and they also have a moral duty to do so.

FHMs have to have good knowledge of effective and efficient management of resources, in particular because the financial resources allocated for care provision has predetermined limits, as well as because of the financial challenges and sustainability of financing health-social care services, as documented for example by NHSE (2014a). It is also a statutory responsibility for healthcare providers to work within the financial resources allocated to them.

The management of resources also include costing of any new or extra human or non-human resources that are required, either in the short term (e.g. use of 'bank' or agency staff) or longer term (e.g. appointment of a specialist nurse, or purchasing new medical devices). Business cases are often required to request additional resources for care delivery, which include details of all costs that they entail, proof of its benefits, an options appraisal and the associated risk assessments.

The management of resources require careful planning, which means deciding in advance, strategically and operationally, how they will be utilised. Doing this includes consideration of the treatment and care that the organisation has been commissioned to provide, the services and activities that the organisation plans to deliver, how this will be achieved and the personnel that will be required to deliver the services. Nonetheless, in an examination of ways in which resources are used and reported on in non-specialist acute hospitals in England, the DHSC's (2016b) Carter Review identifies a number of variations across organisations, in the ways in which treatment and care are provided, and the amount spent on different clinical activities.

The Carter Review indicates that cost of inpatient treatment, for example, varies from £3,150 to £3,850 across service providers; infection rates after surgery varies; and stockholding in the medicine cabinet 'varies from 11 to 36 days, and if everyone achieved (stocktaking) in 15 days this would save £50m' (DHSC, 2016b: 6). The review also found that the mix of qualified to unqualified staff varies from trust to trust; and sickness and absence rates vary as well, etc. It makes a number of recommendations such as adopting a 'single integrated performance framework' with one common set of metrics (2016b: 7) being applied across all service providers, which presently comes under the remit of NHSI.

Productivity refers to the number of units of output (e.g. number of patients seen by a community nurse) resulting from each unit of input (time in minutes per patient, and other resources). It is the ratio or relationship between one or more outputs to one or more inputs, and the quality of the outputs. Productivity formed the basis of the Hawthorne experiments described in Chapter 4 of this book, and the aim is to increase output per 'man-hours' (or person-hours), which is also one of the reasons for the limited amount of time GPs can give to each patient they see in their surgery each day. It is linked to lean methodology which essentially refers to reducing waste and duplication of work.

The next two sections examine the management of healthcare resources in detail under two main parts: (1) non-human resources, that is funding, equipment, etc.; and (2) human resources, which includes recruitment and retention of staff, safe staffing, etc.

Managing Non-Human Resources (1) Budgets

Central funding for health and social services in the UK were identified earlier in this chapter – see Figure 5.1 and the associated discussion. However, there are also other minor sources of finance that healthcare trusts receive and use as appropriate. This section on non-human resources first explores these additional sources of income, then discusses the concept budgets for healthcare, followed by exploration of other non-human resources such as buildings required to provide healthcare, the equipment needed, information technology, consumables, as well as clinical guidelines.

FHMs tend to be made aware of the costs of care and treatment by senior managers, and the requirement to achieve outcomes, the amount of money being spent each month on care services in the work setting and the organisation's requirement to achieve efficiency. With regards to managing budgets as a non-human resource, therefore, this section considers:

- Sources of finance for health service provision
- Managing the budget
- Budgeting techniques
- Additional features of budgeting

Where does money for health services come from?

As noted in the introduction of this chapter, funding for the NHS is derived mainly from general taxation, National Insurance contributions and patient charges, which for England is channelled through the DHSC, then to NHSE and the CCGs. The rest is either generated by the healthcare trust itself, or donated by individuals or other organisations such as charities (trust funds). More specifically, these other sources of NHS trusts' income include mostly:

- *Generated income*: Finance that is raised by care organisations, from the level of NHS trusts to individual wards or departments, including:

- parking charges;
- fees from treating private patients;
- from diverse activities such as lease of space for advertising, or hiring of a room;
- sale of buildings, land and/or capital items.

- *Gifts and bequests*: These can be donations of money to a specific unit, individual or organisation for purchase of equipment or for research. It includes legacies, gifts and appeal funds.
- *Money raised:* Money voluntarily raised by individuals or organised groups, often for specific pre-identified purposes, e.g. cancer research, or very expensive equipment.
- *Loans*: Trusts can borrow money if a monthly shortfall is predicted, especially when approaching the end of the budget year, although interest has to be paid on them.

Funds raised by charities are received and distributed through designation organisations such as NHS Charities Together. An example of outstanding fund raising is the £32 million raised by 100-year-old Major Tom Moore within a month in April 2020 for the whole of the NHS during the coronavirus pandemic (Southworth and Roberts, 2020), which is also the largest amount of money raised by any single individual for a charity. A potential problem with gifts and bequests is that at times they are donated as capital items, e.g. equipment, but subsequently the healthcare provider has to find money for its running costs.

Financial resources are allocated by the government as 'revenue' budget (or expenditure) and 'capital' budget. Of the £178 billion healthcare budget for the UK for 2020/21, £8.2 billion were identified for capital expenditure (capital budget), and £140 billion as revenue expenditure (resource budget) for England's DHSC (HM Treasury, 2020: 28–9). It is noteworthy that the actual amount of money spend each year was usually higher than the initially allocated healthcare budget during 2020 because of extra resources required to manage the corona virus epidemic.

Revenue expenditure (also known as operating expenses) is money that is required for staff salaries, and other day-to-day costs such as cleaning, lighting, food for patients, medications, bed linen, etc. Capital budget (or capital expenditure) on the other hand is the money that is provided to finance long-term spending in the NHS, such as new buildings (for a new outpatients department for a specific group of service users, for example), equipment (for example, magnetic resonance imaging (MRI) equipment, or computed tomography (CT) scanners) and new technology, as well as research to improve workforce productivity for example.

Regardless of sources of funding, healthcare managers are required to spend their allocated money efficiently, except one of the potential dangers of efficiency savings is that it could also impact negatively at provider level through the periodic shortage or incompatibility of certain resources if cheaper poor quality materials are used.

The items on which money allocated to NHS trusts are spent are audited at various levels, and in particular by NHSI. NHS funding has also been changing gradually over the years to 'payment-by-results' as a way of funding that comprises hospitals and other providers being paid for the treatment and care activities actually undertaken rather than the preceding 'block agreements'. The amount of money received by healthcare providers from CCGs and NHSE is based on a standardised national tariff, with some built-in variations.

Managing the budget

Knowledge of budgets involves understanding what a budget is, why budgets are prepared, the different approaches to budgeting, and the likely advantages and disadvantages of each approach in health and care provision. FHMs are required to be cost-conscious, and be watchful of wastage, as suggested in the Carter Report (DHSC, 2016b), and to be aware that there is a set budget for delivering care in their care setting.

A budget is essentially a financial plan allocated for one or more specific purposes and available for a set period of time, e.g. one year. It can be defined as a statement of revenue and cost in financial terms that are anticipated and identified in advance of a period of time for spending on specific activities that reflect the agreed policies and strategies for meeting the objectives of the organisation. The reasons for exploring budgeting is that the management of resources is an essential managerial role for FHMs as identified in Chapter 4, and by Mintzberg (2011) as a 'resource allocator'. It involves deciding where, what and how resources should be deployed, and which other resources are required for effective care delivery.

Budgets are usually prepared by senior managers and administrators of the organisation as they have an overview of the whole organisation's needs, and FHMs are generally only involved when they have to make a case for staff replacement or new staff, or when the budget is overspent in spite of that being due to clinical needs (e.g. extra patients having been attended to). Other reasons for preparing organisational budgets are to:

- determine income and expenditure as precisely as possible with the available information;
- identify organisational objectives and priorities, with awareness that some expectations may not be met;
- communicate plans and co-ordinate activities;
- authorise expenditure and activity; and
- measure performance against objectives.

Budgets also have to be considered in the context of responsibility and ac-countability. After the budget has been agreed, the responsibility for managing components of the budget is delegated, and thereafter each person or depart-ment becomes accountable for details of how the money is spent. Consequently, month-by-month expenditure is monitored, and a monthly statement of ex-penditure for each care setting issued that identifies the exact amount of money spent on each specific group of items, which include pay expenses (e.g. staff sala-ries, agency staff used) and non-pay expenses (e.g. cost of medications, catheters, dressings, equipment). It then shows the total amount spent during the month, and therefore if the care setting is underspent or overspent for that month, and by how much.

Long-term planning also takes budgets into account to ascertain the financial effects of, for example, the plan to purchase and the running of a large item of equipment, or for the provision of a new service. Furthermore, some flexibility needs to be built into the budget in case of unanticipated expenditure, e.g. equip-ment failure and replacement costs, disaster management or delays in the recruit-ment of staff.

Budgeting techniques

Budgeting refers to funding made available to healthcare providers, as a pre-de-termined amount of money is allocated for each provider for the forthcoming financial year. Payment-by-results was noted earlier as the current basis on which the anticipated amount of money needed by a provider is calculated, but there are other ways of calculating how much money each provider will need to deliver its healthcare services. The three basic methods of calculating the forthcoming year's costs the healthcare provider can incur are: activity-based budgeting, incremental budgeting and zero-based budgeting.

Activity-based budgeting

Activity in the context of activity-based budgeting refers to any action or inter-vention that is undertaken by any employee in the course of their duties, those that naturally are taken to meet one or more of the healthcare organisation's aims and objectives. It is an approach to budgeting that the FHM is most likely to be involved in as it entails estimating the volume and nature of the workload for the span of duty. This is supported by identifying the costs involved for each 'unit' of work, calculating total costs and setting the budget accordingly.

For instance, it can involve estimating how many episodes of different opera-tions will be carried out by the Day Surgery Unit during the forthcoming finan-cial year, or how many immunisations need to be performed at a particular health centre, and the cost of the resources that will be required to complete these activi-ties safely and to the highest standard.

When examining budgeting, it is useful to be aware of the advantages and disadvantages of each way of budgeting. The advantages of activity-based budgeting are:

- the budget is set with a clear view of the workload expected;
- it has some flexibility built in to reflect actual workload;
- planned or standard unit costs can be compared with actual unit costs to reflect real costs of the service;
- it enables management to speculate on efficiency (unit costs) and on controlling fixed costs.

Disadvantages of activity-based budgeting include unit/standard costs based on historic costs may not provide a measure of current costs; and identifying simple measures of workload is difficult, as the actual cost of each unit is rarely standard. The NHS LTP (NHSE, 2019a) moots a gradual move away from activity-based funding by CCGs to healthcare providers, to population-based funding ('a blended payment model') in order to reduce transaction cost, and also to support the move towards preventive care models.

Incremental budgeting

An alternative to activity-based budgeting that managers or healthcare commissioners could use is the incremental budgeting method, which comprises first ascertaining the actual budget spent in the current financial year (not the budget set at the beginning of the current financial year), then second, increasing the actual amount of money spent in the financial year by a percentage approximating the prevailing inflation rate, but third, subtracting non-recurring costs. Fourth, any anticipated new clinical activity or agreed changes in service provision is added or deducted, and finally an inflation reserve is created in case the cost rises during the year unexpectedly.

With regards to recurring items, they include all clinical or related activities of the current financial year by the service provider; and non-recurring items include, for example, if a section of the outpatients department will be closed down during the financial year because the specialist services is being moved to a larger hospital.

Additionally, an inflation reserve is created to cater for in case of higher than anticipated pay rises, or rise in the price of consumables for example. Furthermore, 'approved variations' to the budget include income from new contract due to increased private patient workload. They can also include changes to services agreed at some point during the year; new expenses related to previously unrecognised workload; or extraordinary circumstances, e.g. fire, flood damage or increase in infection rates leading to extra costs.

As with other methods of budgeting, there are advantages and disadvantages in incremental budgeting as well. Advantages are that it is easier to operate and understand, and it is less demanding on management and on time. Disadvantages of incremental budgeting include changes in clinical activity are not always reflect-ed in the actual budget, and it can perpetuate inefficient use of resources. There can also be a lack of ownership of the budget by some managers who did not fully agree with the details of the budget in the first place.

Zero-based budgeting

In addition to the above-mentioned two methods of budgeting, another alterna-tive is zero-based budgeting, which entails re-ascertaining the cost of every item of resource, human and non-human, and checking that they are still needed in the forthcoming year. This constitutes identifying the quantity and quality of various services required all over again, and then building up a budget from a zero base with optimum staff numbers and pay bands, consumables, equipment, medical devices, etc.

The zero-based form of budgeting is usually applied, for example, when a new service is being speculated. The advantages of zero-based budgets are that:

- they are directly linked to the quality of service required and the planned level of activity;
- they encourage efficiency and discourage incremental budgeting;
- they are usually realistic and achievable; and
- managers take ownership of them.

On the other hand, the disadvantages are that they can be very time consuming to constitute and therefore costly, there is a danger of 'reinventing the wheel' and it is also difficult to know the exact costs that will be incurred because of increase in demand for certain items such as medications, etc.

Additional features of budgeting

In the inevitable efforts to spend NHS money cost-effectively, efficiency savings are repeatedly advocated and often required. In relation to purchase of consuma-bles and medical devices in particular, one of the most prominent actions being taken by NHSE (2019a) is to centralise the purchase of such necessities. Cen-tralisation involved bulk-buying negotiated through NHSE, instead of each trust negotiating purchase prices separately with manufacturers. It is logical that for these purchases (also known as procurement), the users of these material, that is clinicians, should be involved in choosing which to purchase.

This is because if clinical staff are not involved in discussing changes in clinical product, then they might be just asked to use the new products which could com-promise patient care and safety, which may even be unsuitable, and decisions to buy become based only on cost. Reluctance to engage could be affected by resist-ance to change, organisational culture and structure, personalities, etc. In a study of clinicians' perceptions of changing of clinical products and their procurement,

Donohue (2019) concluded that clinicians should seek to get involved in product selection and clinical product evaluation.

Other important considerations related to budgeting include planning and prioritising. Planning is usually conducted in two stages: strategic and operational.

- *Strategic planning* refers to planning for the long term, usually for five years or ten.
- *Operational planning* is for short term, usually one financial year, or sometimes two years, with monthly breakdown of associated details.

As for prioritising in healthcare, this suggests that healthcare professionals need to be aware that budgeting usually takes into account the activities that are highest priority, and they are allocated monies in preference to those classed as lower priority.

Furthermore, top-sliced money is periodically made available to NHS trusts for a specific purpose or activity, such as appointment of a specialist nurse for stroke care, or a clinical lead for self-harm management programme, which may be available for a fixed number of years after which the healthcare provider is expected to absorb the costs of the service from its normal annual monetary allocations.

To conclude this examination of finance and budgeting, it is apt to note Carter's (DHSC, 2016b) observation related to 'marked variations' in the use of resources across health services in England, citing for example variations in the cost of hip replacement, and that the recommendation to rectify this anomaly is by standardising procedures, being more transparent and working more closely with neighbouring NHS trusts. Some of the recommendations of the Carter Review form the basis for NHSE's (Cripps, 2018) *NHS RightCare* programme, prominent in whose aim in the recommendation to combat variations in care provision (sometimes referred to as the 'postcode lottery').

NHS RightCare's primary objective is to maximise value for the money allocated for healthcare and thereby contribute to the financial sustainability of the NHS, which was also a key priority of FYFV, and is for NHS LTP. It does this by focusing on appropriate intelligence through scrutinising local data on healthcare spending and making recommendations, in order to reduce 'all types of unwarranted variation ... [and] ensuring that the right people are given the right care in the right place at the right time – all while making the best use of available but finite resources across the health service' (Cripps, 2018: 2).

Managing Non-Human Resources (2) Buildings, Equipment, Devices and Materials

After examining the management of finance as non-human resources, this second section on non-human resources ascertains (1) buildings, equipment, information technology and consumables; and (2) managing procedures and clinical guidelines as resources for healthcare.

Buildings, equipment, consumables

In addition to budgets, numerous other non-human resources are required to support the provision and delivery of care, which in the previously mentioned acronym BEICHMM include:

- Buildings
- Equipment
- Information technology
- Consumables
- Medical devices

Buildings – that house hospitals, primary care centres, GP practices and other care organisations, and be they large hospitals or smaller units, they naturally incur running costs and maintenance costs. Often overseen by government policy to deliver a more effective and/or efficient service, new departments and units may be built, and others closed. All buildings, however, have to meet various legal requirements, such as health and safety and energy efficiency.

Equipment – such as beds of different types, special cots, purpose-built armchairs and couches, hoists for moving and handling, those for performing electrocardiographs, tomography, etc., are purchased to aid patients' diagnosis, treatment or recovery. They have to be regularly checked for safety as guided by various health and safety acts and regulations, such as the *Provision and Use of Work Equipment Regulations 1998*, and the *Approved Code of Practice and Guidance* (Health and Safety Executive, 2008).

Information technology – now widely available in clinical settings to support patient/service user care and treatment, and comprises predominantly of computers with access to the internet to facilitate evidence-based practice, and digital devices for monitoring patient progress with their health issue and recovery.

Medical devices – such as pulse oximeter, nebuliser, blood sugar level monitor, blood pressure measuring devices, patient-controlled analgesia device and their attachments also have to be purchased, and also replaced as necessary.

Consumables – are usually single-use items such as dressings, medication, intravenous administration sets, disposable gloves and aprons, personal protection equipment, stationery, etc.

Managing procedures and clinical guidelines

Care providers have to have fully approved clinical guidelines, procedures and clinical protocols available and accessible as resources that support the processes of care delivery, and thereby they ensure that the care activities of the care or-ganisation are performed to the highest standard. Every clinical guideline and procedure have an 'approved date' and a 'review date' to ensure they remain up to date and evidence-informed; and an addendum can be adjoined to the guidelines in line with new evidence or new policies.

The advantages and the issues related to procedures and clinical guidelines is analysed in Chapter 8 in the context of ensuring high-quality care. Inherent with-in clinical guidelines and procedures is person-centred, evidence-based practice.

Managing Human Resources

Having discussed non-human resources so far in this chapter, this section now ex-plores management of human resources, of which in the NHS in England equates to around 1.3 million employees overall (NHSE, 2019a). Of this total number of employees (headcount, not full-time-equivalent), approximately 320,000 are qualified nurses and midwives, 150,000 are doctors, who together represent one-third of the workforce. The remaining two-thirds comprise 320,000 health and care support workers (HSWs), 21,000 ambulance staff and infrastructure support staff (Nuffield Trust, 2019), and 170,000 AHPs in ten professions just in England (NHSE, 2019a).

Furthermore, the NHS is supported by indirectly employed staff who work through private companies to provide particular services, such as laundry, catering and cleaning; and healthcare professionals in the independent sector. Figure 4.2 in Chapter 4 shows details of some of the categories of nursing staff involved, and the staffing structure as an example of different levels of staff involved in direct patient care. The workforce, therefore, includes a large number of HSWs as part of most professions, and a variety of other nursing titles prevail such as nurs-ing associate, nurse practitioner, advanced nurse practitioner, consultant nurse, (modern) matron, occupational health nurse, school nurse, etc.

Additionally, many nurses, midwives and AHPs also have leadership-prac-titioner roles such as infection control nurses, moving and handling trainers, cardio-pulmonary resuscitation instructors, etc., and also supervisor of learning and teaching roles towards all categories of students and other learners such as apprentices, associate practitioners, etc.

An alternative view of this reality is that the NHS workforce costs 45% of NHS's total budget. However, as asserted by Handy (1985), organisations mustn't see their employees as costs (in terms of salaries, etc.), but as assets in the form of human resources, assets that should be valued. Handy referred to this idea about the general workforce as upside-down thinking. Furthermore, Armstrong and Taylor (2020: 9) suggest that employees should be perceived as 'human capital', which is because they 'invest' or contribute their knowledge, skills and abilities to enhance the organisation's capability.

Management of employees of the organisation is often referred to as human resource management (HRM), which constitutes organisations viewing their employees as individuals who contribute to the success of the organisation, and therefore not as costs in terms of wages that are paid to them. This perception largely refers to ensuring that individuals with the right skills (or potentials) are recruited to specific posts, in the right numbers, and at the right time to ensure that the healthcare provider's activities are performed to everyone's satisfaction and its goals achieved (see also discussion on organisations in Chapter 4).

Human resource management refers to 'the function responsible for establishing integrated personnel policies to support organisational strategy' (Buchanan and Huczynski, 2019: 27 and 795). HRM is also referred to as 'personnel management', and this relatively brief and compact explanation with the phrases 'personnel policies' and 'organisational strategy' signify recruiting, training and retaining staff and managing them so that they achieve optimum business performance and productivity. The productive contribution of individual employees simultaneously achieves the employer's business objectives, the individual employee's objectives, and those of society.

ACTION POINT 5.2
Staffing your practice setting

Thinking about the practice setting where you are based, ascertain for yourself all members of staff who contribute to care delivery in the setting. Think of all different categories of staff. Then, as a NRHP, approach a middle line manager and ask them (1) How many of each category of staff (full-time and part-time) are based in the practice setting, and (2) ask about how many should be based in the practice setting in order to ensure the setting's mission or aims and objectives are achieved fully.

Human resources comprise several different staff groups with their own specific skill-sets and knowledge base that are required to deliver safe, effective and compassionate care. They include frontline managers of course with registrants of different healthcare professions such as nurses, dieticians, physiotherapists, etc. as well as HSWs, as noted earlier. It also includes medical staff (including consultants and junior doctors, and Professors in some areas), the hospital chaplains/faith representatives, administrative staff, ancillary staff (e.g. porters, domestic staff), catering staff, as well as estates department employees (site and building maintenance staff, e.g. electricians, plumbers, gardeners, etc.).

All healthcare staff need periodic updating, extra training or continuing professional development (CPD) to ensure their practice is safe and effective, which also involve costs in terms of trainers' time, new devices or equipment, etc.

Healthcare providers often have a training budget, and a small amount of CPD funds are available annually from Health Education England.

However, staff shortfall has been a recurring issue at the turn of the 2020 decade (as also noted in Chapter 1) whereupon care providers have been unable to fill hundreds of vacant posts due to unavailability of appropriately skilled healthcare professionals, according to NHS LTP (NHSE, 2019a). The NHS LTP also indicates for example that 'while vacancy rates are 12.5% for radiologists and 15% for radiographers, etc, the number of patients referred for diagnostic tests has risen by over 25% over the last five years' (p. 105). It argues, therefore, that delivering an effective and high-quality diagnostic service requires increased investment in new equipment and staff, underpinned by a new model of diagnostic provision.

The reasons for shortages include the reduction in nurse training places at universities a few years earlier, which the government subsequently endeavoured to rectify in various ways. Apprenticeship was introduced, for example, for several healthcare professions, which involved individuals remaining salaried workers for a certain number of days each week, and students for the rest of the week. Associates such as Registered Nursing Associate programmes were introduced in 2016 and the first ones to be registered with the NMC did so in 2019, with over 1560 nursing associates on the NMC register by January 2020 (NMC, 2020b).

'The arrival of nursing associates marked a once-in-a-generation change to the UK nursing landscape' assert Traynor and Knibb (2020: 26) on assessing the views of newly qualified nursing associates. A cadet scheme targeting 14- to 18-year-olds was re-initiated in 2020 (Lay, 2020). Other new roles are also being developed, such as physician's assistants, clinical pharmacists and anaesthetic practitioners, and so on, with the aim of further expanding the health service workforce.

One of the first concerns of frontline managers is to ensure that they have sufficient number of staff and skill mix in their care setting. For planning for staffing, there are some time-honoured principles of workforce planning that endure as basic steps that need be taken into account, primarily to ensure that the workforce has the right number of staff, and with the right skills and competences. Skills for Health (2020) identifies a framework for workforce planning that comprise the following components:

Step 1: Defining the plan by identifying the purpose of the plan and responsibilities.

Step 2: Mapping service change by identifying the benefits of change, the drivers of change, and the barriers.

Step 3: Defining the required workforce by mapping service activities, identifying the skills needed, and the types and numbers of staff required.

Step 4: Understanding workforce availability in terms of existing skills and supply options.

Step 5: Developing an action plan to deliver the right staff with the right skills in the right place.

Step 6: Implementing, monitoring the progress of the plan against targets, and revising the plan as appropriate.

Skills for Health (2020) argues that this Six-Step Methodology comprises a systematic practical approach that supports the delivery of quality patient care, productivity and efficiency, and an assurance that workforce planning decisions taken are sustainable and realistic.

The management of human resources includes ensuring that staff comply with the various regulations (e.g. health and safety regulations), legislation and local policies as well as all the professional codes of practice. The next section on managing human resources therefore now addresses specifically:

- Managing human relations in the workplace.
- Recruitment and retention of staff.
- Safe staffing and skill mix.
- Employers' and employees' expectations of each other.
- Gauging staff satisfaction with their work.

Managing Human Relations in the Workplace

As indicated in Chapter 4, the human relations approach to management is naturally the most appropriate approach for managing healthcare staff as it recognises the benefits of acknowledging the social and psychological needs of individual employees and the contribution of each to the organisation's success. It entails taking a humane and caring approach towards healthcare staff, whose very foundation of professional responsibility is based on caring for all, for those who are unwell along with those who are at risk of becoming ill; and for colleagues.

The human relations approach to management is based on the idea that employees are motivated not only by financial reward (which is often based on productivity) but also by a range of social factors in the workplace (e.g. a sense of belonging, feelings of achievement, praise and pride in one's work), and consequently relationships, attitudes and leadership styles all play key roles in the performance of the organisation.

It is an approach based on the consideration of social factors in the work setting, the views of employees about the organisation and the satisfaction of individuals' needs through groups at work (e.g. Mullins, 2019). Productivity tends to increase when employees are comfortable with manager-worker and peer relationships, and if they feel part of a supportive group where each employee's work has a significant effect on the team's output.

Deriving from an in-depth analysis of how effective working relationships can be established between individuals in healthcare, Gopee (2010: 29) defines effective relationship as 'one that comprises acceptance of each other by the two parties involved, establishing a mutual understanding and rapport which might constitute small negotiations and … empathic listening'.

Support with professional development is integral to the overall picture. Staff satisfaction with the working conditions and a motivational, positive atmosphere are the foundations that FHMs and other managers need to sustain to ensure a collective and positive culture prevails in the workplace. Although initiated almost a hundred years ago since the Hawthorne experiments noted in Chapter 4, the human relations approach logically endures in health-social care, and looks set to play a central part of management and leadership despite the prevalence of the technological-digital age and beyond.

Recruitment and Retention of Staff

The FHM needs to have substantial knowledge of the principles of, and be competent in, staff recruitment, in assimilating new recruits into the team, and in staff retention. The process of recruitment of new staff after an existing member of staff leaves can take several months, as the practice setting's managers re-determine the requirements of the post, involve the personnel department for advertising the post, review applications, shortlist, interview, decide on the best candidate to offer the job to, and include the amount of notice the candidate needs to give to their previous employer before they can start the new post. Even then, there will usually be a period of orientation and induction before the post-holder can function fully autonomously.

One of the big concerns for NHS trusts and professional bodies at the turn of the 2020 decade has been difficulty with recruitment of healthcare professionals with the appropriate skills and knowledge, and about 'safe staffing' (e.g. DH, 2000b; RCN, 2019a). The King's Fund (2018: 2), for example, indicates that 'Across NHS trusts there is a shortage of more than 100,000 staff', and that this is partly due to reduction in investment in education and training of healthcare staff since around 2006.

Consequently, retention of staff has become a major issue for healthcare employers to contend with because of ongoing difficulty in recruitment of suitable staff to fill vacancies left by those who have moved on. Cole (2020), for example, reports that various NHS trusts recently noticed that approximately a quarter of NRNs leave their posts through disillusionment and demotivation within a year of being recruited. Trusts then took action to find out why existing staff were leaving by asking questions of those who had left (exit interviews) and those still in post, so that they can decide on solutions.

There are several factors that must be considered carefully to address such challenges related to recruitment and retention of employees, as briefly acknowledged in Chapter 1 under the nature of the twenty-first-century workforce. Considerations also include increasing the total number of healthcare staff in employment, facilitation of continuing learning, career progression, being a valued team member, etc. as illustrated in Figure 5.2.

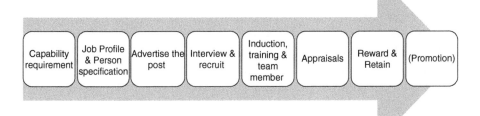

| Capability requirement | Job Profile & Person specification | Advertise the post | Interview & recruit | Induction, training & team member | Appraisals | Reward & Retain | (Promotion) |

Figure 5.2 The recruitment and retention process – simplified

---

ACTION POINT 5.3
Staff motivation and retention

Think of the personal fulfilment that you get from your work as a healthcare professional. Make some notes on this. Then consider the day-to-day and overall steps that your managers and the employing organisation take to keep you motivated in your post, and consequently to retain you as part of their workforce. It might prove useful to discuss this with a more senior colleague.

Consider also, in your experience and view, what can be done to retain staff who may be disillusioned or burnt-out at work.

In *Closing the Gap*, the King's Fund (2019c) identifies a wide range of key areas for action on healthcare workforce, which include the following considerations:

- *Supply of new staff:* providing education and training for them.
- *Pay and reward:* ensuring pay policy supports recruitment and retention.
- *Being a good employer:* making the NHS a better place to work and build a career.
- *Workforce redesign:* the right teams with the right skills and technological support.
- *Supply of new staff:* international recruitment.
- *Social care:* pay, recruitment and retention in social care.

With regards to career progression, note, however, that careers can progress vertically or horizontally (when an employee wishes to move on to a different specialism), and also consideration given to those who wish to have a career break, maybe for family reasons. Other mechanisms for recruiting and retaining staff include routes for returners to healthcare profession, the provision of reasonably priced nurseries for staff with very young children, agile working, etc.

Some of the points you may have made in response to Action point 5.3 include flexible working hours to accommodate family life or being a carer at home (if this is not already established in your organisation), or self-rostering maybe, arrangements for working part-time, job sharing, career breaks, working from home if that is feasible, phased retirement and term-time contracts.

Furthermore, NHSI and NHS Employers (2019) *National Retention Programme* provides guidance for healthcare providers on ways to develop novel ways of retaining healthcare staff through, for example, improved support for NRNs, flexible working to support work–life balance, enabling staff engagement, supporting the more experienced workforce, structured career planning and development, supporting health and wellbeing.

NHSI and NHS Employers, as well as Radford (2019), indicate that the guidance has enabled trusts to improve staff retention and reduce staff turnover. Furthermore, the results of the 2019 NHS England Survey Co-ordination Centre [NHSESCC] (2020) revealed that the national average for staff who are satisfied/very satisfied with the opportunities for flexible working patterns is 54%, which means there is scope for improvement on this.

Moreover, Health Education England (2020a) suggests proactive actions for workforce transformation through redesign based around five key enablers, or domains, namely (1) focusing on supply of workers, (2) up-skilling existing workers, (3) developing new roles, (4) new ways of working, and (5) leadership. As the workforce is pivotal to the success of the NHS, healthcare employers would benefit from heeding these HEE's suggestions.

The NHSE+I publication *We are the NHS: People Plan for 2020/2021 – Action for us all* (NHSE, 2020b), nevertheless focuses mainly on the immediate 2020–21 plans with the anticipation that the principles constitute a blueprint for the future. The document also includes 'Our People Promise' which specifies actions that will be incorporated in the annual NHS Staff Survey. It specifies practical actions that employers, systems and the HEE have to take by devising local People Plans by addressing:

- health and wellbeing for all staff;
- equality and diversity, discrimination and belongingness for every member of staff;
- capturing innovations;
- recruiting, training and retention of staff, including returners and clinical nurse specialists (child and adolescent psychotherapists, for example).

Additionally, *Start Well: Stay Well – a model to support new starter* (NHSI and NHS Employers, 2018) propounds the success of a retention programme that incorporates much more of the human relations approach to management by concentrating on interactions that improve staff experience of working in the trust though direct and sincere consideration of each employee's wellbeing. Furthermore, a

BBC (2020) documentary elaborated on ways in which five healthcare staff who are appointed as mentors (called an 'intern scheme') successfully manage to retain substantial number of NRHPs, those qualified overseas and any nurse experiencing a career crisis at their trust.

Similar perpectives are advocated by Johnstone et al. (2020) who suggest that retention strategies could include redeploying individual staff to another department, where they receive appropriate induction and support from mentors, peer-mentoring, stress reduction programmes, flexible rostering and even short career breaks. The overall impact of these developments can directly show in, for example, more cost-effective care delivery and better use of resources and teamwork, enhanced quality of patient care, improved professional career structures and delivery of care closer to home.

Safe Staffing and Skill Mix

The management of human resources includes ascertaining the staff competence required to deliver the service the organisation offers, and then employing individuals who have those skills. For novel services, individuals might have to be employed and then trained and assessed before the service can be used. In healthcare, safety and effectiveness of care provided is paramount, and therefore appropriate numbers of appropriately skilled staff have to be employed to care for service users, because otherwise harm might come to service users, which is both unethical and illegal.

An appropriate combination of registrants and non-registered staff (also referred to as regulated and unregulated staff) is known as 'skill mix', which refers to the ratio of registrants with different levels of expertise to unregulated staff on each specific ward, unit or department. It is crucial for FHMs to have a very good estimation of the skill mix of staff required for their area of responsibility. However, calculating the precise ratio of registered to non-registered healthcare workers for individual care settings is problematic.

There are top-down methods of doing so, and bottom-up methods, according to Hurst's (2010) analysis, in that top-down methods entail benchmarking against staffing ratio in NHS trusts that are rated highly by the CQC. Bottom-up approaches are based on the professional judgement and consensus of colleagues in relation to bed occupancy, patient dependency, time required for each care intervention, etc.

In the past, actions to ascertain the required skill mix were suspected as having an underlying motive to reduce the number of qualified staff, and allocating more tasks to HSWs. It included quantifying so-called 'unproductive time', which is paid meal breaks and rest periods, and any time when staff engage in conversation that is not work-related.

It is important to ensure an appropriate skill mix of staff because various reports (e.g. Francis, 2013; RCN, 2020c) indicate that quality of care improves proportionately with higher ratios of qualified staff available to provide care, and patient outcomes improve when nurses care for fewer patients. Conversely, a poor skill mix of qualified and unqualified nurses leads to comparatively poorer patient outcomes, job dissatisfaction and low morale, more adverse events and higher mortality rates (Dean, 2012; Griffiths, 2021).

ACTION POINT 5.4
Skill mix in my workplace

Following on from Action point 5.3, now consider the skill mix in your care setting. How many whole-time equivalent (WTE) staff are employed? What is the ratio of registered to non-registered staff? Overall, what is your personal opinion regarding the current skill mix in your care setting or organisation? Identify the reasons for your view.

The skill-mix in different care settings will of course vary, based on patient dependency for example. Therefore, an intensive care unit will require more registrants and specialist nurses than say an outpatients department or a rehabilitation unit. NICE's (2014) guidance on safe nurse staffing levels acknowledges that there isn't one universal correct nursing staff-to-patient ratio for all care settings, and suggests that nursing staff requirements should be determined by, for example, patient factors, ward factors and nursing staff factors, etc. It, however, recommends regular review of nursing staff establishments in all care settings.

On the other hand, implementing the previously commended 70:30 registered to unregistered staff ratio requires a 15% increase in the number of registered nurses, according to Scott's (2015) analysis. Furthermore, staffing ratios for the care setting also requires consideration of other variables including input by AHPs, backfill of staff when they are on training days, etc. Safe staffing levels are also affected by team members now being expected to be more career-minded than before and apply for promotion or higher level posts.

The RCN (2020c) reports that the Scottish Government passed a legislation that sets out the requirements for safe staffing across both health and care services and most clinical professions. Similar progress is being made in Wales and Northern Ireland, but for England the campaign for safe staffing by legislation has yet to be achieved.

Employers' and Employees' Expectations of Each Other

In addition to employers having clear expectations of the staff they recruit, individual employees also have certain expectations of their employer. These expectations are referred to as a 'psychological contract' between employer and employee which might not be in the form of a written agreement, but consists of a range of expectations, rights, privileges and duties that can have a significant impact on both the employee and the organisation.

Consequently, beside agreeing to and signing the employment contract, the organisation expects the employee to adhere to specified organisational rules and regulations, to fully accept the established philosophy of the department and the organisation, contribute to the achievement of their objectives, to be loyal to the organisation when on and off duty, and not to abuse facilities that the employee accesses.

With regards to loyalty to the organisation, Stewart (1993), who was a long-term researcher on management, identified a number of ways in which organisations can acquire employee loyalty (others refer to employee loyalty as 'theory Z') to the organisation, including:

- managers showing concern for employees by spending substantial amount of their time listening to employees about their work;
- an appraisal system that also considers the employee's longer-term or career goals;
- decision-making based on staff consultation.

Furthermore, in addition to employee loyalty towards their employing organisation, there is also the concept of employee engagement or staff engagement (e.g. NHSESCC, 2020). In a cross-sectional study exploring employee engagement at work by different generations of nurses and supervisors, Huber and Schubert (2019) found that generation Y adults (people born approximately between 1980 and 1995) attach less importance to work than did previous generations, but at the same time, professional ambition is seen as more important to generation Y than it is to preceding generations. They, therefore, suggest that it is necessary for employers to know generation-specific differences concerning attitudes towards work.

Conversely, with regards to employee expectations, they are likely to comprise the organisation providing a safe working environment, and:

- personal development and career advancement opportunities, etc.;
- endeavouring to provide job security;
- allocating challenging and satisfying jobs;
- adopting equitable personnel policies and procedures;
- facilitating genuine participation by staff in decisions;
- treating everyone with respect;
- being supportive and providing guidance wherever possible when staff struggle with personal problems.

Individual employees' expectations vary widely, and can change over time, but so can the ability of the organisation to meet them. Consequently, FHMs should also encourage full employee engagement and foster employee loyalty by team members, and be mindful of results of local staff surveys and the CQC's (2020a) in relation to 'Key lines of enquiry'.

Gauging Staff Satisfaction with their Work

Having determined recruitment and retention of staff, skill mix and safe staffing, and employer–employee expectations of each other, this section moves on to explore another essential concept inherent within HRM, namely staff satisfaction at work, which can be a lynchpin for staff motivation and retention, as well as their involvement and loyalty.

Over a number of years, various reports have indicated that healthcare staff are markedly dissatisfied with aspects of their work, and that improvements need to be made in order to retain staff (e.g. RCN, 2015b). The NHSESCC's (2020) staff surveys explore healthcare staff's experiences under 11 themes (covered by approximately 100 questions), which include: staff morale, quality of care, safety culture, staff engagement and team working. Findings of the 2019 survey include:

- 81% satisfied with the quality of care they give to patients/service users ('agree/ strongly agree');
- 69% indicated that they 'agree/strongly agree' to the question about whether they are able to deliver the care they 'aspire to';
- 75% of staff felt enthusiastic about their job 'always/often';
- 80% of staff agreed that they are 'able to do [their] job to a standard [they are] personally pleased with' 'agree/strongly agree'.

However, on the question 'Does the organisation take positive action on (staffs') health and wellbeing?', only 29% replied 'yes, definitely'. Other problematic findings include a substantial proportion of respondents reporting work-related stress in the preceding 12 months, that there should be more staff at the frontline, etc.

It should prove beneficial to take a look through various questions of the most recent NHSESCC staff survey results, and to consider for yourself how your own practice setting would fare against the survey questions. Alternatively, you could look at the content of the most recent staff satisfaction survey conducted by your own employing organisation and view the areas of success and those where improvement are needed.

Furthermore, staff satisfaction surveys also tend to include various other questions such as on harassment and bullying at work, and for this, if respondents indicate that they do experience them, then there can be supplementary questions such as whether it was reported, and what the outcomes were if they were reported.

ACTION POINT 5.5

Staff surveys at your healthcare organisation

Chances are that you will have completed a staff satisfaction survey conducted by your employing organisation in the not-too-distant past. Ask a middle manager who knows you quite well about their knowledge of the results of the latest survey, unless of course if they have already been published for staff to see.

Ask about which specific office initiated the survey, then think for yourself what your views are regarding the results.

Alternatively, access the above-mentioned NHSESCC's (2020) website and view the most recent staff survey for your organisation, and identify its findings.

The level of staff satisfaction can impact on staff retention and quality of care in the long run, and dissatisfaction areas should be followed up rather than be content with overall high levels of satisfaction on survey results. Challenges for frontline care professionals at work was examined in Chapter 2 of this book, along with the formal and informal support that frontline managers can draw on.

Guidance on Management of Healthcare Resources at Clinical and Organisational Levels

The following briefly summarises good practice in the management of healthcare resources:

- Develop detailed knowledge of all resources that are required by your care setting to deliver safe, effective and high-quality care to service users.
- Genuinely value your staff and openly recognise their input towards the success of the care setting and the organisation.
- Familiarise yourself with the content of the monthly or periodic budget statements related to your care setting, and if appropriate for your department.
- When specific areas of overspend have been identified, raise awareness within the team and discuss with your manager and team members the safest ways to reduce the overspend.
- Establish the unit cost of consumable resources wherever possible, and enable team members to review and monitor usage and expenditure.
- Oversee effectiveness of care provided as well as efficiency, and discuss with team members and with your manager how these could be improved.
- Incorporate human relations mode of management in the workplace taking into consideration the organisation's and employees' expectations of each other, and by monitoring staff satisfaction with their work.

- Ensure safe staffing and skill mix in the workplace and participate in staff recruitment and retention as much as feasible.
- Manage non-human resources such as equipment, devices and information technology, and ensure procedures and clinical guidelines are adhered to by team members.

Chapter Summary

A wide range of human and non-human resources are required for the health service to fulfil its obligations, and it simply cannot function without them. Consequently, this chapter has focused on the resources required for effective care provision and delivery, and therefore addressed:

- The necessary human and non-human resources required by service providers for effective care delivery in practice settings, and why resources have to be managed;
- Knowledge of sources of funds required for health services, as well as knowledge of what budgets are, why budgeting is important in health services, how budgets are set and ways of maximising their use;
- The full range of other non-human resources that are required such as hospital or primary care buildings, equipment, clinical guidelines and consumables that need to be managed for effective care delivery;
- Knowledge of multiple components of human resource management, including human relations in the workplace, the recruitment and retention of staff, safe staffing and skill mix; and
- Awareness of the significance of staff surveys in the context of employers' and employees' expectations of each other.

Further Reading

- For details of the *2020 NHS staff satisfaction survey* conducted by the Staff Survey Co-ordination Centre, see: Staff Survey Co-ordination Centre (2020) *NHS Staff Survey Results 2019.* Available at: www.nhsstaffsurveyresults.com/homepage/national-results-2019/trends-questions-2019/. Accessed Date: 31 March 2020.
- For extensive details of changes and adaptations that NHSE+I require NHS employers, systems and HEE to make to reinforce the NHS workforce, see: NHS England (2020) *We are the NHS: People Plan for 2020/2021 – Action for us all.* Available at: www.england.nhs.uk/publication/we-are-the-nhs-people-plan-for-2020-21-action-for-us-all/. Accessed Date: 29 January 2021.

6

Effective Inter-Disciplinary Teamwork and Staff Motivation

Chapter Objectives

The chapter objectives for frontline healthcare managers with regards to inter-disciplinary teamwork and staff motivation are:

- Demonstrate an analytical understanding of the nature of teams in health-care, the differences between groups and teams, inter-disciplinary health-care teams and their characteristics;
- Identify reasons for teamwork in care settings and ways in which inter-disciplinary team performance can be maximised;
- Specify different ways in which effective inter-disciplinary teams operate through team formation identifying team roles, team leadership, compre-hensive multi-professional communication and ways of conducting team meetings effectively;
- Show substantial knowledge of teamwork and different approaches and theories of staff motivation at work, and ways in which they can be applied to inter-disciplinary teamwork; and
- Stipulate some of the different methods of evaluating and monitoring team performance, the challenges and issues related to dysfunctional teams, and how they can improve and harness learning as a team.

Introduction

Co-ordinated, collaborative and cohesive teamwork comprises the foundation stone of safe, effective and person-centred treatment and care. Consider the extensive and detailed co-ordination required to move a patient suspected of head or spinal injury from a trolley to an acute hospital bed, or during major surgery, or when helping a service user with post-natal psychosis. Inter-disciplinary teamwork is an indispensable feature of comprehensive healthcare across all care settings, intensive care to primary care.

This chapter focuses on inter-disciplinary teamworking in healthcare delivery, and therefore starts by first ascertaining the reasons for inter-disciplinary teamwork in healthcare, examining the nature of teams and groups, the characteristics of effective teams, how to create, nurture and lead effective teams, and various methods for keeping individuals and the team motivated (including theories of motivation). The chapter then explores dysfunctional teams and how they can become effective, and finally, ways of enhancing team performance.

Understanding the Nature of Teamwork in Healthcare

Healthcare staff often work as inter-disciplinary teams, and they are supported by more senior and specialist healthcare professionals who are more knowledgeable and provide leadership and function as role models for the more junior team members. This section at the beginning of the chapter analyses what makes teams of workers different from groups of workers, be they ancillary staff or professionals. Thinking across various different occupations, teams are generally more effective at achieving the organisation's aims than are groups of workers who tend to be less organised, and less cohesive, co-ordinated and collaborative.

Furthermore, a group of people or workers usually comprise three or more people with a common interest, but without necessarily the cohesion of mutual trust and established common goals. A group might form informally whereupon members can leave the group at will and maybe others join. On the other hand, a formal group can also be temporary in nature having been brought together in an organisation to plan and implement a particular component, such as guidelines for auditing the application of 'NEWS2', or guidelines for managing COVID-19 or influenza vaccinations for all over-55s within a primary care network (PCN). Informal groups tend to develop more naturally amongst people with similar interests.

A team, on the other hand, in made up of a number of people selected for a particular purpose whose knowledge and skills, and consequently responsibilities, within the team complement each other, and they develop into a co-ordinated unit. The interrelationship between members is also key and comprises mutual respect for team members' views, and acceptance of the organisation's mission statement and the team's goals. All these inherent components of fully formed teams also apply directly to healthcare teams.

An earlier definition of a team offered by the World Health Organization [WHO] (2012: 1) is 'a distinguishable set of two or more people who interact dynamically, interdependently and adaptively towards a common and valued goal/objective/mission, who have been assigned specific roles or functions to perform'.

ACTION POINT 6.1

Do staff in your workplace operate in teams or in groups?

Think of various instances when you meet people in groups, small groups or large, groups that meet only occasionally or frequently, work-related or non-work-related.

Then consider the social dynamics of each of these groups of people when they meet, and for each one decide whether it is a group or a team. Think about the reasons for your decision(s), which may include the explanations of these given in the text above.

Overall, groups are more transient and flexible in terms of their duration and membership than teams, and may be self-selected rather than appointed or invited. Table 6.1. endeavours to differentiate critically between groups and teams, differences that prevail in healthcare as well.

Different types of groups and teams can be identified in organisations, including production groups, service groups, management teams, project teams, advisory groups and action or task groups and performing groups. As for teams in particular, Arnold et al. (2020) indicate that an important feature of a 'true team' is that they have to have been given the authority to make certain decisions, e.g. autonomy in allocation of work to individuals within the team, attendance and absence control, and quality of the work. Teams thereby have autonomy and are empowered.

Furthermore, in healthcare, teams can be uni-professional, that is comprising a single professional group (e.g. nursing staff, social care staff, etc.), or inter-disciplinary teams that comprise a range of disciplines working in collaboration. The mechanics of team-working is also distinctly recognised in the pre-registration programmes of healthcare profession students, and their competence is assessed on their ability to work collaboratively within inter-disciplinary team structures.

Table 6.1   Distinguishing between groups and teams

Groups	Teams
• Made up of larger numbers of people, some self-selected	• Membership is selected and limited
• Existence of cliques/subgroups	• Decisions are made by consensus, after considering all members' views
• Individuals might feel speaking openly is risky	• Individuals feel free to express their views
• Individual accountability	• Accountability rests with individuals and the team
• Skills are random and may be deficient	• Members' skills are complementary
• Has elected or appointed leader	• Shared or rotating leadership
• Political siding	• Have a shared purpose, which is always the focus of everyone's actions
• Individuals might have reservations about the common objectives	• Objectives are reviewed together to ensure they are accepted by all and SMART
• Divergent feelings but focus on leader	• Mutual acceptance; co-ordination

Areas of competence for health and care professionals are identified by the relevant professional regulatory bodies, such as the NMC and the HCPC. For example, under 'Platform 5 – Leading and managing care and working in teams', the NMC (2018a: 19) indicates that RNs across the four fields of nursing 'play an active and equal role in the inter-disciplinary team, collaborating and communicating effectively with a range of colleagues'. It then identifies 12 standards that students must become competent in during their pre-registration programme, including:

• Standard 5.4: demonstrate an understanding of the roles, responsibilities and scope of practice of all members of the nursing and inter-disciplinary team and how to make best use of the contributions of others involved in providing care.
• Standard 5.11: effectively and responsibly use a range of digital technologies to access, input, share and apply information and data within teams and between agencies.

As can be noted, the terms collaborating, communicating and understanding each other's role feature prominently in these standards. Other standards address, for example, demonstrating leadership potential and understanding ways of influencing change. So, NRNs will have developed their ability to work in inter-disciplinary teams by the time they qualify. Similar expectations apply to AHPs and other care professionals. However, interprofessional collaboration and group cohesion and performance may also depend on the work environment and local culture, the group's development stage and maturity, and organisational leadership and support with training, scope for innovation, etc.

Thus, in healthcare, teams can operate mono-professionally (e.g. a team of physiotherapists) or inter-professionally as a member of a team of various health-care professionals. Mono-professionally, for example, a team of tissue viability nurses work as a cohesive team with the common goal of promoting and maintaining healthy and intact skin for service users who are at risk by providing specialist care, advice and maybe equipment to them. However, they may also operate as an inter-disciplinary team if the service user also requires intervention and advice from a physician, a diabetic specialist nurse, an occupational therapist, etc.

Service user care thus often benefits from input from a selection of health-care professions, and various terminologies prevail that include the word profession or discipline, such as the terms multidisciplinary, multiprofessional, inter-disciplinary, interprofessional, transdisciplinary, etc., some of which tend to be used interchangeably, or are ill-defined. However, the word 'multi' usually signifies multiple professionals contributing their specialist interventions and then withdrawing, but the term 'inter' signifies close communication and collaboration between all professions, which enhances service user care.

Health and care professionals in UK are regulated by ten different regulatory bodies (e.g. General Medical Council, General Dental Council, etc.), each with their own codes of practice, and also their professional colleges and their trade unions. With regards to inter-disciplinary teamwork, in the nurses, midwives and nursing associates code of practice, for example, the NMC (2018b: 10) specifies that registrants must 'Work co-operatively ... respect the skills, expertise and contributions of your colleagues, referring matters to them when appropriate'.

Furthermore, in their analysis of models of teamwork, Berlin et al. (2012) concluded that we should be on our guard towards idealistic models (such as inter-disciplinary healthcare models of working), which can be used as a reference standard, but in reality, disciplines function more beneficially and effectively when each is differentiated and the multi-team approach is accepted as reality in most organisations. Therefore, the concept inter-disciplinary is preferable, but the multi-disciplinary outlook is also beneficial in differentiating and valuing areas of expertise.

On analysing teamwork, the NHSESCC (2020) *NHS Staff Survey of 2019* found that nationally 72% of staff indicated that their team had a set of shared objectives ('satisfied' and 'very satisfied'), and 61% indicated that the team often meets to discuss the team's effectiveness. However, it has increasingly become difficult to find time to discuss team effectiveness. One of the negative findings is that 28% of staff are unaware of their team's objectives. Nevertheless, 82% indicated that they were happy ('satisfied', and 29% 'very satisfied') with the support they get from their ward colleagues.

Why Teamwork in Care Settings

The importance of teamwork in enabling service users recover from health issues cannot be underestimated, as the process usually requires input from various specialists each with their own areas of expertise. However, input from differ-ent professionals has been referred to as multi-disciplinary work, which implies that each profession contributes their interventions without necessarily com-municating the details and outcome of their input to other professionals. This suggests disjointed care, and therefore the term inter-disciplinary is used in this book to signify comprehensive communication of service user care amongst care professionals.

Inter-disciplinary care is very much an everyday activity within many clinical specialities, including in mental health care, operating theatres, end of life care, car-ing for individuals with learning disabilities in the community and intensive care. Thereby, in addition to nurses and doctors, care is provided and complemented by dietitians, physiotherapists, radiologists, social workers, psychologists or other pro-fessionals as deemed appropriate by the medical or specialist team (see Figure 6.1).

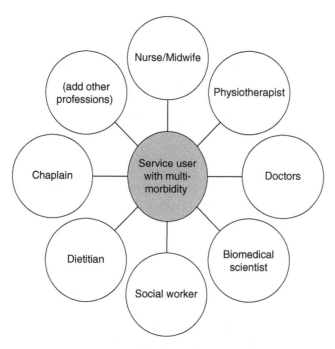

Figure 6.1   Members of the inter-disciplinary team

Healthcare professionals from various other disciplines may be called upon depending on the service user's specific health problem. Speech and language therapists, clinical psychologists, prosthetists, orthotists, specialist counsellors are among those whose specific expertise the core team can draw on. The benefit to the service user drawn from this wide range of input is that they are provided with the specialist knowledge and skills of each discipline based on several years of experience and knowledge base. Each discipline also has its own identified philosophy of care and set of values, but which contribute to the wider, shared philosophy of the inter-disciplinary team.

For service users to benefit fully from inter-disciplinary work, the professionals from different disciplines have to feel they are useful members of the extended team. The benefits of effective teams have been documented by, for example, Havyer et al. (2014) who indicate that team effectiveness is:

- positively associated with improvement in motor function among stroke rehabilitation patients;
- positively associated with patients' perceptions of continuity;
- correlated with lower post-operative complication rate;
- associated with patients' ratings of satisfaction with physicians treating them with respect and nurses listening to them;
- inversely correlated with blood pressure;
- associated with higher mean patient satisfaction;
- negatively associated with patient death or readmission to the intensive care unit.

The added benefits of working in teams is that it also increases clinical effectiveness, job satisfaction for staff, which results in reduced turnover of staff (and therefore reduced costs) and innovation (e.g. West et al., 2011). Conversely, deficient teamwork has been associated with safety failures, including adverse events and errors, according to Dellefield and Verkaaik's (2020) research.

Effective Inter-Disciplinary Teams

Having examined the nature of, and rationale for, healthcare teams in the preceding two sections, this section examines the elements that make teams effective in achieving their aims in the short and long term. Essentially, effective teams first of all need sensitive leadership, which combined with transparent identification of each member's responsibilities, full and open top-down and lateral communication in the organisation, acceptance and respect for each other, and of course provision of training and career opportunities, can enable optimal functioning by the team.

Furthermore, an effective team is one in which team members own the team's common purpose and goals, at both organisational level and team level, and where team members operate in a co-operative environment, maintain effective, mutual working relationships and share knowledge and skills. Attributes that are essential for effective teamwork include:

- *Sense of commitment* – by team members to the team's shared mission statement and objectives.

- *Motivation and engagement* – to ensure team success.
- *Co-operation and full participation* – by all team members.
- *Mutual interdependence* – team members appreciate the benefits of contributing to a positive interdependent team environment wherein individuals promote and encourage their fellow team members to achieve, contribute and learn.
- *Using interpersonal skills* – entails the ability to work effectively with other team members, ensuring a medium wherein team members discuss issues openly and honestly, in a supportive way, and show respect for each other.
- *Conflict resolution* – by team members without the need for intervention by senior managers.
- *Giving and receiving constructive feedback* – supportive feedback as and when requested, knowing that it enhances learning.
- *Open awareness of each other's specific team roles* – to enable members to exercise leadership skills and be a resource on aspects of care.
- *Accountable to the team* – for decision-making that promotes best practice, novel ideas and team learning.

One of the most effective vehicles for enabling cohesive and effective inter-disciplinary teamwork is care pathways (examined in some detail in Chapter 2 of this book). As Scaria (2016) argues, in using care pathways, healthcare professionals from a variety of disciplines contribute their diverse knowledge and competence, which result in enhanced co-ordination, collaboration, communication and decision-making that, in turn, lead to optimal healthcare outcomes for service users. They also enable improved staff knowledge and interprofessional relations, and contribute to person-centred care and increased patient satisfaction.

Furthermore, various tools and questionnaires are available over the internet for assessing team effectiveness, some contain five items, others eleven and others even more. They tend to address common elements for assessing team performance and therefore have to be modified to some extent to assess performance in health and care teams. Emerald Works (2020), for example, provides a 15-question questionnaire for assessing team effectiveness. The areas that they address include:

- *Enabling team development* – as guided by Tuckman's (Agile-Mercurial, 2019) stages on team development that results in setting clear expectations of the overall team and each team member, respect and collaboration between team members, and establishing clear guidelines.
- *Feedback* – to team members on their individual performance, and to the team on their overall performance.
- *Participation and articulating the team's vision* – to motivate and direct the team to reach its goal.
- *Conflict management* – led by team members and leaders.

- *Maximise performance* – by putting team members in the right roles (see Belbin's team roles).
- *Team member development* – for personal improvement and to build and foster the skills in the individuals that are congruent with the needs of the team.
- *Understanding and collaboration* – to enable cohesion, consensus, consistency, in working for the same purpose, and agreement on key issues facing the team.

Question 9 of the questionnaire, for example, presents the statement 'team members are encouraged to commit to the team vision, and leaders help them understand how their role fits into the big picture', and team members have to choose between 'Not at all', 'Rarely', 'Sometimes', 'Often' or 'Very often'. It then provides a total score of 0–75 as the assessment result to work from.

The next section on how healthcare teams can function as effective inter-disciplinary teams now examines the concepts of team formation and team roles, team leadership, teamwork and communication, how to conduct team meetings to the benefit of all members, as well as the prevalence of teamwork and power dynamics in teams.

Team Formation and Team Roles

The words 'consensus', 'mutual' and 'shared' are found in the teams column on Table 6.1 (Distinguishing between groups and teams), which in essence is the result of transition from being a newly formed group of people to a functional team. Tuckman (Tuckman and Jensen, 1977; Agile-Mercurial, 2019) is well known for identifying the process that groups of people generally go through to become teams. The Tuckman model of teamwork includes five stages of development, which are Forming, Storming, Norming, Performing and Adjourning/Mourning. The stages are self-explanatory, but see Table 6.2 for a brief explanation of each stage.

Table 6.2 Brief explanation of each stage of development from group to team

Development stage	Brief details
Forming	Initial meeting of the group, orientation phase, getting to know individual members, poor or no structure at this stage.
Storming	Individuals and group explore purpose of the group; includes questioning, some disagreement, conflicts, taking sides.
Norming	Agree on group objectives, roles allocated/offered, ground rules established.
Performing	The group meet regularly to report on progress with objectives, highlight issues and extra help required, etc.
Adjourning/Mourning	On completion of group task, the group disbands; may have follow up meeting after summative evaluation.

The initial model comprised the first four phases, but following a systematic review of application of the model the fifth stage adjourning/mourning was added by Tuckman and Jensen (1977) for a more complete representation of group development processes. Furthermore, the developmental stages can be completed within one meeting session depending on the length of time available for the meeting, as well as on whether the individuals in the group are already familiar with each other, and of course in the absence of any political or power game individuals want to bring in. The team leader usually facilitates this process of reaching an effective and high-performing state as quickly as possible; that is, into a cohesive team that gets results.

Although the UK's government's cabinet is made of 27 members, which is generally considered a large team, it functions as a team on most government matters, and speaks with one voice as it were. There can easily be that many healthcare professionals staffing a general intensive care unit, and they subscribe to one purpose which is the wellbeing of patients and everyone that uses their services. However, Mullins (2019) suggests that cohesive teams tend to be made up of only ten or twelve members, as larger team sizes verge on splitting up into sub-groups.

Furthermore, from her research on team roles, Belbin (Belbin Associates, 2020) concluded that if all team members were like-minded people and comfortable in their adherence to all the team protocols, then this can be counter-productive by reducing interest in innovations and can dampen creativity. Conversely, when the team includes members who feel they can challenge the status quo and feel free to think differently, then this can be beneficial to the team in terms of divergent thinking and contributing with different ideas.

Belbin then separated the input by each team member as one of nine different team roles (see Table 6.3). However, Belbin added that not all nine roles have to be adopted by different members, as some team members can function in more than one team role. The team roles concept has been applied effectively to teams in a variety of professions over the years. The value of each team role is presented on Table 6.3.

The first three roles – coordinator, teamworker and resource investigator – are also known as 'People Orientated Roles', the latter three as 'Thinking Orientated Roles' and the final three as 'Action Orientated Roles'. Although Belbin identifies the useful qualities of each team role, she also notes likely weaknesses of each role. For example, the weaknesses of the co-ordinator role are that it can be seen as manipulative and might offload their own share of the work. For teamworker, the weakness is that the person in the role can be indecisive in crunch situations and tends to avoid confrontation.

Beyond the strength of each team role identified on Table 6.3, the team leader or the organisation can utilise the concept to gain practical benefits from each role for the organisation. For example, by adopting the 'implementer' role the individual member's asset is in the ability to plan workable strategies and carrying them out efficiently (Belbin Associates, 2020). For a member who adopts the 'shaper' role, for example, they tend to motivate the team and ensure that it

Table 6.3 Belbin's individual team roles

Individual team roles	Advantages of each team role	Workplace orientation
Co-ordinator:	Mature, confident, identifies talent. Promotes decision-making, delegates well. Clarifies goals.	
Teamworker:	Co-operative, perceptive and diplomatic. Listens, builds and averts friction.	**People-Orientated Roles**
Resource investigator:	Outgoing, communicative, enthusiastic. Explores opportunities and develops contacts.	
Plant:	Creative, imaginative, free-thinking, generates ideas and solves difficult problems.	
Monitor/evaluator:	Sober, strategic and discerning. Sees all options and judges accurately.	**Thinking-Orientated Roles**
Specialist:	Single-minded, self-starting and dedicated. They provide specialist knowledge and skills.	
Shaper:	Challenging, dynamic, thrives on pressure. Has the drive and courage to overcome obstacles.	
Implementer:	Practical, reliable, efficient. Turns ideas into actions and organises work that needs to be done.	**Action-Orientated Roles**
Completer/finisher:	Painstaking, conscientious, anxious. Searches out errors and omissions. Polishes, perfects and delivers on time.	

remains focused and has momentum for progress. For a member who adopts the 'completer finisher' role, they could be more effectively used at the end of tasks to scrutinise and refine the work, with a view to achievement of quality assurance.

However, it is noteworthy that not many teams have exactly nine members to adopt each of the roles, which implies some members might take on two roles, or certain team roles just don't get taken up by anyone. Furthermore, in bigger teams, if nine individuals self-profile themselves in one or another role, then some members who are additional to the nine could conveniently marginalise themselves and contribute less. There is also the likelihood of 'role expectation' in that when a team member takes on a role, they may subsequently be expected to fulfil that role(s) for the team again and again.

In addition, research on Belbin's team roles identify both strengths and weaknesses of the model. For example, Aritzeta et al.'s (2007) study identified that in addition to the benefits of the role that each team member adopts, individuals' interaction with other team members can drift into conflict situations between team members, and also in attempts at gaining and exercising power and control. Power, as it relates to control, influence and authority can be subdivided into various cognate areas as identified in Table 3.2.

> ### ACTION POINT 6.2
> ### Individual team roles in your team
>
> As an activity that needs to be performed individually without any discussion, take a moment to see if you can identify individuals in your team who tend to take one or more than one of Belbin's nine team roles identified in Table 6.3. Think also about which team role(s) you tend to assume within the team; and other ones you would like to adopt. Is there any of the team roles not covered by team members?

So, back to the team itself, healthcare teams may be those covering a particular clinical specialist area, or a team of healthcare professionals in a medium-sized GP practice, etc. Healthcare teams could also be broadly classified as care delivery teams, management teams, project teams, estates team, etc. Alternatively, according to the WHO (2012), healthcare teams can be grouped as:

Core teams – consist of team leaders and members who are directly involved in caring for patients, e.g. direct care providers which include nurses, doctors, physiotherapists, etc.

Co-ordinating teams – with responsibility for day-to-day operational management, co-ordination functions and resource management for the above-mentioned core teams.

Contingency teams – with members derived from a variety of core teams and are formed for emergent or specific events, e.g. cardiac arrest teams, disaster management, etc.

Ancillary services teams – comprises individuals not involved in direct patient care such as cleaners, catering staff, electrician, etc. who provide task-specific, often time-limited support services that ultimately facilitate patient care.

Administration teams – consist of the healthcare provider's or unit's top management team along with their support staff, e.g. accountant, medical centre administrator, etc. with responsibility for the overall functioning of the organisation, and monitoring targets imposed by financers (e.g. by the DHSC).

Team Leadership

Inherent within the FHM's roles and duties is team leadership. Effective team leadership is essential to ensure that the team continuously achieves its collective vision. Working in teams has been promoted for at least a century since the Hawthorne experiments in the 1920s (explained in Chapter 4 of this book and later under staff motivation), and implemented widely. Furthermore, the team leader needs to be aware of and allow scope for Tuckman's group processes to develop so that the team can reach the 'Performing' stage and operate more fully as a team.

Additionally, effective team leaders support the achievement of optimal performance by their team members and provide guidance and mentoring as required. Team leadership also entails the FHM as team leader having the skills and knowledge to motivate their staff, which is examined in some detail later in this chapter.

Furthermore, healthcare teams are nonetheless increasingly adopting collective or shared leadership, with the manager's power being de-emphasised, and frontline managers sharing leadership responsibilities, and final decisions being vested with the team. In a systematic review of models of teamwork and team leadership, Chin (2015) distinguished between traditional (usually top-down) and horizontal style (akin to collective or shared leadership) of leadership, and found that shared team leadership is increasingly favoured, and organisations are more receptive to inputs from team members and include them extensively in decision-making processes. Healthcare leadership is explored in extensive detail in Chapter 3 of this book.

Nonetheless, it cannot be assumed that all NRHPs already possess the capability to fulfil their role as team leaders, despite structured opportunities to learn the role during their pre-qualifying programmes. Consequently, they need to be supported to develop their leadership skills, as also concluded in research conducted by Ekstrom and Idvall (2015).

The nine-dimension *Healthcare Leadership Model* (NHS Leadership Academy, 2021) cited in Chapter 3 focuses on individuals' leadership activities, including teamworking. For effective teamworking, the dimensions include 'engaging the team', which involves acknowledging and applying the knowledge and expertise that each discipline contributes for the benefit of all. By engaging the team:

> Leaders [e.g. the FHM] promote teamwork and a feeling of pride by valuing individuals' contributions and ideas; this creates an atmosphere of staff engagement where desirable behaviours, such as mutual respect, compassionate care and attention to detail, are reinforced by all team members. (2021: 10)

As the co-ordinator of care across disciplines, the FHM needs to have a good level of understanding of the roles and functions of each discipline, as well as being fully acquainted with the mechanisms (e.g. forms to complete) to make referrals and transfers to them.

Team Communication

As noted earlier in this section, an essential ingredient for teamwork to succeed is comprehensive and open team communication. Effective team communication is fundamental to comprehensive person-centred care, to ensure patient safety through adhering to policies and guidelines, and achievement of patient outcomes and team goals successfully and efficiently (see analysis of effective communication in Chapter 4 of this book). Conversely, as Gluyas (2015) notes, ineffective communication tends to lead to poor co-operation and co-ordination of care, which results in suboptimal outcomes and adverse events in surgical procedures such as wrong patient, wrong procedure and/or site, retained instruments and infections. Elsewhere, it can compound delayed response to deteriorating patients, etc. Poor communication has also been identified as the cause of about a third of complaints received about acute NHS services (Parliamentary and Health Service Ombudsman, 2015).

Furthermore, for written communication via record-keeping, on and off each inter-disciplinary team enters a brief summary of their interventions and recommendations in the service user's main care pathway or medical files, and then tends to maintain their own patient records by discipline. This essentially is duplication of work and not conducive to teamwork, but it can be rectified by electronic integrated record-keeping systems where a comprehensive account of all interventions can be accessed quickly by different departments of the healthcare provider.

For a structured way of communicating, say at handover reports, see analysis of the SBAR tool in Chapter 2 of this book.

Conducting Team Meetings in Care Settings

As in many other organisations, in healthcare, team meetings are essential to ensure time is set aside for effective communication within inter-disciplinary teams. Meetings can be either formal and fully structured with timed agenda, closed membership and a chairperson, or they can be more informal between individuals or very small groups, which is also known as unscheduled meetings, the purpose of which is to seek or impart information or views. The characteristics of most formal meetings are that they are scheduled beforehand with date, time, venue and agenda identified, members of the group are invited often by email, and asked to indicate if they will attend, and minutes of the previous meeting sent to them.

Newly qualified healthcare professionals will have had some experience of attending meetings during their pre-registration programmes. Everyone is familiar with the handover meeting at the beginning of the span of duty, which centres mostly on members of the team imparting information on patient progress and forthcoming interventions. Individuals may also have had experience of making short presentations at meeting while on practice placement.

Initially, FHMs will not be required to conduct such meetings, but they will likely be required to attend various types of meetings, some of which may be group decision-making meetings, say about a new medical device, or problem-solving meeting when an issue has emerged, or a presentation about an innovation or about new national or local policy. Following attendance at most meetings, FHMs are likely to follow up with certain actions.

Important pointers related to attending meetings are as follows:

- Ensure you have a very good idea about the reason(s) for the meeting.
- Read the minutes of the previous meeting, make notes of any points you wish to query or comment on.
- Read any document that is circulated prior to the meeting.
- Update your knowledge of any key topic area that will be discussed in detail at the meeting.
- Attend with an open mind, and adopt an open posture.
- Ensure members see the point you are making is relevant to the purpose of the meeting.
- If you have an opposite view to one being presented by an attendee, it might be useful to seek the chairperson's permission, so that you can argue your point of view more fully.
- Be aware that the chairperson may go around the table and ask each member their opinion, or ask each member to vote on an issue.
- Be amenable to any post meeting tasks you agreed to participate in, or any point you personally wish to follow up.
- Expect the chairperson to thank everyone present for their contribution at the meeting.

FHMs may be required to lead meetings soon enough, and therefore need a working knowledge of how to lead and manage effective meetings, to ensure everyone attending feels it was useful to attend, and because effectively conducted meetings can enhance the quality of team-working and team effectiveness. All meetings have to be managed carefully to ensure that they are productive and effective, and because of the amount of staff time in hours and minutes that they consume. Meetings that FHMs conduct include handover reports to colleagues, or for discussing patients as part of MDT meetings. So, to maximise the effects of meetings, vital principles that FHMs need to adhere to include:

Begin and finish the meeting on time.
Set a friendly and accepting tone to the meeting so that members can relax, and feel comfortable enough to ask for clarification and to comment.
Ask members to introduce themselves when new members are present.
Draw attention to the agenda, and inform of any guest who is present to provide information based on their particular area of expertise.
Attend to any matters arising when going through the minutes of the previous meeting.
State the progress made since the last meeting and impart information on matters noted in the minutes of the previous meeting.

Ensure all members engage with the purpose of the meeting.

Keep attendees focused on the agenda item being addressed, and verbally sign-post progress.

Ensure strong opposite views are discussed openly and adequately.

Maintain a positive tone throughout.

Prevent any individual member attempting to dominate the meeting.

Restate the key points covered, and the actions to be taken in anticipation of the next meeting.

State the date and time of next meeting.

A more detailed analysis on how to conduct or lead meetings effectively, including involving members, time-keeping, etc., is provided in Harrington's (2019) article, full details of which are provided in the Further Reading section at the end of this chapter. Note, though, that especially after the coronavirus pandemic in 2020, various alternative ways to face-to-face attendance at/or conducting meetings surfaced, both work-related meetings and family meetings. The new methods entailed using videos on computers and mobile phones, examples of software used include Zoom, Microsoft Teams, Big Blue Button, and even WhatsApp and FaceTime on mobile phones.

Team Motivation at Work

One of the more subtle dimensions of the FHM's duties, both as manager and leader, is to ensure that each staff member in the care setting is highly motivated in their job, about the specialism, and in the enhancement of their profession. People are motivated to act to satisfy a personal need, e.g. need to earn money, for self-advancement, for recognition of their actions and re-inforcement, etc. Staff motivation is also instigated to meet these needs, which they do by acquiring employment, and which FHMs meet by acknowledgement and recognition of the individual staff member's contribution in daily duties, and by supporting any scope for further learning that avails itself.

In essence, a highly motivated team member is one who is completely enthusiastic about their job, about the evolving knowledge base and competence required to perform their duties, which they do to the highest standard possible with the resources available to them. The word motivate, according to dictionaries, means to provide with a motive, or a cause or reason to act, to incite, or to impel a specific behaviour. The behaviour might be for someone to start on a weight-loss diet, for a healthcare professional to examine the evidence base for a specific intervention, or to move to work as a healthcare professional in another country.

In the context of weight loss for example, following their qualitative research on motivation for lifestyle change among people with newly diagnosed type two diabetes mellitus, Sebire et al. (2018) identified intrinsic and external motivation (discussed under Herzberg's theory shortly), amotivation (absence of motivation for lifestyle change in this instance) and integrated motivation whereupon practical steps such as diet and exercise are combined with the person's values and broader personal goals. The approaches that healthcare professionals can take to motivate service users to manage their health issues are not addressed in this textbook.

Various work psychologists and behavioural psychologists have endeavoured to define the term motivation, but like many other human behaviours, there is no agreed definition. Work psychologists Arnold et al. (2020: 462) indicate, however, that motivation refers to the factors that determine the 'effort, direction and persistence of a person's behaviour'. Direction refers to the specific action or behaviour that the person is taking or displaying; effort is the intensity with which the behaviour is exhibited; and persistence is the duration of time that the person engages in that behaviour.

For example, motivation to attend a gymnasium regularly, or for someone unemployed to find a job is determined by all three factors: effort to set out to attend the gym or jobcentre; direction means the actions the individual takes to acquire a job (including looking at job advertisements in newspapers, sending their curriculum vitae to potential employers, etc.); and persistence suggests that the activity will not be a one-off or ad hoc, but continue until the goal is achieved.

In relation to staff motivation, on examining why a workforce needs to be highly motivated, *The Times* newspaper reporter Brown (1998) concluded that national productivity and business efficiency could be raised markedly if what was already known about motivation was implemented. For example, ensuring job satisfaction (see Chapter 5) can motivate staff, and thereby increase productivity by 25%, adds Brown (1998: 2), who also quotes a very successful frontline car manufacturing manager saying, 'If you make people accountable as the drivers of the business rather than bit-part players, you have a direct impact on their motivation'.

Conversely, an unmotivated workforce comprises employees who are likely to spend little or no effort in their jobs, avoid the workplace if they can and will leave the organisation if they can secure a job at another organisation with similar pay. On the other hand, making team members the 'drivers of the business' (noted above) is consistent with the prevailing belief and increasing practice of collective leadership (e.g. King's Fund, 2016b), whereupon all team members feel actively involved in enhancing the quality of care in the care setting or the organisation, as noted in Chapters 1 and 3. See Figure 6.2 which summarises the basis for a highly motivated worker and the outcome.

These general principles of motivation apply quite widely, such as motivation to attend fitness classes (a social need and aesthetic need), motivation for obese people to eat excessively more than the daily fuel they need, or to learn to drive a car.

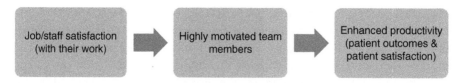

Figure 6.2   Precedent and outcome of a highly motivated team member

Effectiveness as a team requires team members not only to be highly knowledgeable and competent, but also to be highly motivated to work. There are several ways of motivating staff. One of the ten managerial roles identified in Chapter 4 (see Table 4.1) is 'resource manager' which encompasses frontline managers identifying ways of motivating their staff, i.e. their human resource, in their day-to-day work. Drucker (2007: 6) includes motivating staff as one of the five 'basic operations' of management to ensure organisational goals are achieved.

Managers are postholders who have been given responsibility for specific organisational goals identified in the organisation's operational plans. Consequently, they decide on work activities that need to be performed, and suitably motivated personnel to perform them.

ACTION POINT 6.3
Motivating healthcare professionals at work

In your roles as a healthcare professional and as a frontline manager, reflect on the following questions, and think of as many answers as you can, allowing two minutes for each question:

- What motivates me to work as a healthcare professional?
- What are the ways in which my line manager and my organisation ensure that I remain fully motivated to do my work?
- What actions do I take to motivate my team members?
- Are there any other actions that healthcare managers can take to motivate staff?

Hopefully, the questions in Action point 6.3 were easy to respond to, and useful to reflect on to comprehend staff motivation more fully. The factors that motivate employees at work can vary from individual to individual, but common elements include the main source of regular income, the need to have a job or stable vocation, the personal satisfaction gained from helping service users recover from ill-health, etc.

Motivation towards any activity or towards adopting a certain behaviour can be impelled by either intrinsic or extrinsic factors. *Intrinsic* motivation is generated by factors such as feelings and thinking within the individual; *extrinsic* motivation is instigated by external factors such as rewards. The extrinsic factors that direct employees to perform their work are salaries, a job title, socialisation, etc., but intrinsic factors include the satisfaction an individual gains from performing their duties such as helping people recover from health problems, learning new intervention skills and gaining healthcare knowledge, etc.

As frontline managers, FHMs can choose from a number of ways to motivate juniors and other team members at work, many of which can also be applied by the healthcare organisation itself to motivate employees. Ways of motivating staff include:

- ensuring each team member is aware that they are valued and appreciated for the work they do;
- communicating comprehensively by sharing information and involving team members in decision-making;
- openly recognising high standards of care achieved, e.g. reduced incidence of pressure injuries, etc.;
- applying transformational leadership and listening to team members' ideas;
- supporting a learning atmosphere;
- giving responsibility and allowing the use of own initiative;
- being approachable and accessible.

Theories of staff motivation that FHMs can apply at work

Various approaches or theories on how to motivate individual team members and the team as a whole at work are available to choose from, and which care managers apply on a day-to-day basis in order to ensure high-quality care is delivered all the time. This section focuses on specific ways of engendering and maintaining staff motivation at work in the context of published theories and techniques related to staff motivation. It therefore, in particular, examines Drucker's 'management-by-objectives' theory, Herzberg's theory of job motivators and motivation maintenance factors, Maslow's needs-satisfaction approach to human motivation and McGregor's theory X and theory Y. A combination of components of these theories can be applied by FHMs as and when they feel it will be useful to do so.

Management by objectives

Drucker's (2007) management by objectives (MBO) is one of the well-recognised theories of staff motivation, one that enables the employee to contribute to achievement of the organisation's objectives by achieving their own annual objectives, as agreed at their IDPR (staff appraisal). This is because MBO directly links the organisation's goals (corporate mission, aims and objectives) to each individual employee's expectations of the job and objectives at work, and achievement (Herzberg, 2003) is a motivator. IDPR was examined in some detail in Chapters 2 and 4 of this book.

Herzberg's motivators and maintenance factors

Founded largely on employees' satisfaction with components and aspects of their work, and dissatisfaction with other aspects, Herzberg (2003) formulated a theory of motivation back in the 1980s that has been widely accepted, but also provoked discussion. Herzberg's theory of motivation at work is based on findings of previous research conducted before his time, followed by those of his own. It builds on the findings of the Hawthorne experiments conducted in the earlier part of the 1920s and 1930s, the conclusions of which indicated that productivity increases if individuals have stability in their workplace, the purpose of the work is communicated to them adequately, and is a place where they work in collaboration with other people, as well as one where they feel they belong.

Herzberg conducted his own research interviews to explore workers' positive and negative feelings about their jobs that they experienced through events that occurred in the workplace. He concluded that in addition to providing the salaries and good working conditions, employees simultaneously prefer work that is challenging, work which gives them responsibility and a sense of achievement and advancement.

Consequently, Herzberg identified two sets of factors that influence workers' motivation to work. Both sets of factors have to be present for workers to be optimally motivated in their work. The first set of factors are 'motivators or growth factors' which 'intrinsically' motivate employees, and comprise: recognition of the work done, a sense of achievement, having responsibility and opportunities for learning, and thereby personal growth. In addition to these intrinsic motivators, the second set of factors are 'extrinsic' to the individual, referred to as 'maintenance factors', 'hygiene factors' or 'dissatisfaction-avoidance factors'.

'Maintenance factors' comprises the environment and context in which employees work, and are therefore extrinsic to the individual, which Herzberg concluded are as important as motivators (see Table 6.4 for details).

The FHM's role very much includes awareness of motivators and maintenance factors that have been identified by Herzberg, factors that endure over time and across organisations. Furthermore, research conducted by Toode et al. (2015) concluded that the majority of hospital nurses have strong intrinsic motivation towards their work because thereby they gain recognition that their own values and goals are the same as those of the organisation and of society in general. Other motivating factors include opportunities for growth through further

Table 6.4   Herzberg's motivators and maintenance factors

Motivators (intrinsic factors)	Maintenance factors (extrinsic factors)
• Recognition of work done	• Company policies and administration
• A sense of achievement	• Job status and security
• Having responsibility	• The level of supervision
• Opportunities for learning and personal growth	• Doing whole jobs rather than parts of them as tasks
• The process of actually doing of the work	• Relationship with supervisor and with peers
	• Working conditions
	• Adequate salary

learning, empowerment in the workplace, which are also motivators identified by Herzberg.

Needs-satisfaction approach to human motivation

Along parallel lines to Herzberg's motivators such as recognition, advancement, etc., Maslow's (1987) human needs-based theory also comprises a theory of motivation, which incorporates aspects of human relations approach to management. Maslow's theory is based upon the assumption that a wide range of actions that individuals are motivated to take, are taken to meet their own specific basic human needs, upon which the well-known hierarchy of physiological, social and psychological needs was formulated.

The hierarchy of needs theory postulates that individuals take action to meet the more basic physiological needs of food, water, etc., just to survive and thrive in the first place. When physiological needs have been satisfied, then their next priority in life is safety needs (e.g. a house or flat of their own to shelter from potentially harmful weather conditions). Subsequent priorities are social needs, esteem needs and finally their self-actualisation needs.

To meet one's physiological and safety needs, adults are motivated to gain employment with an employer or organisation so that with the salary they are provided they can buy food, and either pay rent or buy a house. Social needs can also be met through employment as individuals make friends through work, etc. Motivation to meet the higher psychological or intellectual needs and goals come afterwards. However, Maslow suggested that if the self-actualisation or self-realisation needs of the individual are not satisfied, then problems of frustration, boredom and apathy tends to ensue.

Consequently, employing organisations and managers can enhance staff motivation by taking action to meet employees' basic and higher needs. Table 6.5 illustrates examples of ways in which these needs are met.

However, on occasions individuals knowingly jeopardise lower-level needs in the quest for higher-level needs of self-esteem and self-fulfilment, and therefore people's major needs centre around realising their full potential as individuals, via creative, worthwhile achievement.

Table 6.5 Applying Maslow's needs-satisfaction theory to staff motivation

Employees' needs	Organisational efforts
1 Physiological needs	• Employee has sufficient income to be able to pay for their food, accommodation, etc. • Refreshment breaks during long spans of duty • Canteen facilities at work
2 Safety needs	• The organisation complies with health and safety regulations • Provision of an employment contract for employee's job security • Policies are instituted to ensure safety for all in the organisation
3 Social needs	• Mechanisms for working in cohesive teams • Supportive supervision by colleagues • Working as members of different sub-groups (non-competitive)
4 Esteem needs	• Being accepted within the team, and adopting the team culture • Reinforcement through recognition of effective practice and for using one's initiatives
5 Self-actualisation needs	• Ongoing development of care intervention skills • Being given scope for creativity • Formal and informal professional development strategies • Professional development plans (PDP) are supported • Career progression and advancement opportunities

Theory X or Theory Y Approach

As a theory of human motivation at work that is not directly based on empirical data (research), McGregor's (1987) theory is based on his observations of managers' practices towards their workers and his conversations with them as Head of institutes of management studies. He observed that management styles are dependent upon managers' attitudes and presumptions about workers in general, and managers consequently used theory X or theory Y. McGregor recommended theory Y as the better way of the two ways of motivating staff.

Theory Y represents a relatively realistic assumption that at work, in addition to the benefits of being in employment, individuals inherently also have a need for self-actualisation (a concept that had previously been suggested by Maslow, 1987) and personal growth. Consequently, managers who apply theory Y tend to believe that employees normally:

Have the capacity, and wish, to exercise a fair degree of self-direction and imagination at work.

Would like to use their ingenuity and creativity as their contribution to resolving organisational issues.

Do not only accept but also seek responsibility, and do not inherently dislike work.

Do commit themselves to contribute to the achievement of organisational aims and objectives.

Readily learn new skills and knowledge, which they hope to be rewarded for under the appropriate conditions.

Only partially use their individual intellectual abilities.

Managers who employ theory Y as their managerial strategy also recognise and support opportunities for personal growth and development of employees as they arise, because they view their employees as resources (referred to as 'assets' by Handy, 1985) with potential for enabling the organisation to enhance its activities. This style of management is dynamic, and is seen as an optimistic view of workers.

Managers who apply McGregor's theory X take the opposite (more pessimistic) approach in their style of management, in the managerial decisions they make and the actions they take. They tend to believe that the average human being's – and therefore employee's – interest in work is limited, and they will avoid work if they can. People tend to avoid responsibility, prefer to be directed at work and have relatively little ambition according to theory X. Consequently, managers utilising theory X believe workers expect and have to be coerced, controlled, directed and threatened with punishment if necessary, to motivate them to perform their duties, and do so effectively.

Clearly, categorising employees under theory X and theory Y is also related to whether the job requires narrowed-down repetitive tasks, or whether the post is based on academic qualifications and is therefore a post with scope for learning. However, it can also be concluded that managing staff based on the two groups of assumptions about workers amounts to a rigid dichotomy, and can lead to ineffective organisational performance, and therefore management education for all managers including FHMs would be highly recommended.

In addition to the four main theories and assumptions just discussed there are other theories of motivation that have been suggested. Social learning theory (research-based), for example, argues that much of our learning in general is triggered by our interaction with other people, direct interaction or indirect via television or electronic devices. Some of these interactions are inspirational and motivate the person to learn new skills, e.g. to learn to play a musical instrument, or a sport, which if rewarded by approval by other people (social re-inforcement) or by material gains motivates the person to continue developing that skill. Drive-reduction theory of motivation is another (not discussed).

Monitoring Team Performance

The attributes that are essential for effective inter-disciplinary teamwork were discussed earlier in this chapter, including good communication within the team, team leadership, etc. From their literature review of team effectiveness, Valentine et al. (2015) concluded that most team performance surveys address communication, co-ordination, respect and use of members' expertise. Consequently, team performance is a concept in its own right that focuses on how effectively or successfully the team is achieving its goals, day in and day out. The NMC (2018b, clause 5.3) indicates that RNs must 'understand the principles and application of processes for performance management and how these apply to the nursing team'.

Team performance is generally assessed using agreed metrics on falls, post-operative infection rates, etc., and FHMs can decide which metrics are appropriate for their own care settings. Team effectiveness tools are generally not designed specifically for care settings, and therefore each specialist can add specific patient outcome measures (for example, patients being pain free, absence of falls [related to patient safety], reduction in post-operative complications or in medication errors, level of motor function among stroke rehabilitation patients, seamless transfer of care, quality of life [in community patients], etc.) to available tools.

Thus, team performance impacts on patient outcomes, which when assessed at hospital level include mortality rates, re-admissions, patient experience, length of stay, etc. However, FHMs have to ensure they are fully familiar with both the

---

ACTION POINT 6.4
Team performance in your care setting

Think about your nursing, midwifery or inter-disciplinary team in your workplace, and consider:

- How effective is your team's performance based on the items or attributes identified by Emerald Works (2020) (Available at: www.mindtools.com/pages/article/newTMM_84.htm)? Base your response on any statistics or audits records that are accessible to you.
- What strategies, both formal and informal, are used to provide both the whole team and individual members with feedback?

healthcare provider's mission statement, and the department's/specialist area's, so that the criteria used can be aligned accordingly. However, the organisation's or care setting-level team's mission statement, which articulates their values and shared purpose, must be reviewed periodically to ensure they are current and acceptable to all team members.

The information that you were asked to consider in the above Action point is not usually easily available, and it requires time being put aside to peruse them. It may, however, provoke further exploration by team members asking the same questions together, and exploring ways of further enhancing teamwork and max-imising outcomes in your care setting.

Effective team functioning needs to be monitored by frontline managers, who are also in a good position to detect any potential or actual lapses in cohesive teamworking. Ensuring supportive and amiable social interaction, harmonious working relationships, maintaining high morale, supported by dynamic distribu-tion of Belbin's team roles, along with well-established collective leadership, can contribute to high team performance.

To conclude this section on team performance, it is noteworthy that the team leader's role is crucial in constructing and maintaining effective teams, which includes understanding of team formation (as suggested by Tuckman), and the role of team building executed through a gamut of team activities. Even the lan-guage used by team members can provide insight into team cohesiveness, in that language such as 'we' and 'us', as opposed to 'I' and 'me', for example, suggests belongingness to the team and a more relaxed outlook.

Dysfunctional Teams and Team Learning

Team leadership and team members always have to demonstrate a commitment to effective, efficient, high-quality care, and willing co-operation within uni- and inter-disciplinary teams. Teamworking is a dynamic process, and although Tuck-man suggested a linear development of groups to teams, Whitehair et al. (2018) suggest that teams can prosper or deteriorate, and therefore need sensitive leader-ship to ensure the team remains functional and healthy.

However, not all teams are equally effective, and even effective teams may not be so all of the time as teamwork issues could surface. Instances of when team-work fails markedly and at times become headline news, include the BBC One *Panorama* (2019) programme related to abuse of people with a learning disability, as noted in Chapter 1 of this book. Deficient leadership and disjointed ineffective teams were identified as contributory causes of the malpractice.

Even more recently, following reports of hundreds of baby deaths at a West Midlands hospital (ITV News, 2020), an interim report identified a dispro-portionately high rate of maternal deaths at the unit, mothers were not risk-assessed properly, at times women were blamed for the death of their baby, staff incompetence, lack of kindness and compassion from some members of the maternity team, etc. They also found that serious incidents were not investigated fully, and consequently there was a lack of record of learning from these incidents and subsequently several recommendations were made for maternity care across the whole country. All these factors reflect instances of poor leadership and dysfunctional teamwork.

Nonetheless, while acknowledging collaboration across disciplines in the care of service users with type 2 Diabetes Mellitus, McDonald et al. (2012)'s research found that professionals from different disciplines make conscious efforts to collaborate with other disciplines. Doctors often assume responsibilities for coordinating the necessary interventions required by service users, but when collaboration is sub-optimal then care interventions can also be delayed or of lesser quality.

Functional inter-disciplinary working is particularly important when the patient journey spans acute hospitals and community care (i.e. different organisations) and shared decision-making in order to ensure a seamless service. To remedy this issue and have in place a more functional inter-disciplinary team, McDonald et al. (2012) recommend that strategies should be instituted to develop trust and respect between disciplines and thereby better interprofessional relationships, and establishing agreed rules that can enhance the efficacy of collaborative care.

Furthermore, barriers such as within-team conflict can hinder teamwork. When conflict occurs but different parties involved are unwilling to collaborate, as noted by Ellis and Abbott (2011), then the team's performance diminishes (conflict management is examined in detail in Chapter 7 of this book). Consequently, knowledge of the processes of team development is important in the formation of effective teams, as is the development of team roles (Belbin Associates, 2020) if they occur spontaneously, and collective leadership.

However, incidence of unforeseen events is a reality of care settings as individual patients' conditions change and new service users arrive. Learning from unforeseen events is an inherent component of teamworking. Additionally, interdisciplinary learning is reinforced by the NMC (2018d: 5) who states that in practice settings there must be a 'learning culture that is ethical, open and honest, and is conducive to safe and effective learning ... [and] inter-professional learning and team working should be embedded in the learning culture'. Previously, the World Health Organization (2010) indicated that it supports the implementation of interprofessional education worldwide in order to foster successful collaborative teamwork.

Interprofessional education (IPE) refers to formally organised inter-disciplinary learning and a widely accepted definition states that IPE occurs when two or more professions learn, with or about each other, aiming to improve interprofessional collaboration and the quality of care (Centre for Advancement of Interprofessional Education, 2020). Research shows that IPE is beneficial, as for example it provides health profession students opportunities to understand the 'roles and responsibilities of other disciplines through IPE co-curricular learning [which] tends to enhance positive attitudes toward teamwork' (Mishoe et al., 2018: 1).

Effectiveness of team performance is often reflected in CQC inspection reports, and teams that are rated as 'requires improvement' or 'inadequate', have to take appropriate action to rectify weaknesses. Over the given time, when required improvements have been made, the organisation should recognise the team's achievement and reward them in some way. There should be some manner of written recognition that is formally documented and the teams directly thanked. If the team wishes to make an occasion of this and wishes to celebrate, the organisation should support this, even if it is verbally or quiescently.

Nonetheless, from their exploratory qualitative study of team processes used by nursing teams in a paediatric hospital unit, Whitehair et al. (2018) summarised that successful teamwork comprises:

1. Aligning and attuning each other's values.
2. Creating psychological safe spaces for relating with team members, with a shared sense of accountability and engagement.
3. Focus on continual monitoring of team performance and detecting signals of breakdown leading to acceptance of any deficiencies in fulfilling responsibilities.

Whether the CQC results are good or not so good, whether adverse events occur or not, effective team leadership with appropriate vision and role models can avert healthcare teams become dysfunctional, and instead proactively take action to enhance team functioning, team learning and team morale.

Guidance for Developing and Maintaining a Coherent and Effective Inter-Professional Team

Drawing on the examination of inter-disciplinary teamwork in healthcare settings in this chapter, the following guidance is directed at achieving effective and high performance teamwork:

Appreciate the substantial benefits of working as collaborative inter-disciplinary teams.

Allow ample time for the group of staff to proceed through the natural developmental stages of becoming a cohesive team.

Ensure team members have a good understanding of the organisation's overall mission statement and (short- and long-term) goals, and the ways in which their individual and the team's work objectives contribute to the achievement of those goals.

Appreciate and support when appropriate the development of different team roles by individual members of staff.

Provide effective team leadership, and ensure comprehensive team communication, which includes conducting team meetings.

Acquire detailed knowledge of staff motivation, especially some of the well-known theories of motivation.

Members and the team leader must strive for a mutually supportive relationship, and informally and formally evaluate team performance and progress with the team's objectives.

Ensure that individual service users are the focus of your team's activities and that they are involved in decision-making about their care and their health outcomes as much as possible.

Appreciate the symptoms of dysfunctional or ineffective teams, and ensure learning occurs from lapses in team cohesiveness.

Chapter Summary

Inter-disciplinary teamwork is absolutely critical in almost all areas in healthcare as healthcare professionals with in-depth expertise in different areas of health problems contribute to the restoration or maintenance of service users' health. Inter-disciplinary team members, therefore, input different areas of expertise to ensure timely intervention with high quality of care, and teams have to function cohesively and collaboratively, which is enabled by establishing good working relationships. Inter-disciplinary teams thereby contribute to the overarching objectives of the healthcare organisation, and FHMs' duties include co-ordinating the care delivery team. This chapter began by differentiating between groups of staff and teams, and delved into:

- An analysis of the nature of teams in healthcare, inter-disciplinary healthcare teams and their characteristics, and the differences between groups and teams;
- The reasons for teamwork in care settings and ways in which team performance can be maximised in healthcare;
- Different ways in which effective inter-disciplinary teams operate through team formation identifying team roles, team leadership in the context of inter-professional teams, team-wide communication, and ways of conducting team meetings effectively;
- Knowledge of teamwork and different approaches to teamwork, identifying models and benefits of teamwork, the characteristics of effective teams;
- Motivating staff at work through knowledge and understanding of different theories of motivation, and ways in which FHMs can apply them beneficially to inter-disciplinary teamwork; and

- Knowledge of different methods of evaluating and monitoring team performance, the challenges and issues related to teams that are dysfunctional or ineffective, and how they can improve and harness learning as a team.

Further Reading

- On how to chair and manage formal business meetings, the following article gives an overview of how to lead and manage meetings effectively, focusing on process, content, managing conflict and how to engage participants fully: Harrington A (2019) Chairing and managing formal workplace meetings: Skills for nurse leaders. *Nursing Management*, 26(5): 36–41.
- For extensive details of the SBAR communication tool, see: NHS Improvement (2018) *SBAR Communication Tool – Situation, Background, Assessment, Recommendation.* Available at: https://improvement.nhs.uk/resources/sbar-communication-tool/. Accessed Date: 6 July 2020.

7

Decision-Making, Problem-Solving and Conflict Management

Chapter Objectives

The chapter objectives for frontline healthcare managers related to decision-making, problem-solving and conflict management in healthcare are:

- Identify a range of day-to-day professional care decisions made by front-line healthcare professionals, and the significance and impact of these decisions;
- Clarify and differentiate between decision-making and problem-solving, and the multifarious macro- and micro-decisions made by healthcare professionals;
- Analyse various systematic ways of making decisions and solving problems individually and as a group, including probability analysis, root cause analysis and creativity in decision-making;
- Analyse the causes of interpersonal conflict in care settings, how they manifest themselves, and consequently the modes or styles of conflict resolution that can benefit the parties involved;
- Feel prepared to engage in opportunities to practise professional decision-making and problem-solving skills with a view to applying creativity and ensuring new learning.

Introduction

Effective management and leadership in healthcare can be based on the ten groups of duties of frontline healthcare managers stated on Table 4.1 (e.g. resource manager) in Chapter 4 and the different forms of leadership FHMs can choose from when making multiple day-to-day decisions throughout the shifts they are on. A range of decisions are made related to assessment and diagnosis of new patients' health problems, and on the range of interventions required to enable their recovery. The service user could be someone admitted to ICU with severe COPD, or one referred to mental health services for substance abuse-related psychosis and malnutrition, or a young person brought into the emergency department with stab wounds-related haemorrhage.

This chapter focuses on FHMs' day-to-day decision-making and problem-solving in care settings, and conflict management when they arise. It starts by identifying various day-to-day decisions that FHMs make, examines the nature of the concepts decision-making and problem-solving, different systematic approaches to making decisions, and solving problems systematically (including root cause analysis). The chapter then examines interpersonal conflict in care settings, how they manifest themselves and the ways in which they are resolved.

The Range of Care Decisions Made by Frontline Healthcare Professionals

A multitude of decisions are made by FHMs during any span of duty, and principally because they are made in care settings during working hours, they could all affect service users' health or their experience of the care received. Consequently, healthcare professionals are accountable for their decisions and for the effects of their decisions. If not in relation to service user care, the decisions might personally affect other members of staff, including care professionals who are involved in care and treatment.

The number of day-to-day decisions that frontline managers make depends on the volume of clinical activities that take place in the care setting, and the number of staff who are based in the setting.

No doubt Action point 7.1 will have reminded you of the many decisions that you make as a FHM during any span of duty, big and small decisions, some of which are made quickly, others needing more careful thought of the implications of the decision; and some made individually, others in consultation with other colleagues. Additionally, several personal decisions are made and maybe problems solved even before coming on duty from the point in time we wake up to the point when we arrive on duty; and several after finishing work.

ACTION POINT 7.1
Examples of specific decisions that frontline managers make

1. As the frontline manager, think of all the decisions you made with one hour of coming on duty, every single one of them, minor ones and major ones.
2. Then, consider all the decisions made over the course of a full span of duty, including delegating specific tasks, caring for the distressed relative of a service user, etc.
3. Allow at least five minutes for this part of the Action point and note all instances of decisions made on a plain sheet of paper, leaving a 5 cm margin on the right-hand side of the paper.
4. Now decide which of these decisions were in fact problems being solved and write 'PS' against them; then write 'DM' against those decisions that were not actual problems.

Examples of the professional decisions made over a particular shift or span of duty that were identified by care professionals studying on management modules include deciding on:

- which patients needs urgent attention;
- which patient/bay of patients to allocate to which team member(s);
- what to do about a HSW who hasn't arrived on duty at the expected time;
- which dressing to use on a wound that is not healing as anticipated;
- what to tell a relative regarding the condition of a deteriorating patient;
- whether to discharge a particular patient because the bed manager says a bed is urgently required;
- whether to agree with a 'Do not resuscitate' limitation on a particular patient;
- whether to have a word with a colleague who sounded abrupt with a student;
- how much time to spend with the new appointee starting on the day;
- whether or when to give more time to listen to a particular patient.

Action point 7.1 suggests that some of the situations involve making decisions while others constitute a problem that needs resolving and, therefore, that decision-making and problem-solving are different concepts. For example, which dressing to use is a decision that has to be made, but what to do about a member of staff who hasn't arrived on duty is a problem that needs attention; and some situations constitute a decision to be made to solve a problem.

The FHM's role as decision-maker and problem-solver is one of the ten management roles of frontline care managers identified in Figure 4.1 (Chapter 4), and similarly four of the ten key roles of managers identified by Mintzberg (2011) are grouped as 'decisional roles' (also noted in Chapter 4).

Decision-making is an activity that all health-social care professionals involved in care delivery engage in by sheer virtue of their contract of employment and their professional body's code of professional practice. For a more junior care professional, an example of decision-making could include when to report a patient observation to the doctor, for instance, and for a more senior care professional, this may involve deciding at which point to increase the dose of a particular patient's medication.

Differentiating between Decision-Making and Problem-Solving

To clarify exactly what the terms decision-making and problem-solving mean, these terms need to be defined and distinguished from each other, examples of the different types of decisions that are made in care settings identified, and also the subsidiary terms micro-, meso- and macro-decision/s explained.

Clarifying the terms decision-making and problem-solving

Inherent within the two terms decision-making and problem-solving are the two different words decision and problem. Yet, these terms are at times used interchangeably because decisions can be straightforward routine decisions, but when problems or issues surface, they also require decisions on ways of resolving them.

The concept problem-solving has a different meaning to decision-making in that in problem-solving obviously a difficult situation has occurred or is about to occur. According to the Cambridge Dictionary online (Cambridge University Press, 2021), a problem is a situation, a person or thing that needs attention and needs to be dealt with or solved. In healthcare, a problem can be seen as an event that has occurred or can potentially occur (e.g. a patient incident or a management proposal) that disrupts or feels threatening to the plans for the shift (or someone's comfort zone).

Decision-making, on the other hand, may involve forward planning without there being an actual problem to solve. It entails considering several components of the situation and finally choosing one specific course of action. It requires accessing and collecting all available information that are relevant before reaching a decision. An open mind is often needed in order to gain a complete view of the situation, considering the availability of evidence, previous experience and the use of professional judgement.

Conversely, problem-solving necessitates making decisions to solve a problem and, as became apparent in Action point 7.1, some activities encompass both notions. However, to distinguish between the two terms, problem-solving entails examining and identifying exactly what the problem is and its detrimental effects, while decision-making can either include a problem or it doesn't.

Furthermore, managerial decisions impact at both individual and organisational levels. That is, it has implications for both individual staff (and service user if involved) and the organisation which has to provide the resources for the decision to be carried out. For example, if a general practice decides to implement a programme of bespoke diets for its type 2 diabetes patients, then individually it will affect individual healthcare professionals' workload, and use up their time at work. At organisational levels, the practice will have to ensure that the staff running the programme are appropriately trained and skilled, and that they have the necessary depth of knowledge to do so.

Decision-making might involve deciding on actions to avert a problem, e.g. when a colleague telephones in sick, then a decision has to be made to avert a potential problem of staff shortage, which can be done by reviewing the workload and patient dependency levels for the shift to establish if cover is required, and maybe borrowing a staff member from another care team, thus ensuring patient safety. On the other hand, decision-making can be forward-looking to something new to be implemented resulting in one specific macro-decision (discussed next) and a number of crucial sub-decisions (that is micro-decisions).

Therefore, as implied above, there can be different types of decisions: routine decisions, adaptive decisions and innovative ones (see Table 7.1).

Table 7.1   Routine, adaptive and innovative decisions

Routine decisions	Applying established guidelines, protocols or policies to routine care and management activities, for example guidelines for performing a care intervention, or for providing a handover report, or invoking the disciplinary procedure. Are usually made by more junior managers as the actions they take are based on well-established, approved protocols.
Adaptive decisions	Made when the issue requiring a decision and the alternative solutions are only partly clear; for example, when a patient exhibits thinking disorder. Ways of dealing with similar previously encountered symptoms may be adapted, and their effects monitored continuously.
Innovative decisions	Made when a problematic situation emerges which is unusual or unprecedented, and creative novel solutions are required; for example, a sharp rise in obesity in children despite public health department's extensive efforts.

ACTION POINT 7.2
Types of decisions

Thinking about the list of decisions that you made in your responses to Action point 7.1, for a random selection of those decisions, identify which decisions were routine decisions, which were adaptive decisions and which were innovative. Then state why each of those decisions were either routine, adaptive or innovative.

Macro-, meso- and micro-decisions

Some of the decisions that clinical staff make requires consideration of numerous inherent factors, but others contain fewer factors to consider. For example, changing the dressing on a wound with reddened and visibly swollen edges require decisions related to several factors including whether taking a swab is advisable as the wound may be infected, which cleansing solution is most appropriate and which type of dressing, whether medical staff would like to see it for themselves before applying a new dressing, etc. However, simpler procedures such as observing a patient's vital signs (pulse, respiration, etc.) on an electronic monitor require fewer decisions.

Decisions that require consideration of several variables tend to be referred to as macro-decisions, while those that are less complex with fewer variables having to be considered in reaching the decision are meso-decisions. Other activities that are simply components of more involved decisions are known as micro-decisions. For example, when a dermatology nurse performs a skin biopsy, the decision about whether to perform the biopsy when they see the state of the patient's skin is the major or macro-decision, but the whole procedure comprises several sub- or micro-decisions. On the other hand, for a practice nurse giving an influenza vaccine to a vulnerable person, there are much fewer sub-decisions, i.e. meso-decisions involved.

Micro-, meso- and macro-decisions have different meanings in different subject areas such as in marketing, economics, space technology, etc. In care settings, meso-decisions refer to the less immediate factors that contribute to making micro- and macro-decisions. They are structural factors (that is the range and types of mechanisms or facilities) that are available to determine the decision, as well as cultural and environmental factors that could be considered such as taking the patient's preferences into account, or the doctor's, or the FHM's.

Many of these micro-decisions are made in seconds in the course of the care intervention. Macro-decisions tend to involve and affect more people, and take longer to complete.

A further example of a macro-decision that involves several micro-decisions is the administration of an intravenous bolus of antibiotics. Gopee and Galloway (2017) identify a number of these micro-decisions, which are akin to reflection-in-action (see Glossary), and which entail continuous thinking about every single action being taken, in conjunction with justifiable rationales for them, and any associated evidence base. Figure 7.1 here illustrates the bare minimum of micro-decisions that an onlooker would make when witnessing a collapsed adult. It doesn't intend to present a complete or exhaustive list of actions, but does provide an inkling into the range of micro-decisions involved in one macro-decision.

The steps and decisions shown on Figure 7.1 are not substitutes for the full guidelines for the procedure when encountering a collapsed individual, as it is intended to merely illustrate the multiple micro-decisions involved in the intervention that a healthcare professional or appropriately trained observer could take

A collapsed adult

Is it safe for you to approach – **If no** > Do not touch the individual, shout for help
If yes

Do you feel competent to intervene? – **If no** > Dial 2222 (in hospital)/999 for immediate help
If yes

Say hello. Ask: Are you alright? If the individual can talk, ask what happened and if in pain
If no

Start systematically assessing for ABCDE (airway, breathing, circulation, disability, exposure). Is the individual breathing? – **If yes** > Record respiratory rate
If no

Can you hear noisy breathing (gurgling)? – **If yes** > Is there an obstruction in the mouth – **If yes** > Remove the obstruction if possible. Are there signs of facial swelling – **If yes** > Consider anaphylaxis, call for an ambulance/help/resuscitation team and ask the individual if they have an auto-injector (Adrenaline)? > **If yes** > Administer Adrenaline into the individual's thigh
If no

Are there signs of life? Can you feel the individual's pulse (central pulse, e.g. at carotid artery)? – **If yes** > Consider the recovery position and await expert help; avoid moving the individual if spinal injury suspected
If no

Lay individual on flat surface, commence chest compressions (place heel of one hand with the other hand directly over the first hand in the centre of sternum and proceed with a ratio of 30 compressions followed by 2 rescue breaths). Continue until either there are signs of life or expert help arrives

Are there any signs of life? – **If yes** > Confirm which signs of life (breathing and pulse) but avoid moving the individual
If no

Continue CPR until signs of life or emergency help arrives, and handover to team.

Figure 7.1   Micro-decisions related to witnessing a collapsed adult

when encountering such as event. For fuller and more precise details of the process of cardiopulmonary resuscitation check your healthcare organisation's clinical guidelines or the national guidelines in *2021 Resuscitation Guidelines* (Resuscitation Council UK, 2021). Further guidelines for clinical interventions are available from, for example, *The Royal Marsden Manual of Clinical Nursing Procedures* (Lister et al., 2020).

Micro-decisions are, therefore, the smaller or sub-decisions that need to be made as part of the bigger decision. So, the healthcare professional deciding whether it is safe to approach the situation (first step in Figure 7.1) may be the first micro-decision they make, as are each of the other items on the algorithm. The decision about whether to actually help the collapsed person is the macro-decision.

Making Decisions Systematically

There are a number of facets to decision-making that need to be considered in relation to ways of making decisions. They include probability of the decision achieving the intended goal, different approaches to decision-making, whether decisions should be based on established knowledge or on intuition, group decision-making and creativity in decision-making.

Probability analysis of alternative decisions

Several organisations have moved on to flatter management structures (noted in Chapter 4), which entails having fewer levels of managers and more decision-making being devolved to the more junior team members. Decision-making in clinical practice, however, is a complex process, and poor decision-making in healthcare results in harm to service users and even death, according an integrative literature review by Nibbelink and Brewer (2018). Complexity of decision-making increases with technological advances, but Nibbelink and Brewer also found that experienced nurses are less likely to make poor decisions as their decisions are enhanced by their self-confidence and intuition based on several years of professional practice. Nonetheless, although several decisions are made with the expectation of a high degree of certainty of achieving the anticipated outcomes, there is almost always some risk of the outcome not being achieved (see Figure 7.2).

Routine decisions (identified in Figure 7.2) made by healthcare professionals usually comprise 'high certainty' of being the correct decisions, and 'low risk' of being incorrect. For example, if a patient is diagnosed with exacerbation of asthma, then a relatively routine decision could be made to instruct the patient to use a specific inhaler in the expectation that it will make breathing much easier. However, despite research evidence, there is no guarantee that this outcome will be achieved because various factors could lessen the effect of the inhaler.

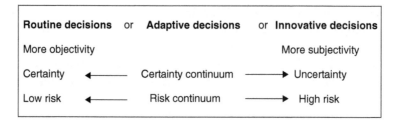

Figure 7.2   Routine, adaptive and innovative decisions – certainty and risks

Adaptive decisions, on the other hand, involve moderate degrees of certainty and risk of the decision being the wrong one. Innovative decisions can involve high uncertainty and high risk, especially because the innovation might not have been empirically rigorously tested. The degree of certainty of outcomes of decisions achieving the anticipated goal is referred to as 'decision based on probability'. Decisions based on quantitative research can be referred to as having 'objective probability', and therefore more likely to be the right decisions; and those not based on research as having 'subjective probability' because they would have been based on individual personal judgement.

Thus, in situations where decisions involve more objective probabilities, as in routine decisions, there is more certainty of the right decision being made, but where they are made with subjective probabilities, as in innovative or adaptive decisions, there would be less certainty. Decisions made under conditions of uncertainty are those for which the consequences and risks are less well known.

Alternative approaches to decision-making

There are further different types of decisions made in care settings, in addition to those discussed above, and include:

Rational or logical decision-making
Clinical decision-making
Informed or shared decision-making
Limited control decisions
Delayed action decisions
Provisional decisions
Optimum decision-making approach
Pessimistic approach
Political decision-making model
Ethical decision-making

In all decision-making situations, it is assumed that the decision-maker examines all inherent perspectives of the issue or decision topic, and then thinks about the different alternative decisions and the consequences of each before choosing which decision will be actioned. This logical decision-making approach is at times referred to as 'rational decision-making', and as 'classical decision theory' by Buchanan and Huczynski (2019).

For clinical decision-making which involves making decisions related to clinical interventions, making decisions with regards to a patient's journey through healthcare are at times made at a broader level, away from the care setting, and it can involve consideration of monetary costs or cost-effectiveness, in conjunction with any prevailing national guidelines.

As for informed decision-making, this involves decision-making that affords the service user a very good degree of information and, therefore, control over the treatment they receive, taking into consideration the known associated degree of harm from adverse effects from a procedure or medication, which are weighed against the evidence of benefit for each individual and their overall prognosis. It is also often referred to as shared decision-making.

On the other hand, there are situations when all information required for making a decision is not available and, therefore, the decision is based on deficient information, which is sometimes referred to as 'limited control decisions'. At other times, decisions about a specific issue can be either postponed for a little while, or the decision is made to take action at a later point in time (delayed action decision), such as whether to perform an operation on a patient while awaiting pathology results.

Sometimes 'provisional decisions' are made; that is, a decision for which the action to be taken is contingent upon certain prerequisites, such as which team members can have the day off on Christmas Day, the prerequisite being, for example, that staff numbers and mix as well as services are unchanged.

'Optimum decision-making' is yet another perspective, which constitutes making a decision which will result in the best possible outcome for all parties involved. Conversely, a 'pessimistic approach' can be taken whereby the worst possible outcomes for each alternative decision are compared and the least objectionable one is chosen. For example, if an older person is being discharged from hospital and wants to go back to their own flat but healthcare professionals fear she is likely to fall and hurt herself; and when other alternatives are to go and live with her daughter's family or in a nursing home, but she objects to both, she might decide going to live with her daughter's family as a less objectionable alternative.

'Political decision-making' is yet another approach, whereby individuals decide to support certain decisions because of who in the group suggested it, rather than taking the 'classical' approach noted earlier on. Finally, yet another dimension in decision-making is *ethical* decision-making, in which the basic principles of ethics have to be fully considered by the decision-maker. The principles of ethics identified by the British Association for Counselling and Psychotherapy (BACP)

(2018) are worded as the core principles of ethical responsibilities, which are: being trustworthy, autonomy, beneficence, non-maleficence, justice and self-respect.

Briefly, they signify:

Being trustworthy: The practitioner can be trusted to tell the truth, and not deceive

Autonomy: Respects the service user's right to choose

Beneficence: Commitment to promote service users' health and wellbeing

Non-maleficence: Commitment to avoid doing any harm to the service user

Justice: Fair and impartial treatment of all service users and in the provision of required services

Self-respect: Practitioner's self-knowledge and integrity enables respect for own values and beliefs and the service user's.

For decision-making in the above-mentioned circumstances, the service user's personal choice, the impact of the decision on others, achievement of national policy/targets and so on must also be considered within the decision-making process. As for research on decision-making, from their relatively extensive research on clinical decision-making by nursing students, Phillips et al. (2021) indicate that students felt that with support from their practice-learning supervisor, they realised that they had more clinical knowledge than they thought they had. Phillips et al. also noted that students' decision-making was based on both intuition and analysis of the situation, which as noted shortly in this chapter, constitutes the quasi-experimental approach identified by Hamm (1988).

Decisions based on facts or on intuition

It is arguable whether all decisions made by healthcare professionals are based on absolute and full facts, and when all the facts are not available then what are the bases on which decisions are taken?

ACTION POINT 7.3
Should care decisions be based on
knowledge or intuition?

Think about your responses to Action point 7.1, especially in relation to the first item, and consider whether each of those decisions were made consciously or subconsciously. Next, especially in relation to 'conscious' decisions, reflect on the range of information on which the decisions were based. Furthermore, think of whether some of the decisions or parts of them were made intuitively, maybe to some extent because of a dearth of information.

Generally, decisions about most situations are based somewhere on a continuum that has knowledge from empirical studies at one end and intuition at the other, according to Hamm (1988). Analysis of situations involves breaking things down into small components for greater understanding, whereas intuition retains wholeness. Decisions also depend on the time available and, therefore, if less time is available, as in a critical situation, for instance, then intuitive approaches might also be incorporated. Figure 7.3 illustrates six sources of knowledge on which decisions are based.

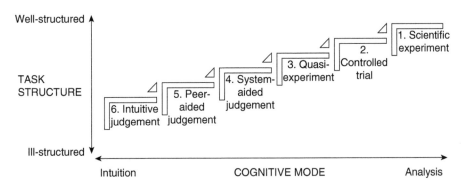

Figure 7.3   Decision-making based on cognitive continuum

Decisions made in health-social care are based predominantly on knowledge from cognitive modes 1 to 4 on Hamm's cognitive continuum; that is, on evidence from rigorous research, quasi-experiments and system-aided judgement (e.g. by receiving and using pathology [system] results). These decisions generally apply to 'well-structured' situations (top left-hand corner of Figure 7.3), and are made after careful scrutiny of available knowledge, and are usually quite accurate.

For less structured, or less clear situations, peer-aided judgement and intuition tend to be used. According to Benner (2001), experienced professionals are inclined to use 'intuitive judgement' more often, and with more self-confidence. The intuitive mode involves rapid unconscious information processing that combines and averages the available information, is low in consistency and is moderately accurate.

Hamm (1988) indicates that a rational-intuitive approach to decision-making is primarily determined by: the complexity of task structure; the ambiguity of the task; and the general presentation of the task. If the task is complex, unfamiliar and the time is limited, then intuitive approaches are used. When ample information is available (well-structured) about the situation, which is therefore less ambiguous, and the situation can be broken down into sub-tasks, then more analytical and knowledge-based decisions are taken.

In problem-solving, on the other hand, problems can be solved using knowledge (including information), experience and intuition. Clearly, FHMs have to base as many of their care decisions on research-based knowledge as possible. However, decisions made by FHMs are also influenced by experience and intuition, which reflect the care professional's own repertoire of extensive and expert knowledge and competence.

Intuitive knowledge refers to patterns of personal knowledge, and sudden perceptions or realisation of patterns as 'cause and effect' in unclear and disjointed situations. Benner (2001) suggests that novices tend to prefer to use rules and guidelines (i.e. practical knowledge) while 'expert' care professionals are comfortable using intuitive knowledge.

Consensus decision-making

In teamwork, decisions that affect the whole team are often made via group decision-making mechanism. When a decision is made to choose from different options (e.g. a multi-disciplinary team meeting to discuss service user's progress and transfer of care options, or where to go on a team night out), then such a decision is better taken as a group after the appropriate discussions, as co-operation by a number of people enhances the likelihood of desired outcomes. For example, when intensive care beds are very limited, consultant doctors could take a consensus decision on which patient to operate on as highest priority, and allocate the intensive care bed to them post-surgically.

One alternative to group decision-making is shared decision-making, whereupon the service user is also involved in the decision-making process, which is a frequent feature in healthcare. Another is group decisions that are made at management or strategic level, which are discussed at structured committees beforehand. However, although such consensus decision-making is preferable because it is also democratic and consultative, and consensus increases commitment, it might also have its limitations or drawbacks in that it is more time-consuming and can lower the decisiveness that leaders are expected to manifest.

Also requiring consideration is the quality of decisions. On evaluating the decision chosen for a particular situation, the FHM might decide that it was not the best decision, the reason for which could have been shortage of time and resources, for instance. The critical elements of decision-making are: choosing and acting decisively; defining objectives clearly; gathering data carefully; generating alternatives; thinking logically; and using an evidence-based approach, indicate Marquis and Huston (2021).

The role of creativity in decision-making

Inherent in decision-making situations is often the scope for reflecting and for learning. They can present opportunities for growth and development, and potentially for changing attitudes, because they normally make us stop and think about the actions or decisions we are about to take, and their consequences. Especially in group decision-making, alternative novel courses of action may be suggested.

Therefore, where decision-making and problem-solving involve dealing with novel situations, novel actions may be required, which would involve thinking creatively. There are different and sequential ways of being creative. Tomey (2009) suggests that being creative entails five stages:

1. *The felt need to be creative*: in relation to a decision or problem situation.
2. *Preparation*: involves exploring several possible solutions.
3. *Incubation*: a period for pondering over solutions after all potential solutions have been identified.
4. *Illumination*: when the most logical or preferred solution emerges.
5. *Verification*: when the solution is implemented, tested, monitored, refined and evaluated.

The preparation stage can entail group or teamwork where appropriate, and uses group techniques such as information sharing, focused case analysis, idea-generation exercises and SWOT analyses (see Chapter 9). Whether situations are dealt with individually or in groups, managers need to be aware that various factors can encourage creativity in care settings, while others can block creativity.

Creative people tend to view problems as new challenges that provide scope for learning, they are always open to alternative views and lines of action, are much more flexible and adaptable, and are enthusiastic about novel situations. They do not see authority as the final, definite, and only perspective, and are keen to be part of new developments. How the roles of individual team members can combine for effective decision-making in care settings is discussed in Chapter 6 under team roles in the context of inter-disciplinary working.

Following on from the notion that novel decision-making and problem-solving situations in particular can present scope for being creative, it therefore follows that some decisions the FHM makes might involve innovative actions. Furthermore, following their quasi-experimental study of creativity, Lui et al. (2020) argue that learning to be creative can itself be facilitated through work-shops and through guidance and re-inforcement of learning.

Solving Problems Systematically

As already noted above, decision-making situations might not involve the presence of a problem, and the actions taken to solve problems entail applying alternative problem-solving methods. Problems related to staff conflict will be discussed shortly. Meanwhile, consider the following situations:

While performing a medical intervention, the new doctor is being rude to a member of your team.

You arrive on duty and find that one of your Band 5 staff who should be on duty has just rung in sick.

What are the processes that the FHM would go through to resolve these problematic situations, and what are the factors that determine the final solution(s)? In management, problem-solving involves taking a systematic set of actions that involve careful consideration of all variables to resolve or to avert a potential problem. Past experiences and intuition can be used to resolve problems, whereupon previously successfully used problem-solving methods might be utilised.

However, if the problem is outside their competence area or their responsibility, then the FHM may pass the problem on to relevant other personnel. Alternatively, they may need to seek expert advice (i.e. further knowledge) before taking any action. They may decide to share the issue with the team to explore the problem and arrive at suitable solutions.

Yet another alternative is that the FHM may decide to delay any action to resolve a less-serious problem (depending on its significance), in the expectation that it will resolve itself. Problems at times solve themselves when they have run their natural course. For example, for the problem when a student is struggling to achieve practice outcomes during placement, the practice assessor may decide to delay assessment of the student, as the student may already be aware of this problem, and is still in the process of learning the outcomes. However, self-resolving problems are rare, as usually some action has to be taken by someone to manage it. Therefore, this is a dangerous problem-solving strategy and in the examples provided above delayed action could result in other repercussions.

At times, the trial-and-error method may be used by FHMs with lesser management experience, whereupon they try different solutions until one works. However, the usual problem-solving method, as identified by several including Marquis and Huston (2021: 7) comprise seven steps, which is presented here as a uni-directional path to solving the problem in Figure 7.4.

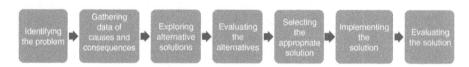

Figure 7.4   Uni-directional path to problem-solving

Although the seven-step path or model looks logical, various interim steps occur when the model is applied. For example, after identifying the problem, the precise nature of the problem needs to be defined, and second, when exploring the causes, other people involved may need to be questioned, and they may or may not be immediately available; and the penultimate step regarding implementation of a solution may comprise a more involved task than is immediately apparent in the model.

Going back to the second step in Figure 7.4, another perspective involves using a systematic method that is referred to as 'root cause analysis' which focuses on both identifying the cause(s), and also the process through which the problem developed. The aim of root cause analysis is also to prevent problems occurring again and learning from them; and is examined in some detail in the next section.

However, on analysing various methods of problem-solving in organisations, Proctor (2020) suggests that a number of factors can interfere with problem-solving and, therefore, might not prove to be a linear and smooth process. These factors are the personality of individuals whom the problem affects, there can be perceptual, cultural and emotional barriers, or intellectual factors and even individuals' ability to express themselves.

Root cause analysis

When problems occur in care settings, such as when patient safety incidents (or an open conflict or uncivil behaviour) occur, in addition to resolving, and then reporting and recording the incident, it is logical to take time to attempt to identify the exact initial cause(s) and the subsequent escalation processes of the problem in order to learn to prevent recurrence of the incident. This tends to take time, patience and impartiality, but is well worth doing so as to restore harmony, and can be performed systematically. Learning from the incident can occur at the individual organisation level and more widely across care organisations to prevent the incident occurring elsewhere.

Systematic analysis of the incident or problem can be performed by root cause analysis (RCA), which entails enquiring about and investigating the problem retrospectively. According to NHS Improvement (2018b), this can be done by repeatedly asking the question 'why?' five times or more, related to aspects of the incident to identify the root cause. A hypothetical example of five whys cited by NHSI are:

- The patient was late in theatre, it caused a delay. Why?
- There was a long wait for a trolley. Why?
- A replacement trolley couldn't be found quickly. Why?
- The original trolley's safety rail was worn and had eventually broken. Why?
- It had not been regularly checked for wear. Why?

Haxby and Shuldham (2018) add that the questions 'what happened?' and 'how ?' should be also be asked. Then, if after the what, how and whys, the cause of the problem is identified, then one or more 'Fishbone diagram(s)' can be used by the team to brainstorm and identify and visually display the specific 'roots' of the problem, that is, the specific contributory factors, as also suggested by NHSI (2020b). This is done to go beyond the apparent cause(s) to identifying underlying sources of the problem. An example of a fishbone diagram, which is also referred to as the 'cause and effect' diagram and as an Ishikawa diagram, is presented in Figure 7.5.

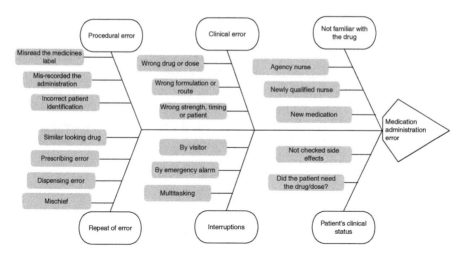

Figure 7.5 Fishbone diagram to identify specific causes of a medication administration error incident

A fishbone diagram is, therefore, a visual tool used by the clinical team to categorise the likely causes of a problem in order to identify its root causes, which is combined with, or partly the result of, brainstorming by the team. Initially, the problem is stated and placed at the head of the fish, and then four to eight major causative factors can be suggested by the facilitator of the brainstorm, or by the team, e.g. the content of the six oval drawings in Figure 7.5, which are then followed by identifying all the potential contributory factors.

When the underlying real causes have been identified by the team, and described accurately in writing, then they can perform a brainstorming session again to agree on potential solutions. Root cause analysis, however, should be followed by action to implement changes in the local healthcare organisation and measuring the effect of the changes. It is also important to disseminate the causes of the incident and the changes made more widely so that lessons can be learned by other organisations throughout the health services.

However, in addition to the local team, RCAs require convening of an appropriately skilled multidisciplinary investigation team that includes risk management personnel, as also suggested by Peerally et al. (2017). Other issues include the team having sufficient independence from the organisation to implement the solutions that they decide on, and time and willingness to disseminate learning from the incident. Furthermore, Kwok et al.'s (2020) review of research on RCA suggests that healthcare professionals lack training, tools and expertise to make large-scale improvements. They suggest that organisations should conduct RCA training for staff and promote an organisation-wide safety culture.

Countenancing Conflict in Care Settings

Despite having numerous rules, regulations and protocols established to ensure organisations function smoothly and coherently, problematic situations do arise and have to be managed, mainly to ensure that the quality of the service or product that they provide is not affected. Issues of human relations between the staff of the organisation, and disagreement and dissatisfaction among staff at times occur and can subsequently develop into interpersonal conflict.

Frontline healthcare managers no doubt realise that disagreements and interpersonal clashes or difficulties do occur in healthcare, and their duties include pre-empting or detecting problems between staff as soon as signs of conflict surface, and start exploring what may be just an issue at this stage, with a view to averting the situation deteriorating. Therefore, they need to ensure that they develop relevant skills and knowledge in this aspect of their work.

What is conflict and how does it manifest itself?

In public service organisations such as healthcare, which seems to have diverse potential for its staff but can be allocated only a certain amount of taxpayers' money, disagreements or conflict of interest about decisions made by those in a position to apportion resources do tend to occur. They result from differences in beliefs about healthcare in their care settings and their priorities, ideas, values or feelings about equity of scope of responsibilities and opportunities between two or more parties. Consequently, conflict is a natural facet of organisations. Such disagreements or alternative strong views can stay as latent dissatisfaction, or manifest themselves as open accusations or allegations.

The noun 'conflict', according to Collins Dictionary (Collins, 2021), means 'clash, disagreement, opposition between ideas, dispute, etc.', and originates from the Latin verb *confligere*, which means 'to fight, combat'. It refers to a definite disagreement or opposition of interests or ideas, and is protracted and felt at an emotional level. It implies different priorities, different attitudes, different perceptions, and they could be due to ineffective or lack of communication. Signs of conflict include open verbal disagreement between individuals, blaming someone without evidence of their guilt, sarcastic comments about individuals, team member becoming reserved and aloof, etc.

Conflict, according to many who have researched the phenomenon, is the feeling about the occurrence of deliberate behaviour intended to obstruct the achievement of another party's goals (e.g. Marquis and Huston, 2021). Conflict, therefore, arises from the incompatibility of goals between two or more individuals or organisations, and from opposing perceptions and behaviours. It can occur at individual level, it can occur within the individual (internal or intra-role conflict), or it could be external at group or organisational level. There can be negative or positive outcomes from the conflict.

Causes of conflict

There are several possible sources of interpersonal conflict in many people organisations, including in healthcare provider organisations. Considering the very wide range of professions (discussed in Chapter 5 under human resources) whose input is required for the health benefits of service users, from healthcare professionals to administrators, ancillary staff to university professors, and the various hierarchies with different levels of skills and seniority, it is conceivable that communication breakdown can occur, which can lead to misunderstanding and suspicions. Aspirations for higher positions and pay in the organisation being denied or delayed can also cause ill-feelings.

The very high workload of many healthcare professionals and the thousands of decisions that they make to ensure patient safety, at times interfere with comprehensive communication, and subsequent feelings of stress compound the risk of conflict further. This situation is further complicated by the inter-dependent ways in which most healthcare professions work, which means communicating referrals (to dietitians for example), who, in turn, must communicate the intended interventions to all-involved, including the service user. Furthermore, different care professionals in different departments make numerous decisions continually related to day-to-day provision of care that can also impact on the staff of other departments.

For example, if a doctor is asked to see a patient urgently, but if after seeing the patient they do not communicate in writing or even verbally the interventions they prescribe, then nurses or other healthcare professionals will be unable to intervene for the good of the service user, which can be frustrating or lead to confrontation. It is not unknown for new care professionals to occasionally carry out a procedure on a patient, but fail to clear packaging, needles, etc. afterwards, i.e. do not follow the trust's protocol.

Yet another reason for conflict in healthcare organisations, as noted above, is that each individual employee and subgroup in the organisation is in some way different from one other, and each have their own beliefs, perceptions, thoughts, expectations and aspirations about the employing organisation, and therefore there are likely to be situations when views differ, and now and again differences are openly vocalised. There can be differences in perception, or perceived inequitable treatment, that can lead to disagreements that, in turn, require attention to restore equilibrium.

An example of inequitable treatment can be a team member not being seconded to go on a professional development university course, another is when a team member asked for a day-off on a bank holiday for a family event, but which is not granted. The FHM can release staff for whatever purpose only after ensuring that service user needs and problems have been addressed as highest priority.

Conflict, consequently, can also occur at different levels in organisations, such as between:

- the healthcare team and the organisation;
- a team member and their line manager;
- two team members in a care setting;
- an employee and the healthcare organisation;
- different teams or groups within the organisation or department;
- informal subgroups in the healthcare organisation and the formal organisation;
- the workforce and NHS leaders.

Furthermore, conflict can also be seen as vertical, or boss–subordinate, or power conflict, when it occurs between an employee of junior status and power, and one in senior employment status; or horizontal conflict when it occurs between employees at equivalent or similar level, that is between peers. Disagreement between healthcare staff and service users is not treated as conflict, and is discussed in the context of complaints in Chapter 8.

ACTION POINT 7.4
Incidence and causes of organisational conflict

Thinking about your own employing organisation or the care setting where you work, can you recall any conflict arising ever, either between two members of the team in the care setting, or between a junior member of staff and their line manager, etc. (see list of sources of conflict above)?

Reflect on one such incident, and the way the conflict developed or escalated. How was the incident managed, and what was the eventual outcome of the conflict?

Unless you are new to the organisation, you should have been able to think of a few examples of incidents of conflict in your workplace. Some of the conflict may have been interpersonal conflict (between individuals), others intergroup conflict (between different teams) or intrapersonal conflict (within the individual), or maybe intra-group conflict (within a group), for instance. Conflict can also be disruptive.

Despite its negative connotations and likely ill-effects, conflict can also prove beneficial if it is well managed. This is because conflict provides an opportunity to check for misunderstandings between colleagues or managers and employees, and new information and knowledge could surface that can result in new learning and the opportunity to apply creativity.

Therefore, too little disagreement could indicate that team members are not being honest and open about their views, but too much disagreement is a symptom of conflict not being dealt with. Conflict that remains unresolved is likely to affect the quality of care provided to service users, it can lower the morale of staff, cause stress and impact on patient safety through, for example, increased incidence of medication errors, falls, etc. (e.g. Johansen, 2012). Individual staff may begin to think about leaving the care setting or the organisation itself.

Conflict can also occur between students and individual staff in a care setting during practice placement. Kim (2018), for example, researched students' experience of uncivil behaviour from registrants, and found that consequently students tend to have difficulty developing appropriate professional values. However, those students who seek social support after such experiences tend to develop stronger professional values than students who rely on their own coping strategies.

How conflict starts and progresses?

Unchecked, when conflict starts it is likely to progress resulting in each party believing with more conviction that they were in the right in the first place. It might escalate silently initially, and could remain like a 'cold war' or develop into 'open conflict'. For both reasons, FHMs need to be sensitive to the beginnings of strong disagreements between team members within the team, if and when they occur, and act accordingly.

A five-stage process of interpersonal conflict has been documented widely (e.g. Almost, 2006) which can be adapted to contemporary conflict resolution in organisations, as represented diagrammatically in Figure 7.6.

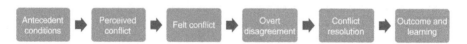

Figure 7.6   Six stages of the conflict process

The antecedent conditions stage of the conflict process, which is also referred to as 'latent conflict', refers to the prevalence of continuing unsatisfactory situations at work, such as when there is staff shortage combined with increasing workload, or withdrawal of overtime pay, which act as the precursor for conflict. The second stage in the process is the perceived conflict stage (also referred to as 'substantive conflict' stage), when questions are asked about the situation, and if there is substantial disagreement between the two parties, then felt conflict (third stage) is experienced as one party or the other feels emotionally hurt or unfairly treated.

In the overt disagreement stage (fourth stage), emotions are expressed overtly, and even hostility is noticed, and therefore action has to be taken to resolve or manage the conflict. In conflict resolution (fifth stage), both positive and negative outcomes could ensue for the two parties, accompanied possibly by creativity and innovation. After the conflict has been resolved and the final stage reached, a new level of relationship could prevail between the two parties, with learning and emotional resilience further developed by each. However, if one party remains partly or fully dissatisfied with the outcome for them, then they might take further action related to their post or occupation.

At the overt conflict stage, there are clear signs of deep disagreement in the work setting, which staff in the setting can detect with the prevalence of such symptoms of conflict as: irritability, mistrust, low morale, suspiciousness, raised voices or shouting, lack of communication, some staff being absent or 'off-sick' frequently and staff being aloof.

How we respond to conflict

A case study follows, with associated analysis of potential outcomes of conflict.

ACTION POINT 7.5
based on a case study: Managing conflict within the team

During the time when there has been a Band 6 (junior sister) vacancy in the acute mental health ward, senior staff nurse Sally has been conducting most of the management duties for approximately four months, but was not appointed to the post. When George was appointed to the post Sally acknowledged George but even at three weeks into the post, whenever they are on the same shift, Sally proactively initiates all management activities, and allocates some of the day's duties to him, despite George being in the more senior position. George didn't object to Sally doing this, but the Unit Manager called George to one side one day and accused George of letting Sally 'run the unit' while HSWs and other staff had complained of Sally's abrupt attitude and bullying to the Unit Manager, who then asked George what he was going to do about that?

For the above case study:

- Identify the actions that George should take to resolve the situation.
- Consider which other actions George could have taken.
- Then consider what might be the possible positive outcomes, and the possible negative outcomes of the particular conflict.

George might initially feel shocked by the observation of the Unit Manager, and by reports of abruptness and bullying that bypassed him and were not reported to him. His initial reaction to the situation might be of hurt and resentment towards Sally, who, in turn, seems to resent his appointment as her senior.

The likely negative outcomes of this conflict when George confronts Sally might be that there is an open argument with accusations flung at each other and which generates more distance between them. Sally might go off-sick, lose motivation at work, foster a social atmosphere of mistrust and suspicion, etc. George might even start to question his capability to do the job he is appointed to.

On the other hand, positive outcomes might include an apology from Sally, claiming that she only wanted to help, and agreement on boundaries of each other's responsibilities, and consequently possibly a stronger team, with the care setting also being back to a full complement of staff. Both parties could learn from each other and gain new perspectives. Furthermore, Sally could see her job interview as a useful experience and go for post-interview feedback to learn more about interviews. It is also an opportunity to identify any continuing professional development needs for Sally, and perhaps guidance on contemporary ways of compiling curriculum vitae with job applications.

Strategies and styles of conflict resolution

Conflict tends to interfere with open communication, it causes stress, hardening of attitudes and leads us to develop habitual ways of reacting to conflict situations. The likely negative outcomes of conflict documented above makes it imperative that action should be taken by the FHM to resolve the conflict as soon as possible. Moreover, the ability to resolve conflict or disagreement within teams is crucial to successful teamwork, as also noted by the WHO (2012). Negotiation often forms the basis for conflict resolution, while appreciating that every negotiation situation is different depending not only on the nature of the conflict, but also on each party's current state of mind, and their respective approach to the negotiation, i.e. whether that be adversarial or non-adversarial, and which strategies (see Table 7.2) they intend to use.

In the endeavour to resolve an interpersonal or a power conflict with the line manager, the individual normally should query the situation with the person whose stance they are in conflict with but need to be economical in putting forward their viewpoint at this stage. They could engage in as much intelligence gathering as they can and could also discuss this with their clinical supervisor in confidence (see Chapter 2 for discussion on emotional resilience and support).

So, conflict resolution depends very much on the stance taken by each party involved, mostly on how co-operative or unco-operative each party is, as well as how assertive or unassertive. At times, the stance (or style) adopted by one side is reciprocated by the other side; i.e. if one party shows that they are willing to co-operate and negotiate, then the other side may also be swayed to react by co-operating. Disjunction and difficulty in resolving conflict might, however, occur if one party is, say, in 'competing' (assertive and unco-operative) mode while the other is in say, 'avoiding' mode. Disjunction can also occur if one party decides to exert power or is unclear of their goals.

Table 7.2   Strategies, modes or styles of conflict management

Strategy or style	Alternating nomenclature and brief explanation of each
Accommodating	Also referred to as obliging or non-confrontation; both parties are highly co-operative and unassertive.
Avoiding	Also referred to as suppressing, or dodging; ignoring the problem; both parties unassertive and unco-operative. Is a dysfunctional mode of conflict resolution.
Competing	Also referred to as dominating, controlling, forcing; both parties assertive and unco-operative; is a win–lose strategy – each party has to win, and the other has to submit or lose.
Compromising	Also referred to as sharing; is based on negotiation, both parties are assertive as well as co-operative to some extent, and each party gains something but also gives up something.
Confronting	The problem is discussed openly by all parties involved, but assertively, to establish the precise disagreement areas, and might result in an agreeable outcome.
Integrating	Also referred to as collaborating, joint-welfare, solution-orientation; both parties are assertive and co-operative; focuses on benefit for both parties; is the win–win strategy that instigates growth, learning, creativity, innovation.
Lose–lose strategy	Neither party wins, no settlement is reached, and is unsatisfactory for both parties.
Negotiation	Some similarity with compromising, as the conflicting parties assert their viewpoints, and then make some concessions on certain aspects.
Partisan choice	Attending to the needs of only one party.
Smoothing/Obliging	Not facing up to the problem, and probably just accepting the other party's decisions.

Thus, with reference to the modes of conflict resolution presented on Table 7.2, if for instance both parties are highly assertive and highly co-operative, then they will be using the integrating or collaborating mode, and therefore the conflict will be resolved and an outcome that is mutually beneficial for both parties should ensue.

However, if both parties are highly unassertive and unco-operative, then they are likely to use the 'avoiding' mode and the issue is likely to remain unresolved. The conflict will also remain unresolved if the goals of the two parties are completely opposed to one another, and they use the competing mode of conflict management, which means both parties are highly assertive but also unco-operative.

Other modes have been identified by Hossain et al. (2018) and others such as confronting assertively, non-confrontation and smoothing. Consequently, when an individual affected by an interpersonal conflict does decide to take action to resolve it, a range of modes of, or strategies (at times referred to as styles) for conflict resolution is available for each of the two parties to choose from.

Moreover, a well-managed conflict can result in growth through creativity, learning and innovation. Appointing a specific independent and unbiased mediator as an impartial referee may prove beneficial if both parties agree to this. However, if unmanaged or unresolved, the conflict causes ill-feelings between team members, lowers morale and quality of care, as already noted earlier.

ACTION POINT 7.6
Reaction to conflict situations

With reference to the strategies of conflict resolution, think about the ways in which you have personally reacted to conflict situations in the past. Which of these strategies have you used? Is there a pattern in the way you generally manage conflict situations? Is your eventual response usually different from your initial reaction?

By identifying any habitual responses that you may have towards conflict situations, you could gain further insight into your modes of conflict resolution, and change them if you feel other strategies could prove more beneficial. Your usual response to conflicts, when they happen, could be adjusted to some of the ways identified on Table 7.2.

It needs to be noted at this stage that when two individuals who are in conflict come together to explain the precise nature of their disagreement, then either party may feel distressed when stating that they have been treated unfairly. In this case, the mediator, who could well be the FHM, needs to be patient and even allow them to express how they feel, which is a form of catharsis.

Based on a literature review of conflict management styles among nurses, Labrague et al. (2018) concluded that nurses tend to use 'integration' and 'accommodation', that is positive conflict management styles, and thereby achieve conflict resolution more effectively than those who use avoiding or competing techniques. They suggested that nurses should be equipped with these styles of conflict resolution through concerted organised facilitation sessions.

Furthermore, the stance that both parties, and the mediator, should avoid if they wish to co-operate (integration) for a win-win outcome include avoiding referring to other previous conflicts, criticising the other party, being condescending and taking a commanding position, according to Ellis and Abbott (2011). When the mediator is of senior status and power to those in conflict, they must also act with integrity and sincerity, and ensure they don't arrive at the meeting with the aim of making one specific party win, maybe because of the other's bad reputation.

On the other hand, especially when the FHM or anyone else acts as a mediator, certain basic communication rules (partly discussed in Chapter 4) and unbiased refereeing rules need to be observed so that the mediation is conducted impartially. These rules include the following:

- Ensure both parties have full airing of their viewpoints (if time doesn't permit this, then a second meeting needs to be scheduled to be held as soon as possible).
- Focus on issues, not personalities or any member's personal reputation.
- If one party is of lower status, ensure the one with more power is not given more say or time, and thereby maintain equity.
- Act as a catalyst to enable participants to think of alternative mutually beneficial solutions.

As noted earlier in this section, conflict is a natural process in organisations as opinions and preferences can differ, but conflict can often be the trigger for improvement. Consequently, FHMs should recognise the precursors and symptoms of conflict early in order to prevent any ill effects. However, when frontline managers find themselves in a situation where team members are in conflict, they should approach the conflict with an open mind, maybe as a challenge to enable both parties to collaborate, analyse alternative outcomes and treat it as an opportunity for learning.

Guidance for Effective Decision-Making, Problem-Solving and Conflict Management

Based on the analysis presented in this chapter, the following comprise guidance on effective decision-making, problem-solving and conflict management.

Accept decision-making, problem-solving and conflict management as normal management encounters, and see issues as challenges and as opportunities for positive outcomes and learning.

Have clear knowledge of the nature and dynamics of decisions and decision-making, problems and conflicts, and examine how they also apply to situations in healthcare.

Acquire as much relevant knowledge as you can and check their accuracy before getting involved in decisive interpersonal interactions with the other party.

Be clear about the goals of the interventional actions that you take when making decisions.

Do not unduly delay decision-making, problem-solving and conflict management, as delays can lead to unnecessary complications.

Use systematic approaches to decision-making, problem-solving and conflict management, such as by performing a root cause analysis of problems that surface.

Decide on the extent to which your decisions are based on empirical or other
    types of knowledge and how far it can be based on intuition.
Allow plenty of scope and appropriate amount of time for team members and
    teams to develop creativity when taking actions to resolve problems and con-
    flicts in consensus decision-making.
If appropriate, complete risk assessments before taking decisions and document
    clinical incidents appropriately with the aim of reducing the likelihood of risk
    occurring.
Appreciate sources and causes of potential conflicts, the way in which conflicts
    progress, how we tend to react to conflict and different modes of conflict reso-
    lution.
Ensure all relevant actions are documented appropriately.

Chapter Summary

When examined closely, it becomes obvious that FHMs' duties include making numerous decisions, even in the course of their routine work. Consequently,
this chapter has explored the decision-making and problem-solving function of
FHMs, which includes conflict management. It has therefore addressed:

- Identification of several day-to-day decisions made by FHMs, and the significance of these decisions;
- Clarifying and differentiating between decision-making and problem-solving,
  and their inherent multifarious macro- and micro-decisions;
- Various systematic ways of making decisions and solving problems individually and as a group, including probability analysis, root cause analysis and
  creativity in decision-making;
- The causes of interpersonal conflict in care settings, how they manifest themselves and progress, and subsequently the modes or styles of conflict resolution
  that can benefit the parties involved; and
- Applying creativity and ensuring new learning in the course of professional
  decision-making, problem-solving and conflict management.

Further Reading

- For further discussion on Hamm's cognitive continuum related to decisions
  based on analysis against those based on intuition, see: Hamm R M (1988)
  Clinical intuition and clinical analysis: Expertise and the cognitive continuum.
  In Dowie J and Elstein A (eds), *Professional Judgement: A Reader in Clinical
  Decision-making* (Chapter 3). Milton Keynes: Open University Press.

- For a literature review of conflict management in healthcare, see: Patton C M (2014) Conflict in health care: A literature review. *The Internet Journal of Healthcare Administration,* 9(1): 9–11.
- For assessing workload related to staffing needs, which is based on the World Health Organization (2010) *Workload Indicators Staffing Need – User's Manual,* see the following research publication: Gialama F, Saridi M, Prezerakos P, Pollalis Y, Contiades X and Souliotis K (2019) The implementation process of the Workload Indicators Staffing Need (WISN) method by WHO in determining midwifery staff requirements in Greek Hospitals. *European Journal of Midwifery,* 3(January): 1–13.

8

Delivering Highest Quality Care

Chapter Objectives

The chapter objectives for frontline healthcare managers with regards to delivering highest quality care are:

- Identify the reasons for the current high level of emphasis on delivering and monitoring quality of healthcare received by service users;
- Define quality of care, and delineate the principal healthcare criteria by which quality is gauged, and enunciate the role of a quality-conscious culture in the care setting;
- Demonstrate knowledge of several of the wide array of quality improvement frameworks and models that can lead to service improvement and service transformation;
- Review and apply many of the quality improvement methods that contribute to enhancement and monitoring of quality of care in practice settings;
- Show knowledge of barriers to quality improvement and of issues related to sub-optimal quality of care.

Introduction

Delivering the highest quality of care requires the appropriate necessary professional knowledge, competence and personal attributes, along with all the necessary human and material resources. As frontline, public-facing care leaders, FHMs have a pivotal role in ensuring highest quality of care and treatment is delivered to service users and achieving best outcomes for them, while simultaneously utilising available resources efficiently.

This chapter begins by examining the reasons for the current continuing strong emphasis on quality of care that is safe, effective, compassionate and professional.

Then, after exploring and defining the concept quality of care, it next addresses the DHSC's three criteria for quality, namely patient safety, clinical effectiveness and patient experience of healthcare, and the various ways in which quality of care is monitored.

Various frameworks and tools for assessing and improving quality are examined, followed by contributory quality improvement mechanisms or tools, including clinical audits, patient surveys and metrics, and how they apply to your care setting. Managing complaints is discussed next, followed by clinical negligence issues and their implications for health services. Learning from patient incidents and 'near misses' is integral to high-quality healthcare, and is addressed in the context of learning in Chapter 10 of this book.

Why So Much Emphasis on Quality in Health Services?

Quality consciousness has been present in healthcare provision and delivery in the UK and other countries for several years. Various standards and criteria for quality have been published and researched. Conversely, in the twentieth century, quality of care has also often been questioned whenever mistakes by healthcare professionals have become headline news, including incidents of abuse of service users. Reports on low-quality care and malpractice leading to death or long-term suffering include, for example, the Francis (2013) Report on malpractice at a UK NHS trust hospital. Some of the most recent national publications urging improvement in the quality of care include:

- *High Quality Care for All (Darzi Report)* (Department of Health, 2008a);
- *Improving quality in the English NHS A strategy for action* (King's Fund, 2016c);
- *NHS Long-Term Plan* (NHSE, 2019a);
- *NHS Outcomes Framework* (NHS Digital, 2020a).

Quality of treatment and care was highlighted with striking emphasis in the Darzi Report (DH, 2008a), which focused on various ways of accelerating improvement in quality of care by further reducing waiting times, lengths of patient stay in hospitals, etc. It was followed by the then government's White Paper for healthcare in *Equity and Excellence: Liberating the NHS* (DH, 2010a: 13) whose aim included quality of care that 'achieve healthcare outcomes that are among the best in the world … [by] involving patients fully in their own care, with decisions made in partnership with clinicians'.

Most recently, quality care and outcomes at national level has been detailed in the *NHS Outcomes Framework* (NHS Digital, 2020a) with a range of quality indicators for NHS trusts. The framework also comprises an accountability mechanism between the Secretary of State for Health and NHSE, and thereby also acts as a vehicle for questioning and enhancing quality of health services. Quality indicators in the outcomes framework focuses on improving health and reducing inequalities, and they are identified under five domains, which are (NHS Digital, 2020a):

Domain 1: Preventing people from dying prematurely (e.g. Indicator 1.1: Under 75s mortality rate [per 100,000 population] from cardiovascular disease).

Domain 2: Enhancing quality of life for people with long-term conditions.

Domain 3: Helping people recover from periods of ill health or following injury.

Domain 4: Ensuring people have a positive experience of care.

Domain 5: Treating and caring for people in a safe environment; and protecting them from avoidable harm.

For indicator 1.1 for England, as an example, there was a significant decrease in the number of deaths from cardiovascular disease in the under 75s since 2003, a decrease from 138 per 100,000 population in 2003 to 71 per 100,000 population in 2018 (NHS Digital, 2020a), which represents evidence of improving quality of care.

For indicator 5.6 however, which addresses 'patient safety incidents' (PSIs) this includes the rate or number of PSIs reported involving harm or death and incidence of medication errors causing serious harm, and for this more than 1100 were reported between October and December 2019, and has been increasing over the years. NHS Digital, however, indicates that the figures need to be interpreted with caution because the increase might mean more incidents are being reported rather than more occurring.

Key health and social care organisations that also lay the spotlight on quality of care include:

- NHS Improvement (NHSI)
- Local authorities through Health and Well Being Boards and Healthwatch
- National Institute for Health and Care Excellence (NICE)
- Care Quality Commission (CQC)

Ultimately, it is also each individual healthcare professional's own professionalism that determines the quality of care received by service users. Having identified the reason for quality consciousness in healthcare in the UK, the next section endeavours to define the concept 'quality' and then disentangles the key components of quality in healthcare.

What Is High-Quality Healthcare?

This section focuses on defining quality of care and unravels its constituent components. Specifically, it explores the concepts patient safety and safeguarding vulnerable people, followed by clinical effectiveness, service users' experience and views, as well as the very important role of approved clinical guidelines, protocols and procedures in assuring quality care.

Defining quality of care

Overall, the healthcare professional chooses to become an occupational therapist, a midwife, a doctor, a speech and language therapist or a nursing associate to apply their professional knowledge and competence to provide the highest quality of care they can to service users. There have been several endeavours to state precisely what high-quality care is. Manufacturers and service providers generally have identified criteria or specifications to identify high-quality product or service.

Explanation of the word quality in dictionaries also tends to include 'degree or standard of excellence' and 'having or showing excellence'. Therefore, applied to health services, 'quality of care' would mean that care is provided and delivered to a 'standard of excellence', a standard that both healthcare staff and service users perceive and feel as being of high quality. In manufacturing, high quality also refers to a measure of excellence or products being free from defects, deficiencies and significant variations from the company's statement of their standards.

Accordingly, over several decades various researchers have attempted to define quality in relation to healthcare, which include:

- A process which seeks to attain the highest degree of excellence in the delivery of patient care (Lang, 1976);
- Provision of care that exceeds patients' expectations and achieves the highest possible clinical outcomes with the resources available (Ovretveit, 1992).

The definition by Ovretveit is one of a few that are widely accepted definitions of quality in healthcare. An array of terminologies that include the term quality thereafter evolved over time; for example, quality assurance, quality improvement, quality control, quality circles, etc. Quality assurance, for example, implies a process of assuring high quality, with the word assurance meaning guaranteeing or pledging to fulfil specified standards. It therefore signifies certain criteria will be met, and the endeavours to achieve those criteria consistently comprise 'quality assurance'.

When quality is being judged for manufactured products (e.g. mobile phones, televisions), that is implements made by humans (or robots), it is fairly straightforward to assess their quality because the criteria that they have to meet are tangible, visible and often measurable. When quality of care is being judged, this can be less straightforward because it involves human perceptions and behaviour towards patients, which can be subjective and interpreted differently by different judges.

ACTION POINT 8.1
What does high-quality care mean to you?

Reflect on this question, then write the answer using your own words.

Staff's perceptions of high quality tends to depend on two groups of factors: (1) intrinsic factors – which relates to each individual's values, beliefs, attitudes and self-knowledge; and (2) extrinsic factors – mostly refers to resources such as the time available for each clinical activity, money, staff and their level of training and education, etc. However, it can be argued that the best judges of quality of care has to be its recipients, that is service users, and consequently should be involved in healthcare providers' definitions of high-quality care.

Quality of care being subjective also denotes that individual perceptions of high quality is based on the individual's own personal values such as valuing treating service users with respect, dignity, compassion and equality, improving their lives and wellbeing by educating them, etc. Usually, these personal values are also shared values within a team, which are also guided by national requirements through the NHS Constitution (DHSC, 2019a), for example, and from regulatory bodies (e.g. NMC) together with initial and continuing professional education. Furthermore, team values are guided by the care setting's mission statement (or written philosophy) and annual and long-term aims.

Additionally, according to Health Education England [HEE] (2016), values motivate people towards their goals and influence their behaviour, and, therefore, ways in which care is delivered and patient experience. In expounding on values-based recruitment of healthcare profession students, the HEE asserts that 'The workforce will have the skills, values, behaviours and support to provide safe, high quality care wherever the patient is, at all times and in all settings' (2016: 13). This statement directly links personal values to quality of care.

As for applying these values to care settings, the National Quality Board [NQB] (2016) identified the parameters of high-quality care, which is also consistent with those identified in FYFV (NHSE, 2014a), in the NHS Constitution (DHSC, 2019a) as service users' rights under 'Quality of care and environment', and prior to them by the Darzi Report (DH, 2008a: 47). These parameters are patient safety, clinical effectiveness and patient experience (see Figure 8.1).

- *Patient safety:* Signifies ensuring we do no harm to any service user by making care settings safe and clean, preventing errors, preventing healthcare-associated infections; and ensuring the care we provide is evidence-based.
- *Effectiveness of care:* Signifies monitoring and enhancing the success rates of care interventions, and scrutinising clinical measures such as mortality or

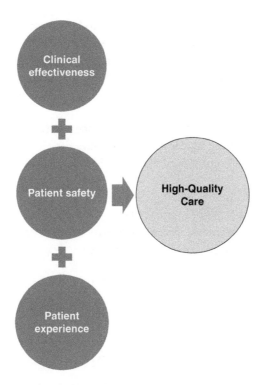

Figure 8.1   The three interrelated parameters or dimensions of quality

survival rates, complication rates and measures of clinical improvement; extends to people's wellbeing and ability to live independent lives.

- *Patient experience:* Signifies personal care with compassion, dignity and respect for service users being treated; and by acing on the findings of patient satisfaction data.

All three parameters are interrelated, and must be present for best quality care to have been achieved.

Applied to, for example, a person who attends Day Surgery Unit for cataract surgery, *clinical effectiveness* signifies that post-surgery the service user's vision is improved markedly soon after any trauma and swelling has subsided, colours appear sharper, ability to see at night is improved, and consequently improved quality of life. For *patient safety*, this means the patient doesn't suffer any harm in the Day Unit, nor surgery-related harm, e.g. post-operative eye infection, and appropriate advice is given to the service user. For *patient experience*, this means the service user reports a positive experience of care, e.g. treated with dignity, respect and compassion, and that they feel they can recommend the service to their acquaintances.

Prior to these parameters being declared in the UK, the Institute of Medicine (2001) in the USA specified six dimensions of quality to specify the meaning of high-quality care that continues to apply today; these being safe, effective, patient-centred, timely, efficient and equitable. The RCN (2019b) endorses these aspects or parameters of quality in healthcare by specifying six aspects which are also consistent with USA's Institute of Medicine's dimensions of quality in healthcare (at times referred to by the acronym STEEP), which are:

1. Safe, and therefore prevent any harm to service users.
2. Timely care, that also reduces waste and delays.
3. Effective by providing services that are evidence-based and beneficial to service users.
4. Efficient, which signifies making the best use of available resources.
5. Equitable, that is care does not vary because of a person's characteristics.
6. Person-centred, based on a practitioner–patient partnership that ensures service users' needs and preferences are respected.

Following an integrative review, Beattie et al. (2012) suggest adding two more dimensions to quality, which are 'caring' and 'navigating the health care system'.

ACTION POINT 8.2
High-quality care in your care setting?

Consider the NHS Constitution (DHSC, 2019a) and several other documents that concur with the three parameters of high-quality care: patient safety, clinical effectiveness and patient experience. Then, consider from the viewpoint of service users who receive care in your care settings. What are the specific different ways in which the team monitors or evaluates the achievement of these quality parameters?

It is no doubt useful to pause and consider some of the ways in which concepts of quality laid down in policy documents apply to day-to-day frontline care. However, the FYFV (NHSE, 2014a), as well as the NHS LTP (NHSE, 2019a), indicate that a comprehensive high-quality health service is represented by actions stated in the NHS's 'triple aim', which are better health for everyone, better care for all and sustainability (money management) (as discussed in Chapter 1).

Patient Safety

As noted in the preceding section, patient safety is central to the quality of care provided in health services. 'Safe, effective and compassionate care', 'safe, effective and personalised care' are phrases that occur repeatedly in publications by national healthcare-related organisations that include the NMC, GMC, NHSE, etc. Clearly, then, service users' safety is one of the highest priorities in healthcare provision and delivery, safety from healthcare-associated infections, for example. Ensuring safety consequently signifies that no harm should occur to any service user whenever in contact with health services, which requires commitment from clinicians and from Board-level managers.

Ensuring no harm occurs to service users is also central to both 'Personal moral qualities' and the ethical practice of 'non-maleficence', that is 'a commitment to avoiding harm to the client' asserted by the British Association for Counselling and Psychotherapy (BACP) (2018: 9–10). Consequently, as could be expected, all sections of all healthcare professions' codes of practice address patient safety (as well as wellbeing) which are often developed from principles of ethics. The clauses of the section specified, for example, in the HCPC's (2016) *Standards of Conduct, Performance and Ethics* includes:

6.1 You must take all reasonable steps to reduce the risk of harm to service users, carers and colleagues as far as possible.
6.2 You must not do anything, or allow someone else to do anything, which could put the health or safety of a service user, carer or colleague at unacceptable risk.

Nonetheless, a quick search of patient safety-based items in just one journal of nursing for the period January to August 2020 showed 188 items, almost all of them highlighting possible concerns over patient safety in UK health services (Nursing Standard, 2020). This includes one news item indicating that between 2017/18 and 2018/19 the number of whistleblowing claims made by nurses related to patient safety went up by 68% (from 2,223 allegations to 3,728).

Another dimension of patient safety is for those service users who are cared for in their own homes within the community. This includes two groups: (1) those who need after-care following hospitalisation or under GP prescribed care; and (2) people who are identified as vulnerable or at risk and require health and/ or social care interventions. Caring for vulnerable people is also referred to as safeguarding.

Safeguarding is fundamental to high-quality health and social care, and is everyone's responsibility, states the CQC (2018a: 1), who indicates that 'Safeguarding adults means protecting the rights of adults to live in safety, free from abuse and neglect', and that people and organisations should work together to prevent and stop both the risks and experience of abuse or neglect. Individuals who need safeguarding are often elderly and frail, or adults with mental or other disability who may be unable to protect themselves against harm or exploitation. They might be living either in institutions or at home.

The CQC's role includes monitoring how well providers are safeguarding those who are vulnerable or at risk by assessing the quality and safety of care they provide, and by checking that care providers have effective systems and processes to help keep vulnerable children and adults safe from abuse and neglect. Thereby, the CQC also gauges whether individuals are receiving very high standards of care. Frontline managers and team members in care organisations should, therefore, ensure they are acquainted with their roles, responsibilities and policies related to safeguarding the vulnerable.

Patient safety incident reporting will be explored in detail in Chapter 10 of this book in the context of learning from incidents and 'near misses'.

Clinical effectiveness

In essence, the term clinical effectiveness denotes the effect or impact of clinical interventions. Before the impact of each intervention is ascertained, however, clinicians or healthcare professionals need to assess the service user's health problem accurately, have the knowledge and competence to do so, and ensure that the recommended intervention is evidence-informed. According to the King's Fund (2017), clinical effectiveness entails preventing people from dying prematurely, enhancing quality of life and helping people to recover following episodes of ill health. The King's Fund's explanation is broader and less specific than the one given above, but they do explain it further subsequently.

Clinical effectiveness or efficacy, therefore, signifies that patient care interventions undertaken by healthcare professionals are successful in achieving the goal(s) set in the care plan or care pathway for the service user. Success rate can be gauged by conducting audits.

Service users' experience of health services

Much has been published about ways of gaining insight into service users' experience of the care they received while hospitalised and after discharge from hospital. Often, service user feedback is obtained through patient satisfaction surveys using online or postal questionnaires that are conducted nationally and locally at healthcare provider level. Nationally, for example, the CQC conducts such surveys, and the findings are published for anyone who is interested in them. Often the results are quite good, in that service users are generally satisfied with the care they received. (More information on specifics of survey questionnaires is provided later in this chapter.)

However, good results from surveys may not always reflect service users' views accurately, according to Trueland (2019), which is because they might have adjusted their comments based on their awareness that healthcare professionals are often working under pressure of staff shortage and healthcare financial constraints. It is suggested, therefore, that use of survey questionnaires may be limited and so qualitative data should also be obtained through, for example, patient and staff stories of their experience of receiving and providing care respectively.

In their endeavour to capture patient experience with the aim of improving healthcare services, Goodrich and Fitzsimons (2019) argue moving away from the concept patient satisfaction because if a service user has low expectations of the health service, or is in a low mood, they are likely to indicate they are highly satisfied. Patient experience is, therefore, different from patient satisfaction, and consequently needs to be assessed not by tick-box survey questionnaires, but by asking the service users open-ended questions about their experience of hospitalisation for instance.

Sufficient time needs to be allocated for obtaining patient experience data by encouraging service users to verbalise in their own words and in depth the actual care that they received (or didn't), and incorporating active listening when gathering information by 'patients' stories' method, as Trueland suggests, or by conducting focus group discussions, and by following up complaints and compliments, for example.

Ultimately, the purpose of gauging service users' experience of the care they received while hospitalised and after discharge from hospital is for healthcare providers to learn from the feedback from these surveys and other empirical methods, from both positive and negative comments, and to work on things that need improvement. Quality improvement entails endeavouring to provide service users with a positive experience of the care they receive.

ACTION POINT 8.3
What is a positive patient experience?

Consider for a moment what constitutes a positive patient experience for someone who is hospitalised with multiple injuries following a serious road traffic accident, and jot down your answers.

As already highlighted, the patient experience is a key component of high-quality care. The response to Action point 8.3 related to a positive patient experience probably include timely attention to health problem, timely management of pain, and also being treated with respect, kindness, dignity and compassion, and being provided with emotional and psychological support to relieve or reduce service users', family members' and carers' fears and anxiety. However, as the Health Foundation (2013) notes in its extensive review of different methods that can be used for assessing patient experience, there are pros and cons of each method such as low return rate of survey questionnaires but producing empirical data, and patient in-depth interviews being time consuming but less generalisable.

Current Quality Improvement Concepts

As a relatively enduring concept, quality improvement (QI) in healthcare according to the King's Fund (2017) refers to the systematic use of methods and tools to try to continuously improve quality of care and outcomes for patients. The NHS LTP (NHSE, 2019a: 111) asserts that QI provides 'an evidence-based approach to improving every aspect of how the NHS operates'. As already noted earlier, high-quality entails ensuring patient safety, clinical effectiveness and patient experience. One way of meeting all three criteria and their components is to adhere to the healthcare provider's established and locally approved clinical guidelines, procedures, policies and protocols in full, which are normally readily available in clinical settings, through the organisation's intranet or in paper-form.

Clinical guidelines (e.g. for leg ulcer management, suturing), procedures (e.g. for hand washing, intra-muscular injection) comprise step-by-step actions for care interventions based on systematic appraisal of the best available evidence. These care intervention methods are essential resources at the disposal of FHMs to support highest quality, safe and effective practice. They are also reviewed regularly as well as by pre-determined dates to ensure their evidence base remains valid. NICE provides a wide range of clinical guidelines for several health problems on its website. They are often presented as algorithms, with associated detailed information on key components, and can be adapted for local utilisation.

However, for quality improvement, a wide range of frameworks (or models), tools and methods are available to QI leaders to utilise, to either enhance or monitor quality of care (see NHSI, 2020b for examples), which will be explored in the next section of this chapter, followed by specific widely applied methods (or techniques) and tools that contribute to quality management (including patient surveys, and 'lean' care methods). Before doing so, the following inherent popular concepts related to QI will be briefly explored:

- service improvement and service transformation;
- a quality-conscious culture in the care setting;
- organisational governance and clinical governance;
- total quality management; and
- management of quality.

The evidence base for the impact of QI through the successful implementation of QI in mental health services, its outcomes and recommendations, is provided by Davies et al. (2020), for example, who indicate that the outcomes of the programme include reduced readmission rates and increased accuracy of electronic transfers of care. Their recommendations include developing staff skills to implement QI, engaging with service users and carers, nominating frontline staff who are enthusiastic about developing ideas for change to become QI champions, who can work as a small group to identify areas of improvement, etc.

Care setting managers are involved in leading or participating in QI programmes. Therefore, it is important to both adopt a systematic approach to improvement through the application of appropriate models or frameworks and selected tools and methods to retain focus on service improvement.

Service improvement and service transformation

The concept service improvement in healthcare has prevailed for some time. It signifies proactive planned actions to improve health services. The NHS LTP (NHSE, 2019a: 111) recommends 'a reorientation away from ... performance management to supporting service improvement and transformation across health systems'. Complementarily, the Chartered Society for Physiotherapy (2018) distinguishes between service improvement and service transformation by indicating that improvement is about making service user care and treatment better, and transformation is about changing them in their form, appearance or structure, signifying more radical change of the service.

Service improvement is also a substantial component of the work of NHS support mechanisms GIRFT – Getting it right first time, and Rightcare, whose functions include generating and ensuring adoption of innovations and service improvement (NHSE, 2019a: 77, 104–5, 108).

Although service improvement is a term widely encountered in relation to health 'services', the term quality improvement is preferred in this book because it denotes quality as an already prevailing feature, which healthcare professionals endeavour to 'improve', while service improvement can imply starting from a poor-quality baseline.

A quality-conscious culture in the care setting

For high quality to prevail in care settings, an organisation-wide quality-aware culture needs to have been established. The importance of organisational culture was noted in Chapter 4 in relation to the voice of informal groups within employing organisations. The word culture and sub-culture refers to the individuals as well as the team collectively having shared values, norms and assumptions as well as being guided by certain rules of their own, beliefs that they hold in common, myths, behaviours, thoughts, and specific words, abbreviations, etc. that they use.

Different occupational groups are likely to have their own identifiable values, beliefs and attitudes, much of which tend to co-exist with those of other care professions. Nonetheless, these inherent features of profession-specific cultures endure over time, and team members feel they are beneficial and achieve success for them.

On the other hand, in the endeavour to urge everyone involved in health services to become much more quality-conscious, the Darzi Report (DH, 2008a: 48) asserted, 'make the achievement of high quality of care an obsession within the NHS', which suggests an enduring and omnipresent way of thinking, that is part of the culture of care settings. Consequently, if QI is to be achieved, then it follows that the culture and sub-culture of organisational units and sub-units have to value and believe in them for it to be ingrained as part of the culture.

In a review of the literature examining 70 instruments that were available for exploring organisational culture, Jung et al. (2009) concluded that none of them were ideal for assessing organisation culture. However, following work done previously at King's College London, NHS England (2017b) has published an online tool to enable healthcare teams to assess their workplace's culture of care, and thereby to identify areas of strength and weakness that can inform planning for improvements.

The development of a culture of care 'barometer' was instigated by major failings in healthcare organisations that had previously resulted in harm to service users, which when investigated revealed deficiencies in care, compassion and dignity for service users. Items in the Likert-type culture of care questionnaire include:

- I feel respected by my co-workers.
- My concerns are taken seriously by my line manager.
- The organisation listens to staff's views.
- I get the training and development I need.
- I am able to influence how things are done in this organisation.

These items clearly address features of cultures and sub-cultures in organisations. Following assessment, the online tool expects the team to take action to improve quality of care in health services as and when necessary. Another tool to assess sub-culture in healthcare organisations is the organisational values questionnaire used by Johansson et al. (2014) which was utilised with the aim of assessing the feasibility of change implementation in care settings (also referred to in Chapter 9 of this book in the context of management of change).

ACTION POINT 8.4
Culture of Care Barometer

Download the NHS England (2017b) Culture of Care Barometer from www.england.nhs.uk/wp-content/uploads/2017/03/ccb-barometer-rep-guide.pdf.
   Then perform a self-assessment of your care settings to gain an impression of the readiness of your workplace to implement changes to improve the quality of care being provided.

Research suggests a shift from a quantity-conscious culture to one that is quality-conscious (Sarre et al., 2020). Despite the general culture barometer noted in Action point 8.4 implying that there might be a model of quality culture, it is questionable whether the concept of 'cultural uniformity' and the 'cultural prescription' recommended by Francis (2013) is achievable.

A culture change that is effective and endures can be supported by the collective mode of leadership, along with a listening and trusting management. Furthermore, there is a direct link between ineffective leadership and compromised patient safety, as observed in several recent national high-profile reports on suboptimal care in the NHS, and collective leadership is recommended for a change of culture where high standards of care is valued (e.g. Nightingale, 2020). As noted in Chapter 3, collective leadership comprises developing and maintaining a leadership culture where several members of staff have designated leadership responsibilities.

Collective leadership is acknowledged in the NHS LTP (NHSE, 2019a: 89) which asserts that 'Great quality care needs great leadership at all levels. Evidence shows that the quality of care and organisational performance are directly affected by the quality of leadership and the improvement cultures leaders create.'

Moreover, team members can be asked to form a group, on a rotating basis, to monitor and suggest ways to improve quality. They could use appropriate QI tools and techniques, which they can choose from those published by NHS Improvement (2020b), some of which are discussed shortly in the next section under 'Contributory Quality Improvement Techniques'.

Organisational governance and clinical governance

A quality-conscious organisational culture in the care setting, as just noted above, refers to a collective and shared set of values, beliefs and behaviours, which new frontline staff assimilate progressively and get to own the culture. However, QI needs to be valued and supported by the organisation for it to be more fully effective, which is often performed by appointment or designation of top management level senior nurse or other appointee whose remit includes enhancing and monitoring quality of treatment and care at the healthcare trust. This is Board-level appointment, who essentially oversees 'organisational governance'.

The British Standards Institute's (2020) BS 13500 standard indicates that organisational governance constitutes of the organisation's rules and its defined sense of direction and purpose, and therefore is a framework that aims to continuously improve and assess its development. As a generic explanation of the concept, the word improve applies to QI in healthcare and the word assess suggests full awareness of its staff's level of knowledge and competence base, and subsequent learning to ensure they are up to date and current.

In healthcare, organisational governance has been known as clinical governance, which has been instituted in health services since around 1995. Healthcare trusts may even have a clinical governance building or section at its main site. The Royal College of Nursing (2020b: 1) has adopted the definition of clinical governance previously publicised in the BMJ by Scally and Donaldson (1998: 61), which identifies it as 'a system through which NHS organisations are accountable for continuously improving the quality of their services and safeguarding high standards of care by creating an environment in which excellence in clinical care will flourish'.

The above definition of clinical governance is referring to 'a system', which when translated signifies having structures and processes with a number of essential components or activities, which the RCN refers to as five key themes that are interconnected and constitutes a framework for looking closely at how to improve the quality of care. These themes are said to appear repeatedly in policy documents about healthcare quality, and they are:

- Patient focus – how services are based on patient needs;
- Information focus – how information is used;
- Quality improvement – how standards are reviewed and attained;
- Staff focus – how staff are developed; and
- Leadership – how improvement efforts are planned.

Structures, processes and activities comprise facilities for conducting risk management, audits, information management and patient surveys as and when required, and are discussed later in the chapter in the section on 'Contributory Quality Improvement Methods'.

Total quality management model

As a quality assurance model that has been derived primarily from industry, total quality management (TQM) has provided a holistic basis for QI that has been applied very successfully to production industries. In the purchaser-provider ethos that prevailed mostly until around 2008 in UK health services, the model was deemed fully appropriate to apply to healthcare. Although much of quality monitoring in healthcare now is dominated by CQC's national standards, the underpinning influence of TQM still prevails in terms of, for instance, the organisation's TQM philosophy of 'doing things right' and 'doing the right things', and use of such tools as lean methods and patient surveys.

Total quality management has been defined as the continual process of detecting and reducing or eliminating errors in manufacturing, streamlining supply chain management, improving the customer experience and ensuring that employees are up to speed with training by holding all parties involved in the production process accountable for the overall quality of the final product or service (Investopedia, 2020: 1). The definition suggests focusing on the customer needs, effective communication and involvement of all employees (total in TQM), and a highly trained and motivated workforce that continually seeks better ways of working (quality in TQM) which are all overseen by the management team (management in TQM) of the organisation.

The concepts in the definition resonate with approaches in healthcare in that customer needs equate with service users' needs, and involvement of all employees across all occupations in the organisation equates with inter-disciplinary working in health services. However, one of the primary flaws with the TQM model is its prime focus on the ongoing process of detecting and reducing or eliminating errors, while healthcare prime focus is on preventing errors and patient safety. Often referred to as 'quality management' (without the word total), the application of TQM as a model is only partly visible in healthcare, as more healthcare-specific QI models that apply more directly to healthcare such as CQC's standards, RCN's QI framework, etc. have been instituted.

Management of quality

In addition to the four QI concepts discussed above, the National Quality Board (NQB) (2016), which is supported by the FYFV (NHSE, 2014a) and builds on the recommendations of the highly regarded Darzi Report (DH, 2008a), identifies a seven-step framework for systematically addressing how to improve quality, as illustrated in Figure 8.2. The framework builds on already

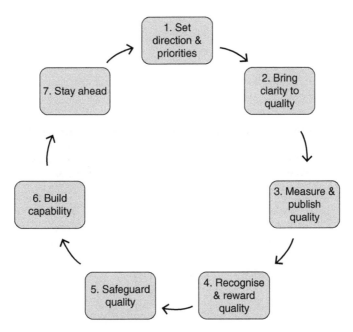

Figure 8.2   The seven-step framework for commitment to quality (National Quality Board, 2016: 8)

existing activities that are part of local clinical governance. To access further explanation of the NQB framework, see details in the Further Reading section of this chapter.

How to Improve Healthcare Quality – Models and Frameworks

Having discussed some of the key perspectives on QI, such as service improvement and service transformation, etc., the next section examines some of the most widely used models and frameworks of quality assurance. The term quality assurance denotes assuring or endeavouring to ensure that the quality of care provided is of the highest standard known, and is therefore a proactive approach, as different from quality monitoring activities conducted by the CQC and other organisations. It refers to assuring the service user of a high quality of care, and that actions will be taken to remedy any deficiency.

A range of published frameworks or models of quality management are available for measuring, monitoring and improving quality, and those discussed here are (see also Table 8.1 for brief details):

CQC's five headline questions model;
RCN Quality of Care framework;
Maxwell's elements of quality;
Donabedian's structure, process and outcome model; and
The Plan, Do, Study, Act (PDSA) cycle.

Table 8.1   Quality Improvement Models and Frameworks

CQC's five headline questions	RCN Quality of Care framework	Maxwell's elements of quality	Donabedian Model	The PDSA Cycle
• Are they safe?	• Patient focus	• Acceptability	• Structure	• Plan
• Are they effective?	• Information focus	• Accessibility	• Process	• Do
	• Quality improvement	• Appropriateness	• Outcome	• Study
• Are they caring?	• Staff focus	• Effectiveness		• Act
	• Leadership	• Efficiency		
• Are they responsive?		• Equity		
• Are they well-led?				

The CQC's five headline questions

Most healthcare professionals are likely to be familiar with the quality reviews conducted by the CQC using standards that come under the five headline questions. However, quality of care is monitored informally all the time, and formally periodically. How far a culture of quality care prevails in care settings is gauged in various ways, including by evaluation of care given, patient feedback, the healthcare professional's intuition, etc. Health and social care services are also externally monitored to ensure that standards are achieved, and outcomes are met. This monitoring function is provided through a number of channels in addition to the CQC, including local authorities (LAs), CCGs and NHSE+I.

The CQC monitors care quality formally regularly. It was established in 2010, when it replaced preceding organisations with quality of care monitoring roles, as an integrated independent regulator that monitors the quality of care in both NHS and non-NHS health and care sectors in England. Its role is to ensure that national standards of quality and safety are met by health and care providers, including acute and independent (private) hospitals, dental services; GP practices and out-of-hours or mobile doctor services, walk-in centres, minor injury units and urgent care centres (UCCs); homecare agencies providing care to people in their own homes; community-based services for people with learning disabilities, acute or chronic conditions; community and inpatient mental health services; family planning clinics; residential care homes and nursing homes; etc.

ACTION POINT 8.5
CQC activity at your workplace

Find out when the CQC last visited the care setting where you work as a FHM, and the specific results of their visit to monitor quality of care.

You could visit the CQC website and view the full detailed report from the latest inspection of your workplace at: 'Find a hospital | Care Quality Commission (cqc.org.uk)' and type in your organisation's name in the search box.

As noted in Chapter 1 when perusing the contemporary context of healthcare, the CQC's role includes inspecting quality of care and patient safety, and to become the recipient of inspection, care services in England have to register with the CQC. The standards by which the CQC inspect services is transparent and publicly available on its websites (CQC, 2020a), and come under five headline questions aimed at all care services:

1. Are they safe? – i.e. protected from avoidable harm and abuse.

2. Are they effective? – i.e. care, treatment and support result in outcomes related to quality of life for the service user, and is based on the best available evidence.
3. Are they caring? – i.e. service users are treated with compassion, dignity and respect.
4. Are they responsive to people's needs? – i.e. to individual service user's needs.
5. Are they well-led? – i.e. the management and governance (quality monitoring) are focused on providing high-quality care and promotes an open and fair culture.

After inspection, the CQC rates the service inspected as outstanding, good, requires improvement or inadequate, and takes action as they see appropriate to protect vulnerable people as the baseline.

The CQC also conducts patient surveys 'to find out what people think of the NHS healthcare services that they use' (CQC, 2020b). Its survey of maternity care services exploring the experiences of women who had a live birth in 2019, for example, found that women feel they are listened to by midwives and their concerns taken seriously, that staff respected their feeding choices, but that there was still scope for improvement in post-natal care which was consistently poorer than the care they received during pregnancy and labour. Other examples of surveys conducted by the CQC include adult in-patients, community mental health, children and young people, urgent and emergency care, ambulance, outpatients, etc.

RCN quality of care framework and clinical governance

The RCN's (2019c) Quality of Care framework comprises five key themes that it states repeatedly appears in policy documents on healthcare quality, as identified on Table 8.1, and details were given in the preceding section entitled 'Organisational governance and clinical governance'.

The 'information focus' theme is placed at the centre of a circle containing the other four themes, indicating the high significance of information management and communication in healthcare organisations and care settings. Ample details of the RCN framework are available in the publication for it to be applied to implement quality improvement in care settings.

Maxwell's elements of quality framework

As a quality framework that can be applied to most product and service organisations, Maxwell's (1984) six-element quality framework is comprehensive, and can easily be applied within healthcare. It comprises three 'A's and three 'E's, namely Acceptability, Accessibility, Appropriateness, Effectiveness, Efficiency and Equity.

Applied to the care setting, for pain management for example, if the care standard is that all patients should be pain-free within ten minutes of complaining of pain, then Maxwell's model can be used to monitor whether:

this standard is 'acceptable' to the patient and staff;

they have 'access' to the healthcare practitioners to obtain pain-relieving interventions;

the means of pain relief is 'appropriate';

the method of pain relief is 'effective' from the patient's and the healthcare professional's viewpoints;

the pain relief is administered 'efficiently' (without wasting time or any materials); and

all patients are afforded the 'same standard' of care (equity).

Donabedian's structure-process-outcome model of quality improvement

As a straightforward and simpler but highly effective model of quality improvement in healthcare devised by Donabedian (2005) in the 1980s, this model consists of three sets of criteria: structure, process and outcome. The Donabedian model is also discussed as a model of evaluation of change in Chapter 9 of this book.

Structure criteria comprise the main physical structure and infrastructure required to deliver care. It therefore represents the buildings that house the healthcare provider; the employees (including staff numbers, skill mix, training, expertise); the equipment, medical devices and consumables; ancillary services – e.g. laundry, pharmacy, paramedical services, catering, laboratory services; the agreed policies and procedures, rules and regulations; etc.

Process criteria refers to the care and clinical activities performed by healthcare professionals and team members, and therefore involves assessment of patients' health problems, planning and implementation of care, and evaluation and making changes where appropriate. It encompasses the staff's knowledge and competence; training to apply the healthcare organisation's procedures and clinical guidelines; clinical interventions and education of service users and their carers and relatives;methods of documenting; and ways in which resources are used.

The *outcome criteria* represents the specific benefits or positive results experienced by the patient, which encompass indicators of patient outcomes such as health status, wound healing, patient satisfaction, immunisation uptake, patients' knowledge of their condition, behaviours such as successful use of medical devices by patients, as well as evaluation of the competence of staff delivering care.

The Donabedian model has been widely and successfully applied in the contexts of both quality improvement and evaluation of change (e.g. Gardner et al.,

2014). The PDSA Model (e.g. IHI, 2020b) presented on Table 8.1 is discussed and applied in Chapter 9 in the context of management of change.

Contributory Quality Improvement Techniques

Having examined some of the popular forms of QI (e.g. service transformation), followed by QA frameworks and models that can be applied, this section now focuses on a number of specific QA techniques or methods that can be applied to monitor quality of care and service improvement on a smaller scale, which contribute to the implementing of QA frameworks that lead to a fuller and more comprehensive implementation of the chosen framework. The following techniques are addressed in this section, which also addresses potential barriers to quality improvement:

- Quality of care patient satisfaction surveys;
- Quantifying quality of care through the use of metrics;
- Healthcare or clinical audits; and
- Process mapping, care bundles, benchmarking.

Quality of care surveys

Patient satisfaction surveys is one of the earliest techniques used to gauge service users' experience of healthcare that they received, mostly in acute hospitals. Previously, a questionnaire was posted to patients' home addresses after discharge from hospital asking about noise on the ward during their hospital stay, quality of meals, waking up times, etc. This technique is now more instantaneous through the use of fewer and simpler questions that service users are asked while still an in-patient.

There is a variety of these surveys, an analysis of which was presented earlier in this chapter under service users' experience of health services. The CQC (2020b) is an example of national patient surveys that are conducted regularly to assess service users' experiences of different areas of healthcare services and the findings are publicly available over the internet.

Such surveys can identify both areas of satisfaction and areas of dissatisfaction with healthcare experience. For example, in their cross-sectional study of patient satisfaction ratings, Perneger et al. (2020) concluded that patients who are generally satisfied with the service and are also eager to please others are likely to both complete and return the questionnaire and to rate the care received highly. Conversely, those who do not return questionnaires are the ones who are dissatisfied. It seems logical, therefore, that service users who do not return questionnaires should be followed up, with a view to obtaining not just ratings, but also qualitative details of areas of their dissatisfaction.

Quantifying quality of care

On the one hand, healthcare is awash with statistics gathered continuously either to justify actions or to demonstrate accountability for money spent on specific care interventions or to monitor how far government quality of care targets for healthcare (such as patients' waiting times in A&E departments) are being met. Several attempts have been made over the years to quantify episodes or items of care, which have been known as key performance indicators, quality indicators, nursing metrics, patient outcome indicators and similar terms, so that they can be costed, and finance made available to the healthcare provider or team based on the data collected.

The use of these mechanisms, especially metrics, peaked by around 2010 and then gradually receded into the background but indicators and outcomes have remained prominent. Healthcare metrics are specific quality indicators on such items as incidences of patient falls and injuries, hospital-acquired infection rates, etc. As a quality indicator, metrics tend to feature as numerical data from bespoke data collection tools and comprises a point of reference by which performance in the provision of services or care can be measured, as also noted in the *Health and Social Care Act 2012* (Legislation.gov.uk, 2012).

There has been endeavours to quantify most aspects of care. However, when it comes to quantifying such care interventions as 'being compassionate' or being respectful to patients, or maintaining their dignity, these have proved problematic. Such quantification of care tends not to feature as highest priority when there are peak demands on the health service, such as during an influenza epidemic, the coronavirus pandemic, etc.

Furthermore, as Griffiths and Maben (2009) noted, although there are many benefits for keeping healthcare metrics, they are problematic because, for example, three macro-interventions – patient safety, effectiveness and compassion – are not delivered in isolation, and are therefore quite challenging to quantify separately. Furthermore, Nursing Standard News (2009: 11) also indicated that staff feel 'bamboozled and alienated by metrics jargon' as nurses felt confused by indicators introduced to measure the quality of their care, which is accompanied by difficulties in collecting data.

Nonetheless, data and statistics have to be collected for all interventions that can be quantified for purposes of allocation of resources, accountability and monitoring quality of care, and progress that has been made with this process. Examples include incidence of pressure injuries during hospital stay, availability of psychological therapies, re-admission rates, childhood immunisations, drug administration errors, etc.

Evidence of the benefits of metrics as quality indicators include research by Radecki et al. (2020), whereupon metrics (numerical information) collected using a patient fall assessment tool through collaborative safety conversations with patients and engaging each as 'experts' in the development of their own safety plan. Patient participation in the development of the safety plan resulted in 25% reduction in falls and 67% reduction in injury from falls.

Healthcare audits

Often known simply as audits, or as clinical audits, healthcare audits are very useful tools for gauging quality of care. A clinical audit comprises a systematic assessment of the process or outcome of a care activity to determine whether it is:

Effective:　making progress towards particular goals.
Efficient:　achieving a particular target with the least effort.
Economic:　achieving a successful outcome with the minimum cost.

Audits measure the extent to which healthcare workers adhere to approved guidelines in the course of their daily duties and whether agreed best practice is being followed. There are two types of audit: (1) *retrospective*, which examines what happened after the episode of care has been completed; and (2) *concurrent*, which examines what is happening at the time of the care activity.

An example of a retrospective audit is a scrutiny of monitoring charts such as fluid balance charts to establish that they are being completed in full; and an example of a concurrent audit is hand washing, where the auditor monitors whether approved handwashing techniques are being followed when performing this task. A range of methods are used to collect audit data on the quality of care, including observation, checklists, questionnaires, interviews, documentation checking and case reviews.

Process mapping, care bundles, benchmarking

A number of other QI methods and techniques that contribute to assuring or monitoring quality of care have been documented including process mapping, care bundles, benchmarking and lean methods. These and other tools can be viewed in the NHSI (2020b) publication *Quality, Service Improvement and Redesign (QSIR) Tools*.

Process mapping refers fundamentally to delineating the service user's journey (NHSI, 2020b) through the health system, whereupon the process mapper diagrammatically identifies every step of the journey from the point in time when they first make contact with healthcare (often the GP), and the amount of time spent at each intervention, and the time span between each intervention, etc. Thereby, a clear picture of all care activities and interventions are identified (which are represented in the service user's care pathway), and undertaken by whom, so that any blocks and delays in the system can be identified and action taken to prevent them in future.

Care bundles generally apply to critical care settings. A care bundle is a straightforward structured set of three to five evidence-based interventions which, when performed together, have better patient outcomes than if performed individually. It is normally related to a particular condition or event in patient care, and is a means of assessing quality of care, and is known to prevent avoidable morbidity and mortality (e.g. Horner and Bellamy, 2012). Examples of care bundles with specific components include sepsis management bundle, resuscitation bundle and ventilator bundle.

Benchmarking comprises a quality improvement technique based on peer-learning whereupon when a change or innovation in care methods has been reported in a specific aspect of care at a particular health service provider as 'best practice' and is evidence-informed, then peers (healthcare professionals) from other healthcare providers in the same specialist area might contact the former to obtain detailed information on ways in which the innovation or change was achieved and how it improves patient outcomes or quality of care. Thereafter, the practice can be adopted at the latter's healthcare organisation or care setting, maybe in collaboration with the former.

These tools form part of the overall QI techniques, and therefore an appropriate combination of them can be applied. Rowson and McSherry (2018), for instance, report on a locally constituted unique integrated QI framework that is based on the CQC's (2020a) criteria that uses benchmarking among other tools, and which enables the framework to act as an internal accreditation system.

Issues Related to Improving Quality

With regards to issues that can surface when endeavouring to improve quality of care, this section explores potential barriers to quality improvement, managing service user complaints, duty of candour, and clinical negligence and its implications.

Potential barriers to quality improvement

As noted near the beginning of this chapter, there is no universal definition of the terms quality and quality in healthcare, because perceptions of quality are subjective to individual healthcare professionals. At organisational level, there is a range or sets of criteria utilised by different organisations for quality assurance and for monitoring quality – see, for example, Table 8.1 'Quality Assurance Models and Frameworks' above.

> # ACTION POINT 8.6
> ## Which QI techniques are applied in your care setting to monitor or assure quality of care?
>
> Ponder on the ways quality of care is managed in your care setting by the care team, by the healthcare provider organisation and by national organisations, and make some notes. If you are a relatively new FHM, it might prove useful to discuss this with a peer or colleague with whom you share mutual trust and respect.

Detailed records of quality monitoring and assurance are often filed away (in paper-form and/or electronically) in practice settings, which is probably because quality is relatively rarely achieved at the optimal level. Whether they are audit results or the result of a CQC inspection, the highest awards or grades (e.g. 'Outstanding' by CQC) are only sporadically achieved. Frontline staff and FHMs' lack of detailed knowledge of CQC's criteria for quality or criteria in local audits is therefore a barrier to quality improvement. Other barriers could be lack of appropriate resources, human resources and non-human.

Barriers to quality improvement were explored through the use of surveys and interviews by Feary (2012), for example, who identified lack of leadership (note 'well-led' is one of the five sections of criteria currently used by the CQC) in delivering quality as one of the most prominent barriers. Feary found that managers saw effective running of the organisation and quality of service as high priority, while frontline care delivery staff felt patient outcomes and patient experience are the best indicators of high quality. In other words, managers and healthcare professionals had different priorities in healthcare.

Other barriers to quality improvement noted by Feary include time available to focus on quality, lack of training in quality sensitiveness, staff morale and government targets. Lack of time and managers and healthcare professionals having different priorities in healthcare has also been identified by Zoutman and Ford (2017) and others as barriers to quality improvement, which they indicate can be rectified by enabling more staff engagement in quality than is generally prevalent, and by 'daily time allotted to QI activities'.

Managing service user complaints

The service user or their relatives might complain about the care or treatment that they received either during a care intervention or soon after. The complaint might be made verbally, or maybe in written form afterwards if they feel that the standard of care has been below the standard they expected. The NHS Constitution (DHSC, 2019a) asserts that every patient has the right to expect competent and safe healthcare from care professionals employed by the service provider. There-fore, when this doesn't happen, then service users have the right to complain formally about any malpractice if they choose to do so.

The FHM has to have knowledge of the procedure that the complainant should follow, and has to guide them to the complaint form they need to complete, and inform them of who to send the complaint to. Complaints can be seen as one of the vehicles that reflect standards of care from the recipient's viewpoint, and con-versely it should not be assumed that service users are satisfied with the care they receive merely because the care setting does not receive any formal complaint.

Service providers and healthcare managers, therefore, need to be comfortable with the idea that when a complaint is received, the complaint reflects the actual experiences of the service user, and ensure that root causes are investigated and resolved. In some instances, the component requiring redress is confined to one care setting or area, while in other instances organisation-wide changes may need to be made to review policies, clinical guidelines and leadership.

ACTION POINT 8.7
Why are service users reluctant to complain?

It has been suggested in the past that generally service users are unwilling to complain formally when the care they receive is below the standard they had expected, particularly for aspects that they consider to be less significant than their main health problem, such as noise at night that disturbs their sleep or delays in receiving information about their prognosis.

1. Is this suggestion consistent with your experience as FHM, and if so, then why are service users reluctant to complain? What are the likely reasons?
2. If they do complain, what actions could be implemented in the care setting or organisation-wide to resolve the complaint and to share the learning from them?

Information on ways in which service users can raise a complaint about a ser-vice are generally visible in clinical settings. Often the care area has a leaflet prom-inently placed that indicates how to do so, and of course such information is also available on the trust's website. The advice to service users generally is to address the complaint to the care staff in the care setting, who would normally investigate and endeavour to resolve the issue. However, if the service user feels their con-cern has not been resolved, or they are not comfortable discussing the issue with the care setting staff directly, then they are advised to contact the Trust's Patient Advice & Liaison Service (PALS), or email, telephone or write to the trust, and a letter template is likely to be available on the website for the complainant to use if they wish to do so.

The reasons why service users do not complain about healthcare could include the following:

- Do not want to relive an unpleasant experience.
- Unaware that they are allowed to complain.
- Feeling grateful enough for any care received.
- Fear of lapsing into aggressive behaviour if complain is not heeded or understood.
- Do not know who to complain to.
- Do not want to, or are unable to, write letter of complaint or fill complaint forms.
- Fear of being ill-treated or labelled 'complainer' or 'moaner' after complaining.
- Feel they might not receive good care if re-admitted to the same team in future.

Subsequent to receiving the complaint, the trust investigates the problem and often aims to resolve it in around three weeks. If the service user is still unhappy with the outcome, they are advised to contact the Parliamentary and Health Service Ombudsman (2015) to review the complaint, who in 2014-15 reported receiving 21,371 complaints about different NHS organisations which were unresolved locally, and which they group under such headings as staff attitude, not acknowledging mistakes, poor apology/remedy, etc. Health service providers are normally willing to listen to service users' complaints, respond to them and learn from them, and they are also required to do so.

Clinical negligence and its implications

The NHS LTP (NHSE, 2019a: 107) acknowledges that in addition to reducing harm to service users, strategies for improving patient safety will also reduce costs substantially. These costs are in terms of claims of clinical negligence made by service users or their relatives, which has been a significant issue for several years leading to scarce NHS money being wasted. To monitor and provide healthcare providers with support on this issue, the NHS Resolution and the NHS Counter Fraud Authority have been established. A part of the role of the NHS Resolution (whose predecessor was the National Health Service Litigation Authority) is to handle negligence claims and also help service providers learn lessons from claims to improve patient and staff safety.

Simultaneously, the NHS Counter Fraud Authority was established to investigate and manage suspected fraudulent claims and corruption related to service users claims, payroll and procurement (NHSE, 2019a).

On evaluating the current position on clinical negligence costs, researchers Yau et al. (2020) observe that spending on clinical negligence is escalating, which constitutes a major threat to the sustainability of the NHS in England, especially as payments for negligence awards are drawn from the funds that are allocated for providing care. The NHS paid £2.4bn in clinical negligence claims in 2018-19 (Yau et al., 2020). Maternity care accounted for 50% of the total amount of money claimed in 2018–19, according to NHS Resolution, mostly because of injury to the child at birth.

Yau et al. indicate that improvements in quality and patient safety might help to reduce litigation costs but requires system-wide effort, engagement and co-ordination. They recommend four areas of fundamental principles for safer care and actions to take when mistakes occur: (1) invest in staff and infrastructure (structural problems); (2) a real commitment to learning; (3) learning from high performance; and (4) enable and support system-wide safety improvements.

Guidance for ensuring high-quality care

The following comprise guidance for ensuring delivery of highest quality of care:

Acquire detailed knowledge of the wide range of instances that have led to marked emphasis on quality of treatment and care in health services.

Take time to enable team members to reflect on what constitutes high-quality healthcare, arriving at a definition of high-quality care, a definition that incorporates the national requirements for quality to address patient safety, clinical effectiveness and service users' experience of healthcare delivery.

Be knowledgeable about your organisation's quality metrics against which quality performance of your practice setting is monitored and reviewed regularly or periodically.

Ensure you have knowledge of major current quality improvement concepts such as service improvement, and organisational governance and clinical governance.

Be conversant with prominent published quality improvement models and frameworks, as well as contributory QI techniques and methods.

Create an environment that supports a quality-conscious culture in the care setting, and during meetings discuss safety issues and ways in which quality can be ascertained and further improved.

Reflect on your leadership in relation to service improvement, and review progress regularly to explore how you can strengthen your approach.

Monitor team members' compliance with policies, procedures and guidelines.

Informally ask service users about their experiences of quality of care and whether they have any suggestions regarding how care could be improved.

Be aware of issues related to improving quality and have full knowledge of the management of service user complaints, including the implications of clinical negligence claims.

Chapter Summary

The actions that FHMs take to check that the quality of care being delivered in their practice setting meets expected standards are crucial for both staff satisfaction and patient satisfaction. The focus of this chapter has been on high-quality care, that is on what high-quality care is, why we have to be quality conscious, how to improve or enhance quality, and what are the consequences of not monitoring the quality of care healthcare professionals provide. Consequently, this chapter has addressed:

- The reasons for the current high level of emphasis on delivering and monitoring quality of healthcare received by service users;
- Definitions of quality of care, and the principal healthcare criteria including patient safety, clinical effectiveness and service users' experience by which quality is judged, as well as analysing the role of a quality-conscious culture in care settings;
- Knowledge of several of the wide array of quality improvement frameworks and models such as National Quality Board's seven-step framework for commitment to quality, clinical governance, Maxwell's elements of quality and Care Quality Commission's criteria for quality that applies to care settings and to service improvement and transformation;
- Application of multiple quality improvement methods and techniques that contribute to enhancing and monitoring quality of care in practice settings such as quality of care surveys, metrics and healthcare audits;
- Knowledge of barriers to quality improvement and of issues related to suboptimal quality of care;
- Ways in which FHMs support quality monitoring and quality improvement in care settings or in the organisation, which includes the application of evidence-based practice through the implementation of approved clinical guidelines and policies.

Further Reading

- The National Quality Board's (NQB) (2016) seven-step framework for systematically addressing how to improve quality, which is supported by the NHS England's (2014a) *Five Year Forward View*, see: National Quality Board (2016) *Shared Commitment to Quality from the National Quality Board*. Available at: www.england.nhs.uk/wp-content/uploads/2016/12/nqb-shared-commitment-frmwrk.pdf. Accessed Date: 3 September 2020.
- For a detailed account of quality improvement (QI) in healthcare which includes the systematic use of methods and tools to try to continuously improve quality of care and outcomes for patients, see: King's Fund (2017) *Making the Case for Quality Improvement: Lessons for NHS Boards and*

Leaders. Available at: www.kingsfund.org.uk/publications/making-case-quality-improvement#:~:text=The%20term%20'quality%20improvement'%20refers,Healthcare%20Improvement's%20Model%20for%20Improvement. Accessed Date: 25 March 2021.

- For recent guidance on quality improvement, see: Health Foundation (2021) *Quality Improvement Made Simple What Everyone Should Know About Health Care Quality Improvement* (3rd edn). Available at: Quality improvement made simple (health.org.uk). Accessed Date: 19 July 2021.

9

Managing Change, Improvement and Innovations

Chapter Objectives

The chapter objectives for frontline healthcare managers in relation to managing change, improvements and innovations are:

- After identifying recent changes in care and treatment methods in your area of practice, enunciate reasons for continuing changes in healthcare delivery;
- Explain systematic ways of managing the implementation of change, using well-informed alternative management of change frameworks or models;
- Demonstrate knowledge of the application of project management as a form of change management for quality improvement, and the associated risk assessment and management activities;
- Ascertain ways of ensuring team members recognise, analyse, prepare and apply strategies for change taking into account the sub-organisational culture and users' perspective;
- Demonstrate knowledge of planning and leading the change which incorporate applying contributory strategies initiated by the change leader for implementing change;
- Show knowledge of means of evaluating and sustaining the change.

Introduction

As most healthcare professionals know, changes in the ways in which we deliver care is an integral feature of clinical practice, which is driven partly by the requirement for evidence-informed practice. Often only small changes are made, such as forms or charts to be filled, which catheter to use, which dressings to apply, procedures to be followed, etc. Health and care organisations in particular are subject to ongoing change, which is at times due to the need for efficiency, such as cheaper medical devices, or communicating with patients over the telephone rather than face-to-face.

Ongoing change is an important feature of forward-looking organisations, and for profit-making organisations including those who manufacture medications or medical devices, it is unavoidable either for growth or just survival. This chapter focuses specifically on the several reasons for changes in healthcare organisations, and ways in which to 'manage' change both systematically and effectively, and therefore the role of FHMs in managing and leading change, and also evaluating the impact of change and then embedding them in clinical practice. Project management as a way of introducing major changes is also examined.

Recent Changes in Care Delivery Methods

Numerous research studies in healthcare are conducted each year and their findings and recommendations for changes usually disseminated, frequently published, and some get applied to practice depending partly on the quality of the research. Furthermore, new national and local policies initiated by government directives as well as new technology also prompt changes in healthcare practice. The aim of these triggers for changes are usually quality improvement, but can also be related to cost-effectiveness and productivity.

ACTION POINT 9.1
Recent changes in your care setting

Thinking about your own place of work or your specialist area of healthcare, think of any changes that have been made to care interventions over the past few weeks, or few months, or in the last year or even going further back. Think of specific methods of delivery of care, or the ways in which staff and work are organised, or of any innovations. The change may have been initiated bottom-up or directed by more senior managers.

Next, think of an aspect of practice in your work setting that you feel would benefit from change. This may have been triggered by a research article that you read, a discussion with colleagues regarding perhaps a new way of resolving an issue, or an innovation that you came across at a study day or conference.

Depending on the range of patient care activities required in your specialist area, you should have been able to identify some, or several, changes or innovations made or encountered in the last 12 months, smaller changes or major ones. Some of the changes or innovations you mentioned might include the following:

- National Early Warning Score (NEWS2) or 'Track and trigger' scoring systems for assessing deterioration in patients.
- Bedside shift handover.
- Enhanced recovery after surgery.
- Cognitive Stimulation Therapy – a NICE-recommended psychosocial intervention for people with mild to moderate dementia.
- GPs prescribing gymnasium exercise to patient with mobility problems.
- Meals served on a colour-coded tray to identify patients who require encouragement to eat.
- Diabetes patch implant for more effective monitoring and management of type 1 diabetes.
- New pain scales, e.g. for non-communicative children.
- Improving access to psychological therapies (IAPT) programme for anxiety disorders or depression.
- Health MOTs at GP's practice for people over 75.
- Single-handed care supported by equipment and technology to enhance patient privacy and dignity.
- Robots and artificial intelligence to help elderly people in their own homes reminding them to take medication, to trying to mimic human interaction for companionship.
- Admiral nurse – specialist nurse with expertise in supporting people affected by dementia and their family/carers who experience difficulties.
- Vanguards for new model of healthcare provision.

Various other examples of innovations and change can be added to the above list based on the reader's own professional experience. More details of these innovations are widely available through the internet. For example, for NEWS2, Skills for Health (2019) explains that following its early beginnings in 2012 as 'Early warning systems', latter versions have been led by the Royal College of Physicians, which after extensive user feedback is now in its current form and very widely used. Training for NEWS2 can be more focused, with NEWS2 for sepsis, for hypercapnic respiratory failure, etc. Other published tools for assessment of physiological deterioration in hospital patients include Maternity Early Warning Score (can be modified by adding 'obstetric' for example) and Paediatric Early Warning Score.

Another innovation is virtual reality therapy that is applied to help people with mental problems, especially focusing on exposure-based intervention for anxiety disorders such as phobia, post-traumatic stress disorder and stress relief. Yet another is single-handed care which refers to providing equipment that enables specific interventions to be performed by only one healthcare practitioner, rather than by two staff members up to now. It is, however, useful to remember that such tools are only as good as the healthcare professional's competence and willingness to use them.

Change, however, is a different concept to innovation in that change occurs to something that is already established (e.g. change from EWS to NEWS2), by changing certain components of the intervention. 'Innovation' refers to something new, a method of care delivery, or area of care provision that is largely unprecedented. Innovation is defined by West et al. (2017: 5) as:

> the introduction and application of processes, products, treatments or procedures, new to the team, department, ward, pathway, organisation or system and intended to benefit patients, staff, the organisation or the wider society.

Changes to ways in which care is managed include: Integrated care systems (ICSs); assistive technology; virtual wards for patients who are at risk of emergency hospitalisation; electronic records; telehealth/telemedicine; outreach work; and new roles, e.g. physician assistants and nursing associates. With the use of assistive technology, for example, people with increasingly complex health and social care needs can be supported to have their needs met in their own home, where previously they may have required monitoring in an inpatient or residential setting.

Digitalisation in Health Services

New electronic devices are increasingly facilitating access to health services, which is one aspect of digitalisation of care provision and an example of NHS-wide change. Digitalisation has been increasing consistently, and an example of one of the landmarks has been the establishment of Health and Social Care Information Centre in 2016, which had been set up as part of the HSCA 2012 as the national provider of information, data and IT systems for commissioners, analysts and clinicians in health and social care in the UK.

The centre was replaced by NHS Digital (2020b), who indicates that it is the national information and technology partner for the health and social care system that helps healthcare professionals (including doctors and nurses) to improve efficiency and make care safer, by for example:

- Creating and maintaining the technological infrastructure that links systems in the health service together to provide a seamless service.
- Providing information to the health service to support more effective planning and monitor progress.

Examples cited by NHS Digital (2020c) include:

- Child protection information system – for helping health and social care staff share information securely to better protect society's most vulnerable children.
- Electronic Prescription Service – that sends electronic prescriptions from GP to pharmacies.
- Bowel cancer screening invitation – by identifying people who are eligible and inviting them to participate in screening (also has a separate system for breast screening, and other forms of screening).
- Hospital Episode Statistics – a data warehouse containing details of all admissions, outpatient appointments and A&E attendance at NHS hospitals in England.
- Summary Care Records – an electronic record of important patient information, created from GP medical records, which can be seen and used by authorised staff in other areas of the health and care system involved in the patient's direct care.

Furthermore, the NHS is making significant advances in 'digital diagnosis' with the use of artificial intelligence imaging technology to speed up the diagnosis and accuracy of illnesses like cancer, and thereby also free up more staff time (DHSC, 2020c). They will, according to the DHSC, lead to more personalised treatments for patients, and consequently improve survival rate.

Digitalisation in health services has been evolving gradually, but research on this is still very limited, both in numbers and in quality. A review of research on healthcare students' experience of using digital technology in patient care by Wilson et al. (2020) revealed that their autonomous use by students is relatively limited (due to their student status) and therefore their learning needs in their use during practice placements. Furthermore, regarding the use of personal digital assistants, although beneficial for students, they could be seen as having a negative effect on nurse–patient relationship. Examples of digital technology students are exposed to include wearable devices, smartphone apps, e.g. personal digital assistants, telemedicine and electronic health records (EHRs).

Additionally, NHSX (X stands for user experience) (2021b) is a parallel but separate organisation to NHS Digital that was instituted in 2019 as part of NHS LTP to focus on improving patient experience in the therapy areas of cancer and mental health by providing staff and service users with technological devices that can be used for more video consultations and thereby improve the speed of access to clinical staff.

Why Make Changes in Healthcare Delivery?

New research findings and government-based policies for improvement in healthcare consistently drive changes in health and social care services. Change is also enabled through clinician changing practice to improve care for service users which is also referred to as clinical practice development, and it can also be triggered by service users' expectations of health services. However, for these changes to be successfully implemented, they need to be managed and led systematically, step-by-step.

In other words, changes in care are driven by innovations and service improvement as well as evidence-informed practice. Changes also occur in response to evaluation of effectiveness of care given, complaints received and suggestions. At other times, change seems to evolve naturally in practice settings. The role of frontline managers, including FHMs, involves managing change, as noted under the 'Evidence-informed clinician' role on Tables 4.1 and 10.1, as well as in Mintzberg's (2011) management role theory as 'entrepreneurial roles'. Consequently, FHMs need to have good insight into and developed expertise in the management of change.

Yet another trigger for change in nursing practice has been the proliferation of 'Nursing Development Units' at a handful of healthcare sites where improvements in nursing practice were successfully implemented at the turn of the millennium and where most of the changes were implemented accompanied by action research or the Donabedian (1988) model of evaluation. Such changes have been referred to as practice development (e.g. England Centre for Practice Development, 2021) (at Canterbury Christ Church University).

Practice development refers to experimenting with new ways of delivering everyday patient-related care interventions, or for providing new care services, in order to enhance person-centred, safe and effective care delivery. Healthcare professionals always endeavour to improve the care they provide, and under the 'service improvement' domain, the NHS KSF (NHS Employers, 2019b) indicates that every team member can be a practice developer.

Service improvement itself is defined as 'a systematic approach that uses specific techniques to deliver and measure sustained improvements in quality' (Gage, 2013: 52), and is often used interchangeably with the term quality improvement (discussed in Chapter 8 of this book).

Another avenue for change is through 'nurse entrepreneurs', who systematically implement radically new care intervention initiatives locally or nationally for specific groups of individuals with one or more common health problems (e.g. malnourished homeless people); a role often initiated by health visitors, nurse or AHP consultants, and non-NHS healthcare practitioners working in alternative medicine.

Innovations and Service Improvement

Several instances of transformation of patient outcomes through innovations and service improvement by nurses, midwives and AHPs have been documented (e.g. Council of Deans of Health [CODH], 2014). One example is related to improving recovery in mental health services which has resulted in a reduction in the use of mainstream services and has enhanced the quality of life enjoyed by people with mental health problems. Another is related to the training delivered to several health and social care practitioners on promotion of self-management methods for service users that has led to improvement in quality of life and self-efficacy following stroke rehabilitation.

Other examples cited by CODH include preventing pressure ulcers, people with long-term conditions being supported to self-manage their conditions, etc. Further key publications on practice development and innovations are available from the RCN, NHSE and other organisations, including NHSE (2020c) and NHSE (2014c).

Additionally, health and social care journals, professional trade union organisations, as well as the CQC and other professional organisations, frequently publish information publicising and promoting innovation and examples of best practice. They document examples of good practice and projects where vision and focus by individuals and teams have had positive results in terms of care outcomes. Areas of good practice are also highlighted by various organisations such as Royal Colleges, the DHSC; and also through professional award initiatives such as the Nursing Times Awards for recognising 'exceptional work' by healthcare professionals.

Evidence-Informed Practice

As already noted earlier in this chapter, one of the notions that prompts changes in healthcare is new evidence from research, which is referred to as evidence-informed practice (and also evidence-based practice [EBP]). It constitutes care and treatment based on best available evidence being applied to patient care, resulting in improved quality of care. Evidence-informed practice is also often included in a clause of healthcare professionals' code of practice (e.g. NMC, 2018b).

An associated term is evidence-based healthcare, which is evidence-informed best practice related to groups of patients with a specific long-term condition, while EBP refers to single care interventions. Best evidence, however, needs to be applied in conjunction with healthcare professionals' vocational experience, and the actions taken are continually appraised.

Several sources of evidence that support improvements in care can be accessed. These include research findings from randomised controlled trials (RCTs), for example, and from qualitative studies; findings from systematic reviews and meta-analyses available from electronic databases, e.g. Cochrane Library; clinical guidelines; colleagues' and other healthcare professionals' knowledge; service user and their family; suppliers' information, etc.

Evidence that have been extracted from these sources can be categorised as grades or levels of evidence to identify the strength of evidence supporting the care intervention. Five levels of evidence can be identified, which are usually presented as a hierarchy of evidence (see Figure 9.1) with the strongest evidence placed at the top of the hierarchy. Some sources also identify a number of sub-levels.

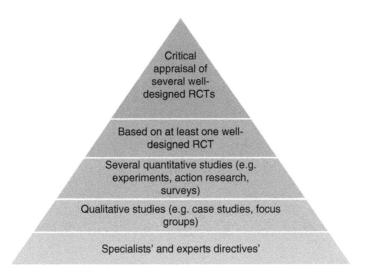

Figure 9.1   Hierarchy of evidence for EBP

In addition to the Cochrane Library website where evidence constituted from systematic reviews of research are available, other electronic sources include NHS Evidence, Joanna Briggs Institute, SIGN and other organisations. However, when considering applying evidence to practice, the service user's preferences also needs to be taken into account whenever this is feasible and beneficial.

The Management of Change

New research findings and recommendations, new medical devices, digitalisation and other service improvements (e.g. in management of sepsis) are examples of reasons for changes in the ways in which healthcare professionals deliver care to services users. Instances of change generally surface when they are either:

- presented as an initiative by senior managers or at national level (i.e. imposed);
- instituted after brief discussions (i.e. introduced);
- developed (evolved) over time;

- personal change due to life circumstances, e.g. bereavement, being diagnosed with a long-term illness; or
- systematically managed as a process.

Consequently, change could be applied at organisational level, team or individual level, but for the change to be fully effective, owned by the users and continued following implementation, they have to be managed systematically, as a step-by-step process. Some changes can be relatively minor and require just one or two amendments to existing procedures or guidelines (e.g. changing one or two components of a pressure injury assessment scale or a pain assessment scale). Other changes can be more substantial, and others major changes.

ACTION POINT 9.2
How change is implemented in your care setting

Thinking of the above-mentioned ways in which change is introduced in care settings, consider a recent change in your practice setting, and make some notes on the ways in which the change was made, implemented or managed.

The NMC (2018b: 19, clause 5.12) identifies the ability to influence change as one of the standards in which NRNs should be proficient by the time they qualify as RNs, stating that at the point of registration, the registered nurse will be able to 'understand the mechanisms that can be used to influence organisational change and public policy,'.

Thus, the different ways in which change can affect individual users can vary depending on whether they feel involved and feel they have ownership of the change, whether they are excited about it or stressed, and whether they feel it will increase their individual responsibility, or they feel it will improve patient care. Furthermore, for more major changes, such as changing to use of a new computer program or to manage an anticipated surge in a viral infection, the management of change is often executed at three levels:

Level 1: Steering group/management committee, which include senior officials, heads of departments, finance officer, specialist services representatives, etc. to initiate the change idea, and then designate a group of selected professionals to plan and implement the change.

Level 2: The selected professionals act as a 'task force' who meet and agree different individuals' roles in the implementation of the change; and they report to steering committee periodically.

Level 3: Appropriately qualified or trained individuals who will execute or use the change, including users of the service.

Before moving on to discuss the dynamics of the management of change, the next section explores introducing change at a macro level, which is generally referred to as project management.

Project Management

Major changes in organisations are often treated as projects that require substantial planning and careful monitoring of expectations, particularly so when the change is an innovation, a new activity or way of thinking, and therefore the concept 'project management'. This section on project management begins by defining what a project is, and then moves on to provide details of how to start, proceed and complete projects to the satisfaction of all concerned.

A project is often explained as a temporary, time-limited venture to achieve a one-off single specific, new and unique end-product, service or result. The service or product can also be for a limited time, or for the long term. So, in healthcare, a service could be influenza vaccination for everyone aged 55 years or over, or to provide all newly diagnosed diabetics at one GP practice with a diabetic (electronic) patch. General examples of projects include: a new design vacuum cleaner; electric-powered 'black cabs' cars; HS2 (High Speed Rail 2); designing and producing a new computer game from scratch.

Projects are instigated by organisations or individuals whereby the product or the service will benefit the particular organisation or individual(s). Designing a new computer game or a new type of vacuum cleaner will benefit the manufacturing organisation financially. An influenza vaccination campaign will benefit the government financially based on reduced hospital admissions, as well as popularity maybe, but more importantly in avoiding the illness for many.

The Project Management Institute (2020: 1) defines project management as 'the application of knowledge, skills, tools, and techniques to project activities to meet the project's requirements'. Complementarily, the Association of Project Management (2020: 1) defines project management as follows:

> Project management is the application of processes, methods, skills, knowledge and experience to achieve specific project objectives according to the project acceptance criteria within agreed parameters (such as) a finite timescale and budget.

Project management is also the step-by-step, systematic process in many ways akin, but not identical, to the RAPSIES change management model (Gopee and Galloway, 2017) discussed later in this chapter. One difference is that in the management of change, the change leader may be an integral member of the team who will actually use the change afterwards. Another is that projects are usually large-scale ventures, while change can also be large-scale, it can also be much smaller, and therefore incur much less costs.

Additionally, a key factor that distinguishes project management from 'management' in general is that a project has a finite timespan, from initiation of the project to the final delivery date, while management is a never-ending and ongoing process. Consequently, a project manager needs to be capable of a wide range of skills, often technical skills, and certainly people management skills and good business awareness.

Furthermore, effective teamwork (discussed in Chapter 6) is vital to the successful completion of the project (also referred to as a 'venture'), and teamwork needs to be sustained by considerate and caring project leadership to ensure it is effectively implemented. Figure 9.2 identifies the usual logical stages of project management (e.g. a project to provide an outpatients clinic exclusively for patients with sickle-cell disease).

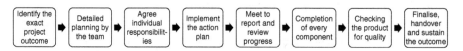

Figure 9.2   Stages of managing a project

A similar sequence of actions which is constituted in the form of a framework for improvement in health services has been published by NHSE (2021), the six stages of the framework being:

1. Starting out by identifying the opportunity or problem, and the service, area, or process that needs to be improved.
2. Defining the scope of the project based on the current situation.
3. Measuring and understanding the benefits and impacts of the project and determining whether the change is an improvement.
4. Designing and planning with a clear and shared understanding of the process and agreed action plan of clearly identifiable tasks.
5. Implementation of the improvement plan after presenting it to stakeholders.
6. Handover and sustaining the service, with benefits realised, shared learning from any arising issues.

For the second stage in Figure 9.2, 'Detailed planning by the team', it is worth noting the process that a group of people go through before they become a functioning team, which include forming, storming, etc. identified by Tuckman (Agile-Mercurial, 2019) as discussed in Chapter 6 of this book. Brief details of the stages of managing a project are given in Table 9.1 below.

Risk assessment and risk analysis are regularly conducted in healthcare. For example, when a course of a specific antibiotic is prescribed, it is not 100 per cent certain that it will kill the bacteria causing the infection, and meanwhile the patient's health condition could deteriorate. Furthermore, there are risks of side effects associated with antibiotics in terms of nausea, diarrhoea, allergy, etc.

Table 9.1   Brief details of the stages of managing a project

Defining the exact nature of the outcome (often by the initiator/instigator of the project)	Appoint project leader/manager Identify in full detail the precise nature of the final product or service, and the terms of reference Ethical considerations Risk assessment/analysis Budget for the venture Project completion date
Detailed planning by the team	Project Leader convenes project team Project leader/manager creates a vision of the outcome Root cause analysis of the problem SWOT/PESTLE/forcefield analysis Stakeholder management/engagement Identify all success criteria – SMART criteria Tasks and times of completion of each component – on Gantt chart Business plan with details of costs defined for both human resources, and equipment and materials How will the expected benefits or outcome of the project be recognised
Agreeing individual responsibilities	Which team member will oversee which component/system? Team meeting dates to report on actions taken and to check progress Support by project leader and others – for the project and team members
Implementing the plan of action	Execution of every single system/component of the venture Ensure staff implementing each component has the necessary skill to execute the activity and provide training Risk register and risk management Monitor costs in detail
Meet to report and review progress	Evaluation plan – formative and summative Monthly budget statement Ensure steps required to minimise risk are adhered to
Completion of each component	Sign off every component completed Quality control
Checking the product for quality	Assess fitness for purpose and discuss product with stakeholders Final risk and ethical assessment Ensuring all materials, equipment is removed from site
Handover and sustaining the outcome.	Handover to users of the venture Mechanism for troubleshooting after the project aim is up and running Mainstreaming/sustaining the implementation (of the venture)

Therefore, the decision to prescribe it is based on cost-benefit analysis (in terms of health recovery) (more on risk analysis and risk management shortly).

Other factors to decide on are the quality of the project, procurement (purchase of materials or equipment) routes and stakeholder management (and good people management). Quality of the product or service refers to its fitness for purpose (e.g. the running of HS2 without breakdowns; the prevention or substantial reduction in the incidence of influenza), that is with high stakeholder and recipient satisfaction with the product or service.

Projects cost money and the outcome of the project must show that it was money well spent. To do this, a business plan has to be written at the proposal stage, which includes a breakdown of all monetary costs. The project proposal would therefore have to have the following:

1. Executive summary, to include the main aim and total funding of the project.
2. Introduction, background and context of the proposal.
3. Theoretical background and review of any research, audits on similar projects.
4. Project aim, objectives and success criteria.
5. Project plan and project milestones.
6. Breakdown of financial costs, of each component, in full detail.
7. Evaluation plan; recognising/evaluating success.
8. Mainstreaming the project (implementing and sustaining the product/service).
9. Supporting material/appendices.

ACTION POINT 9.3
Applying the project management process

Think of any major project conducted by your team, your department or your employing organisation, and identify one that you have some insight into, one that you might even have been part of.

Then using the eight components of the process of project management detailed in Figure 9.2, identify as many actions as you can that would enable the successful completion of the project. You can use a copy of Table 9.1, and either remove the items in the right-hand column, or you can add a third column to the right for your responses to this Action point.

From their research on the necessary communication skills of project managers for the success of projects, Zulch (2014) ranked the communication skills of effective project managers from those of highest importance to lesser important ones. At the top of the list of these specific communication skills are:

1. Developing trust, collaboration and teamwork.
2. Allowing team members to take responsibility for their work.
3. Sharing the vision of the project with the project team.
4. Etc.

The least important item in Zulch's list is 'Following the rule book'. However, Zulch also identifies leadership, motivating the team, problem-solving, stress-handling skills and presentation skills as those essential skills that project managers need to exercise for the success of the project.

Risk Assessment and Risk Management

As noted earlier, risk assessment, risk analysis and risk management are integral components of project management, as they also are for patient safety, quality of care and of organisational governance. It is often said that risk to people is everywhere, especially in healthcare settings. Risk features in our everyday life activities as it is all-pervasive and therefore also prevails substantially in care activities. In daily life, people make several decisions that have some level of risk associated with them, such as eating at a restaurant, visiting the hairdresser's salon and going on a bicycle ride.

The word 'risk' itself, as a noun, according to the *Cambridge Dictionary* (Cambridge University Press, 2021), means the possibility or threat of something bad happening, danger of damage or loss, a difficulty a hazard that can cause injury or damage, a dangerous situation. The verb 'to risk' means to expose (someone or something valued) to danger, hazard, harm or loss. The words injury and harm in the meanings of the word risk applies to service users, that is to 'patient safety', and it is each healthcare professional's responsibility to protect service users from harm. Loss can signify financial penalties to the healthcare organisation in terms of settlement of clinical negligence claims paid as a result of litigation by service users who have suffered harm while hospitalised.

In order to minimise or preferably eliminate risk of harm to people, that is to service users or to staff, a risk assessment is often indicated or is necessary. A risk assessment is the process of identifying what hazards currently exist or may appear in the workplace, and workplace hazards that are likely to cause harm to employees and visitors, according to UNISON (2020). It is, therefore, a systematic process of evaluating the potential risks that may be involved in a projected activity or undertaking. Kaya et al. (2019) indicate that risk assessment aims to identify, analyse and evaluate risks that may have a negative influence on the quality and safety of the care delivered

Risk assessment is also usually an activity conducted as part of management of change to ascertain if the proposed change poses any level of likelihood of harm or loss to anyone. However, a range of risks are assessed regularly on daily basis especially in acute hospitals, and examples of instances of risk assessment include risk of:

- wound infection post-surgery;
- pressure injuries/ulcers;
- effects of incorrect manual handling;

- venous thromboembolism;
- suicide attempt or self-neglect by a person with mental health problems.

In relation to risk assessment prior to manual handling, for example, a range of different types of manual handling equipment, in particular trolleys, beds and patient platform support surfaces, all need to be assessed to identify and reduce or eliminate manual handling risk to care staff. Often a validated risk assessment form is completed for a certain level of precision in the assessment. For risk management to promote person-centred dementia care, for example, in addition to the traditional focus on preventing physical harm, action must be taken to risk assess and manage their social and psychological wellbeing as well, according to Clarke and Mantle (2016).

Although various appendages are associated with the word risk in relation to quality of services (e.g. risk identification, risk analysis), a number of these work in a logical sequence, as illustrated in Figure 9.3, which is somewhat similar to the step-by-step process of risk management in general identified by Health and Safety Executive (2020).

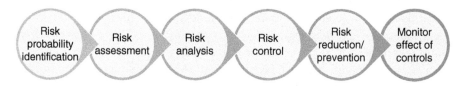

Figure 9.3 Sequence of risk management

Risk assessment is, therefore, a proactive and preventive action, as different from the reactive process of investigation of patient safety incidents. *Risk probability and risk identification* refers to identifying the particular hazard(s) that have the potential to cause or result in harm to the individual(s). *Risk assessment* is normally conducted using a bespoke tool (a checklist), which is then analysed to ascertain to whom the hazard could cause harm, and its likelihood, severity and frequency. *Risk control* incorporates making changes to *prevent* the risk, to *reduce* the likelihood of the risk occurring or to reduce its effect.

The outcome of the actions taken needs to be *monitored* regularly afterwards and the level of risk reassessed if necessary. However, on evaluating user requirements for risk assessment, Kaya et al. (2019) conclude that risk assessment as a patient safety activity is underutilised for various reasons, including insufficient guidance for healthcare professionals on how to perform them.

Risk assessment is performed using a risk probability tool which usually entails completing a form with focused questions, which when completed gives a score or percentage risk of harm. The score from the form will indicate the patient is at

> ## ACTION POINT 9.4
> ### Risk assessments you know of in your clinical setting
>
> With regards to the care setting where you work, think of which risk assessment activities have been formally conducted recently, even today, or within the last month or so. Precisely in relation to which care activity or service user were the risk assessment activities conducted?
>
> Which assessment tools were used to identify and manage the risks? Peruse one or two of the tools to check how you feel about the questions asked in the tools.

high risk (of e.g. developing pressure ulcers), medium risk or low risk. However, a systematic review of randomised controlled trials of risk assessment tools for pressure ulcer risk conducted by Moore and Patton (2019), found that the three tools that they tested, and also compared to not using a risk assessment tool, were all almost equally good and made no difference to patient outcomes in terms of reduction in the incidence of pressure ulcers.

If risk assessment suggests there is a probability of risk of harm, loss or damage, then the next step is risk management, which refers to both the overarching process of conducting risk assessments, and to managing the risk after the assessment.

For example, when during the coronavirus pandemic in 2020 it was observed that NHS workers from black and minority ethnic backgrounds were disproportionately more adversely affected by the virus, NHS Employers (2020) and NHSE+I (2020b) issued guidance to healthcare organisations to take specifically sensitive action when conducting risk assessment of colleagues from those backgrounds. Employers were also asked to publish a number of metrics of assessment of at-risk groups of staff and include the data in board-level reports. A risk assessment template adapted from Health and Safety Executive (2020) is presented in Figure 9.4.

Models of Change Management

Depending on the various individuals who the change will affect, and their reaction to the proposal indicated earlier on in this chapter (i.e. excitement, etc.), the process of change tends to take a more or less predictable route that endures, although every change is different in some way and follows its own unique process.

Risk assessment template							
Company name:				Assessment carried out by:			
Date of next review:				Date assessment was carried out:			
What are the hazards?	Who might be harmed and how?	What are you already doing to control the risk?	What further actions do you need to take to control the risks?	Who needs to carry out the actions?	When is the action needed by?	Action completion date?
1.							
2.							
3.							

Figure 9.4 A risk assessment template (adapted from HSE, 2020)

Whenever practical, change should be managed systematically and therefore not imposed on staff at short notice. Systematic management of change therefore entails taking a carefully planned, team-based approach for the change to be successful. Dawson and Andriopoulos (2021) indicate that change that is led through 'dialogue' is a change that is more likely to 'take root'. Note the word 'dialogue', which signifies two-way communication between the change leader or co-ordinator and all parties involved; and the term 'take root', which signifies that there needs to be a plan in place to ensure the change endures.

As determined earlier in this chapter, differences in the way organisations operate is not new, and change will not stop happening, which is a reality that also applies to health service organisations. For change to be implemented systematically, step-by-step and in a logical coherent manner rather than ad hoc, or imposed, the change can draw on a known framework or model of change management. A number of published frameworks for managing change are available to select from, including the *NHS Change Model* (NHS England, 2020d), and Kotter's (2012) 8-stage change model.

For the *NHS Change Model*, it has been developed over a decade through consultation with numerous NHS staff at all levels and prevailing research. NHS England (2020c: 1) asserts that the model comprises 'a framework for any project or programme that is seeking to achieve transformational, sustainable change'. It consists of eight components:

1. Shared purpose
2. Leadership by all
3. Spread and adoption
4. Improvement tools

5. Project and performance management
6. Measurement
7. System drivers
8. Motivate and mobilise

Shared purpose is placed at the centre of a septagonal diagram, implying its high significance, and is designed in such a way that it ultimately benefits the recipients of the change. An alternative to the *NHS Change Model* is Kotter's (2012) eight-stage change model, as identified on Table 9.2. Kotter's model has been adapted and applied to various settings. For example, Lv and Zhang (2017) describe how the model is combined successfully with collective leadership to manage barriers to change and create an effective environment for sustaining changes.

Table 9.2 Components of three models of management of change

Gopee and Galloway's (2017) seven-step framework for management of change	Kotter's (2012) eight-stage change model	NHS England (2020d) eight-component framework for management of change in healthcare
1) *Recognition* of anticipated benefits of the change	1) Create urgency	1) Shared purpose
2) *Analysis* of change options, the environment, and the users of the change	2) Build a guiding team	2) Leadership by all
	3) Create a vision for change	3) Spread and adoption
	4) Communicate the change vision	4) Improvement tools
3) *Preparation* for the change	5) Remove obstacles	5) Project and performance management
4) *Strategies* for implementing the change	6) Create 'short-term' wins	6) Measurement
5) *Implementation* of the change	7) Consolidate gains	7) System drivers
6) *Evaluation* of the impact of the change against initial goals	8) Anchor the new approaches in the culture	8) Motivate and mobilise
7) *Sustaining* the change		

However, models in healthcare and in social sciences in general are rarely perfect for all situations and for all teams, and therefore published models may have to be adapted or slightly modified so that they can be more effectively applied to local organisational cultures and circumstances. For a model that can be applied to healthcare directly and that is based on numerous years of experience in healthcare, as well as on the extensive literature on the management of change, Gopee and Galloway (2017) offer the 'seven-step RAPSIES model for effective change management (see Figure 9.5). See also Table 9.2 for a comparison of the components of each of these three models of change.

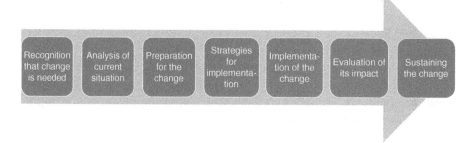

Figure 9.5   The seven-step RAPSIES model for effective change management (Source: Gopee and Galloway, 2017)

Despite quite a few common elements in the three models of change outlined on Table 9.2, the RAPSIES model is designed to work by full involvement of the users of the change, but works well in a top-down approach as well (see Figure 9.5). The seven-step model comprises the crucial components of the management of change, and although the RAPSIES model is illustrated as a linear model in Figure 9.5, it requires reflexivity throughout the process, constantly evaluating progress and making adjustments if appropriate. See Table 9.3 for further brief details of the components of the RAPSIES model, and thereafter each component is discussed in further detail.

Table 9.3   Components and details of the RAPSIES model of change

Components	Comprises
Recognition	Making staff, as users of the change, aware of the need for change, e.g. to solve a problem for instance, or to improve an element of practice, and to provide knowledge of choices
Analysis	Of the change includes performing a SWOT analysis, PESTLE analysis or forcefield analysis, of the setting where change will be implemented, and of the users of the change
Preparation	Planning the change by initially appointing a skilled change leader to lead its implementation, education of the users of the change, defining intended outcomes
Strategies	Contributory strategies implemented by the change leader, e.g. PDSA
Implementation	Signifies all the planning has been done, and a date chosen for the change to come into force, including piloting the change beforehand
Evaluation	Formative (ongoing and continuous) and summative (at predetermined dates) evaluation against anticipated outcomes
Sustaining	Ways of ensuring that all required resources are available for the change to 'be firmed up' and endures

Applying a model of change management

The main purpose of implementing change is usually to enhance or improve the provision and delivery of care. However, the change also has to be compatible with the care team's current philosophy of care, that is their existing beliefs and values related to caring, as well as their practice. Also useful to consider is how easily the change can be understood by users of the change. Its 'trialability' (i.e. the possibility of piloting the innovation) must also be part of the deliberation.

Recognising, Analysing, Planning and Applying Strategies for Change

The application of the RAPSIES model of change includes recognition of the proposed change, analysis of the change, planning and leading the change which includes applying known contributory strategies for change.

Recognition of the proposed change, and analysis

The first stage of management of change entails healthcare leaders and team members recognising the need for change, and then acquiring detailed knowledge of the change. As noted above, the change may have been requested by senior leaders and a steering committee, or it has evolved, and a named change leader designated. Otherwise the team may be in a position to explore alternatives together before deciding on implementing a particular change.

Several examples of change have been cited throughout this chapter, but the basis for the change has to be that there is a need for the change for improvement or enhancement of practice. Moreover, the likely advantages and disadvantages of the change also need to be considered, which can be executed in systematic ways through forcefield or SWOT analyses (discussed shortly).

Users' perspective and sub-organisational culture

In considering the users of the change (e.g. team members using a new bandaging technique for leg ulcers), the planning part of the change also includes 'selling' the change to the users, and exploring any training and education needs of individual team members or for the whole team. Users of the change are normally the staff who deliver care in the care setting, and for successful implementation, as change leader the FHM must actively involve the entire team, so that each member develops ownership of the change. They need to become active advocates of the change rather than passive recipients, which essentially comprises the bottom-up approach.

Staff members get accustomed to established ways of working and feel secure with them. However, concluding from research conducted some time ago, Rogers

and Shoemaker (1971) identified six categories of users of change, as also identified by Yun (2020) and which apply to many work settings (see Figure 9.6).

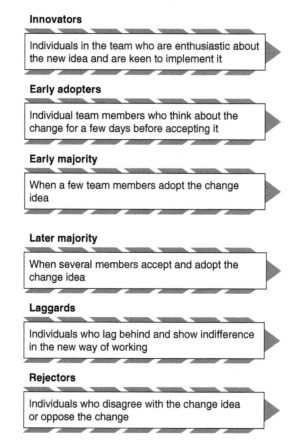

Innovators
Individuals in the team who are enthusiastic about the new idea and are keen to implement it

Early adopters
Individual team members who think about the change for a few days before accepting it

Early majority
When a few team members adopt the change idea

Later majority
When several members accept and adopt the change idea

Laggards
Individuals who lag behind and show indifference in the new way of working

Rejectors
Individuals who disagree with the change idea or oppose the change

Figure 9.6   Innovators, laggards and rejectors of change

ACTION POINT 9.5
Innovators and rejectors in my workplace

While avoiding stereotyping or labelling team members, see if you can identify team members who are innovators in your workplace or organisation, and those individuals who tend to oppose all proposed changes.

As noted earlier, the change leader's actions are pivotal to the implementation and consolidation of the change. With users of the change who are 'innovators', the change leader can build on their enthusiasm and energy by affording
them responsibilities for aspects of the change. The remaining categories of users

comprise those who resist change either momentarily or longer term. Early adopters should be welcomed to the change and their participation acknowledged, whereas those who form the later majority are staff who need more time to assimilate the new concept, and should be afforded a reasonable amount of time and knowledge to comprehend the change.

For users of change who can be seen as 'Laggards', the team should make a concerted effort to provide them with extra support and time to enable them to understand the change more thoroughly, and thereby prevent disillusionment. As for those who can be deemed 'rejectors', the change leader or the line manager will need to explore their stance further with them to identify possible reasons for this. The employee might, for example, have had negative experience of the change previously, or be undergoing temporary personal upheaval that may be clouding their judgement.

Furthermore, it is not just the laggards and rejectors who resist change; it could be several members of the team, some of whom may appear on the surface to go along with the change, but because they feel the change is directed by managers, they therefore feel they cannot do other than comply with it. Their stance can come under the umbrella term 'resistance to change', which the change leader should endeavour to anticipate and then manage.

Additionally, at times the culture in care settings might itself propagate resistance to change, because by nature sub-organisational cultures are enduring and have widespread support within the subgroup. A cohesive adequately staffed team who are encouraged to be innovative and creative, and a supportive leadership are also important components.

Resistance to change is measurable using a resistance to change scale, which Johansson et al. (2014), for example, utilised to assess the likelihood of a specific change succeeding in a mental health care setting. They concluded that the instrument constitutes a fairly good predictor of the team members' 'change preparedness' based on the team's subculture. It was used in conjunction with the 'organisational values questionnaire' to assess the sub-culture in the healthcare setting to gauge if the values in the sub-culture could change, and if that would lead to improvement in the care provided. Individuals' natural personal disposition to resist change has also been established through extensive research by Oreg et al. (2008).

Planning and leading the change

From the point in time when the change is being contemplated, one of the most important actions is to consider and select an appropriate person to lead and co-ordinate the change, i.e. the change leader, at times referred to as the change agent, who, in turn, must be wholeheartedly interested in the change and fully motivated to implement and maintain the change.

The FHM's role in the management of change may involve being the change leader, although admittedly, change leaders are often a level or two more senior to recently qualified frontline managers. The change leader role could also be taken by a facilitator who is another employee from within the department, or from the healthcare trust or even external to the organisation. Their duty would include promoting, implementing and managing the change, and they could even be the initiator of the change.

The change leader needs to be completely clear about the final form of the outcome, and about the present state of readiness for change. The nurse leader's role is paramount in co-ordinating and sustaining changes, for which the leader must create a supportive culture and environment in the practice setting, and be seen as a practitioner of the specific change themselves, as Bianchi et al. (2018) concluded from their integrative review of EBP.

The change leader must also have thorough knowledge of the dynamics and processes of systematic change management and be cognisant of the components of the seven-step RAPSIES framework, for example. Other components of the change leader's role also include:

- planning the change thoroughly;
- promoting ownership of the change by the team;
- determining and deciding on relevant change strategies;
- identifying team members' with development/training needs;
- monitoring and supporting change users throughout the process; and
- problem-solving to address any challenges that are experienced.

For change leaders to be fully effective, they need to have transformational leadership capability, and the Carter Review (DHSC, 2016b: 9) recommends 'significantly improving leadership capability from "ward to board"' so that trans-formational change can occur. Chapter 3 of this book provides detailed analysis of transformational leadership.

Suitable strategies for the particular group of users would include taking time to explore staff knowledge and understanding of the nature of the change, and then detailed analysis needs to be done by the group of staff using popular tools such as SWOT (strengths, weaknesses, opportunities, threats) analysis, PESTLE (political-economic-social-technological–legal–ethical/environmental) analysis and forcefield analysis.

It needs to be acknowledged that change can cause anxiety and feelings of resistance to the change. These happen because the users of the change might:

- feel their current practice is being criticised as below acceptable standard;
- lack knowledge of the change, and therefore fear of the unknown;
- feel loss of power and influence;
- be unsure if they will be supported if the change doesn't work, or cause harm.

Staff might also resist change if they feel overburdened by too much change at a particular point in time. However, for each of these factors, the FHM or change leader can take specific proactive and reactive actions. For feelings of criticism of current practice, the change leader has to convene a meeting of all involved to provide evidence of poor practice, or to persuade the anticipated users of the change that it will improve practice further. For lack of in-depth knowledge about the change, the answer is obvious, which is to provide knowledge directly or by sending staff on relevant study days or workshops, and subsequently to discuss the change openly within the team.

Furthermore, the change leader has to be capable of exercising resilience and make time for reflection as and when progress with the process of change may feel slow or hitting obstacles. Additionally, however, the change leader should consider undertaking empirical work in the form of action research for example, with the venture.

Contributory strategies initiated by the change leader

Planning the change also involves considering which contributory strategies to incorporate in the venture. To promote ownership by the users of the change and by the organisation, communication by all parties involved is essential. Relevant change strategies that require communication include:

- Plan–Do–Study–Act;
- Lewin's three-stage process;
- Empirical–rational, power–coercive and normative–re-educative strategies.

The Plan–Do–Study–Act cycle

As a widely applied model of quality improvement, the Plan–Do–Study–Act (PDSA) model may initially look too simple to be applicable to healthcare, but a closer look at the model indicates its value in its simplicity. The PDSA cycle, which is also known as the Deming Cycle, is a continuous quality improvement model based on sequences of four steps as illustrated in Figure 9.7. The steps include:

Plan:　　　　 how you will implement the change and break it down into steps.
Do:　　　　　 implement the plan.
Study (check): study the results and outcomes.
Act:　　　　　 standardise or further improve the process.

The PDSA cycle is also a quality improvement strategy that is endorsed by England's NHSI (2018c) and is also recommended for healthcare by the IHI (2020b)

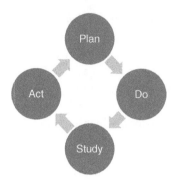

Figure 9.7   The PDSA cycle

based in North America. Its four components are straightforward in that the change component needs careful planning, then the plan is implemented, its impact observed, and if the change functions as intended then it is adopted in the setting. It is sometimes referred to as PDCA, which stands for Plan–Do–Check–Adjust. Furthermore, Reed and Card (2016) indicate that the PDSA is a 'sophisticated' QI tool (and change strategy) that might reveal related issues, minor or major, that need to be addressed in order to achieve the improvement goal.

Lewin's three-stage process of change

Another very useful strategy that the change leader can usefully implement is Lewin's (1951) three-stage process of change implementation entailing unfreezing, movement and refreezing, which is presented in Figure 9.8.

Like the PDSA cycle, Lewin's model may also appear simple, but it is a realistic and usable change strategy, except to note that each step comprises a number of sub-steps. Unfreezing can be performed through discussion within the team

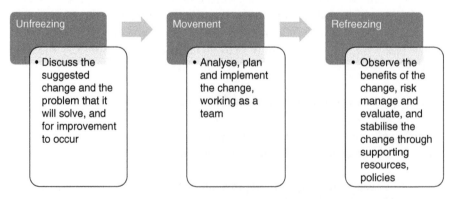

Figure 9.8   Lewin's (1951) three-stage process of change implementation

and use of systematic tools like SWOT analysis, forcefield analysis, or PESTLE analysis.

So, in SWOT analysis in relation to strengths and opportunities related to implementing flexible shifts or e-rostering, for example, these comprise the positive effects of the change. As for threats and weaknesses, as the team would now become aware of these, they can think of actions to take to resolve them, although they might need manager support to help them do this. Strengths and weaknesses are factors that are internal to the team or the organisation, while opportunities and threats are usually external to the individual or team.

Forcefield analysis entails the team collectively identifying factors that support the change and those that comprise obstacles. There might be several factors driving the change, and several that are blocking it. Lewin (1951) indicates that individuals' behaviour in organisations tend to develop into a pattern, and forcefield analysis can facilitate 'unfreezing' the forces that maintain behaviour in its present form. After unfreezing, the change leader can instigate actions to: (1) increase the driving forces by adding new ones or strengthening existing ones; (2) reduce or remove the resisting forces; and (3) convert one or more resisting forces into driving ones.

In addition to resisting forces, inherent within the organisation itself there could be 'barriers to change'. This concept refers to such barriers as insufficient staff or non-human resources, too concerned about efficiency savings to consider novel ideas, introducing the change too quickly without fully planning and managing the implementation, etc. On the other hand, organisations that tend to have less barriers to change are treated as 'effective organisations' according to Beckhard and Harris (1987), which are organisations that manifest such characteristics as having a strategic or longer-term view, having relatively open communication, valuing differences in team members' views, willing to learn, etc.

Some of the barriers to implementation of research findings can also apply to implementation of change, including insufficient resources to implement new practice, and lack of skills to critically appraise research reports. A change endeavour can succeed or fail depending on the various factors discussed above, but if the change implementation is managed using one of the frameworks cited (e.g. the RAPSIES framework), then the change should be effective in achieving the desired improvement.

Empirical-rational, power-coercive or normative-re-educative strategies

Other alternative strategies that the change leader can utilise are: empirical-rational, power-coercive or normative-re-educative strategies, although a combination of these three strategies may prove more productive.

1. Empirical-rational

Empirical broadly refers to research-based knowledge, and rational means what sounds like a logical or reasonable thing to do. It suggests that if team members can be given detailed knowledge and rationale for the proposed change, then they are more likely to accept it. Thus, this strategy is based on empowerment. Government health warnings or guidance are usually based on this strategy.

2. Power-coercive

Implementing change by virtue of management's right to do so. Implicit within this strategy are threats of sanctions by seniors if the change is not adopted. This strategy is unlikely to appeal to most employees and is rarely owned by the users of the change. It could be applied though if other strategies fail.

3. Normative-re-educative

As a strategy that suggests that the proposed change is normal activity at other successful organisations, and stating the benefits of the change to the service and the users, then team members could be willing to consider the change proposed. This strategy suggests opportunity to learn new ways of working, and therefore personal growth.

Any of the strategies cited above could suffice to implement the change efficaciously, but may not depending on the numerous other impinging factors identified above. If visible beneficial effects of the change can be sensed by the team, then they are more likely to feel more positive towards it. Following application of the abovementioned strategies, the change then can be implemented, evaluated and embedded.

Implementing, Evaluating and Sustaining the Change

Starting implementation of the change

Following exploration of the users' perceptions of the change and selection of the strategies to be utilised, the change leader makes a decision on whether all the consultations have been completed, that they have all the resources the change requires, and then set a date for implementation of the change, that is the date from when the change comes into force. As for all preceding components of change management, the implementation date itself also requires careful planning.

When the change leader and the team decide on the timing of implementation, they have to take various factors into account, including any other initiatives being started, other changes that have recently been implemented, and whether to recruit additional staff members. The right time coincides with the time when the users are ready, and the setting is 'ripe for change' for successful implementation, which includes when there is openness and trust amongst staff, two-way effective communication prevails and morale is good.

Implementation must, however, be avoided during periods of high annual leave, when there are staff vacancies or long-term sickness, or when other major managerial changes are imminent, or when there is organisational resistance to the change.

ACTION POINT 9.6
Plan of a change in your workplace

Thinking of your own care setting or the organisation where you work, consider a change that you feel would be useful to implement for the benefit of either service users or the staff. Then, identify a full set of step-by-step activities drawing on the models and strategies of change management discussed above that should ensure that the change is successfully implemented, and that will endure.

Using any of the models of change management discussed in this chapter should result in successful change implementation, which then needs to be evaluated, adjusted if necessary and maintained.

Evaluation of the change implemented

However apt and promising a change might seem initially, its impact has to be assessed and continually monitored to check on its enduring success and continuing suitability, and ensuring no harm is occurring to anyone particularly when its effect is on people. The effect needs to be evaluated continuously as well as at predetermined end-points. This needs to be done both informally and in more structured ways.

General impressions of the effect of the change can be gauged by observation and by casual questioning. For structured evaluation, a known framework such as the Donabedian (1988) model can be applied (more details in Chapter 8). Evaluation of the impact of the change can entail comparing anticipated outcomes against actual ones, utilising specific indicators, e.g. healing rates of wounds, reduction in injury, reduced length of hospital stay, etc.

Embedding the change

For the change to last, 'grassroots' staff need to feel empowered and supported, be it changes in the time of ward rounds, limiting visiting during mealtimes, or other. This is also because in her report from different NHS trusts, Moore (2017) indicates that initiatives are often imposed by senior managers and they tend to fail due to lack of such support and empowerment. Grassroots staff such as Band

5 healthcare professionals and non-clinical staff should be in a position to suggest changes in the first place and be part of the discussion and analysis of the proposed change as they will also be the users of the change.

So, following implementation, the change leader has to ensure that the change endures in the care setting; that is, the change remains in place as originally intended. This can be achieved through open recognition of the achievement by senior managers, and support provided in terms of any extra resources that are required. Users of the change also should be able to see tangible benefits of the change following mainstreaming. Furthermore, progress should be checked continually, for which the PDSA cycle (Reed and Card, 2016; IHI, 2020b) method can be applied.

The plan for mainstreaming and sustaining the change will have been established at the very beginning of the change implementation, which includes:

- having adequate staffing;
- any extra finances required, for devices, etc;
- staff expertise development for utilisation of any new equipment or devices;
- monitoring mechanisms, such as regular concurrent and retrospective audits;
- staggered evaluation of the effects and impact of the change;
- time for dissemination of the change and learning from feedback;
- users retaining ownership of the change (active user participation);
- managing emerging issues and maintaining team motivation; and
- support and leadership of senior managers.

When the change has been successfully implemented and mainstreamed, then it should be disseminated to interested parties.

Publicising the change

Following successfully implementing and embedding of the change, it is useful to bring it into the public domain by disseminating the change. Publicising the change gives the change implementers the opportunity to be proud of and celebrate their achievement as well as their contribution to quality improvement.

Publicising the change is a collegial activity which constitutes sharing knowledge of benefits of the change, as well as the strategies that have been applied for successful implementation of the change. The change can be publicised by several means, such as by presenting a report locally to colleagues, by local or national conference presentation, writing up as a journal article, maybe in a peer-reviewed profession-specific journal, reporting at journal clubs and even creating educational materials.

There are various add-on benefits to each chosen route of dissemination. When doing a conference presentation, for example, this affords the presenter the opportunity to work diligently to perfect the content of the presentation to fit in with the time allocated and the theme it belongs to, to make the presentation interesting so as to hold the audience's attention, to polish their presentation skills in terms of voice production, pacing, etc. In addition, comments and questions forwarded by the audience can comprise avenues for further learning for the presenter.

Having examined the RAPSIES change management framework, it has to be acknowledged that there is no universal model of management of change that applies to all situations, as also noted by Dawson and Andriopoulos (2021) who indicate that we need to be aware that change is often also a political process. Therefore, organisations or change leaders can choose the most appropriate model for their circumstances, but adhere as closely as they can to the model chosen because they are almost always developed over several years and with extensive deliberations. This argument provides further rationale for choosing the RAPSIES model, as it reflects a logical, unbiased and coherent framework for managing change in healthcare.

Guidance for managing change with impact and effectiveness

For the systematic management of change, improvement and innovations, the following constitute related good practice guidelines:

- Be open-minded about changes such as digitalisation in health services that are being promoted centrally by the government.
- Support and implement innovations and service improvement activities, particularly if they enhance evidence-informed practice.
- Be amenable to heed change-related activities such as risk assessment and risk management, and project management.
- Acquire knowledge of different models and frameworks of change management so that you have a view on the most plausible and proven models for your care setting.
- When opting to apply a model of change management, check to ensure its compatibility with the team's existing values and practices that currently prevail in the care setting.
- Only apply a model of change management after careful thorough planning in advance and in detail, which includes deciding on a change leader and involving team members at key stages.
- If opting for the RAPSIES model or any other model cited in this chapter, ensure the planning includes systematic implementation in the sequence identified in the model, and by incorporating all its components.
- Ensure you have detailed knowledge of various change strategies, which may include providing team members detailed knowledge of the change or innovation, and ways of overcoming any resistance to the change and any other arising problem.

- Institute education and training as a means for team members to acquire knowledge and skills, followed by updating and upskilling as necessary.
- Support active participation by intended users of the change, implementing empirical action research if that is viable.
- Apply ongoing and summative evaluation of progress with the change, which also includes providing a medium for team members to share experiences, for questioning, providing feedback and support, and possibly refinement.

Chapter Summary

The management of change, improvements and innovations have to be planned very carefully and thoroughly in order for the change to have intended impact and to endure. Frontline healthcare managers are the most appropriate staff members to implement change, which has to be executed systematically and with full participation by the team. Consequently, this chapter has addressed:

- Identifying recent changes in care and treatment methods in various areas of practice, along with the reasons for continuing changes in healthcare delivery;
- Systematic ways of managing the implementation of change, including project management using well-informed alternative management of change frameworks or models;
- Knowledge of the application of project management as a form of change management for quality improvement, and the associated risk assessment and risk management activities;
- Ways of ensuring team members recognise, analyse, prepare and apply strategies for change taking into account the sub-organisational culture and users' perspective;
- Knowledge of planning and leading the change which incorporate applying contributory strategies initiated by the change leader for implementing change; and
- Knowledge of means of evaluating and sustaining changes.

Further Reading

- For evaluation of vanguards as a major nationwide change to a new care model, see: Davis S F, Hinde S, Ariss S (2020) Complex programme evaluation of a 'new care model' vanguard: A shared commitment to quality improvement in an integrated health and care context. *BMJ Open,* 10 (2020): e029174.
- For details of hierarchy or levels of evidence in EBP, to access critically appraised resources related to healthcare, view the content of the Joanna Briggs Institute website: Joanna Briggs Institute (2021) *JBI EBP Resources.* Available at: https://jbi.global/ebp. Accessed Date: 14 February 2021.

- For an example of management of change utilising a change model, and including root cause analysis and forcefield analysis, see: Thorpe R (2015) Planning a change project in mental health nursing. *Nursing Standard*, 30(1): 38–44.

10

Managing Healthcare Professionals' Continuing Development

Chapter Objectives

The chapter objectives for frontline healthcare managers in relation to managing continuing professional learning for team members are:

- Be cognisant of ways in which frontline managers manage and facilitate team members' continuing professional development (CPD), starting with managing structured preceptorship development programmes for NRHPs, then covering ways of facilitating team members' professional revalidation requirements, which includes various formal and non-formal practice-based learning activities;
- Enable team members to appreciate the significance and ways of engaging in continuing learning, followed by focus on management training and development programmes for frontline managers as well as funding for staff development;
- Managing supervision of students' practice learning while maintaining a learning culture in care settings as learning organisations;
- Manage issues related to learning and development, in particular those related to management of poor practice, and learning from clinical incidents.

Introduction

Healthcare interventions performed by healthcare professionals are evidence-informed or evidence-based, and as new evidence of more effective or efficient practice as well as innovations emerge, healthcare professionals have to harness these and incorporate them in their day-to-day work if and when appropriate. To do so, they need to update their knowledge and competence, which essentially constitutes their CPD. Having addressed almost all aspects of leading and managing in healthcare in the preceding chapters, this final chapter of the book explores frontline managers' duties as a facilitator of team members' learning, as well as those of healthcare profession students.

Frontline healthcare managers' role with regards to facilitating team members' CPD is the main focus of this chapter, mostly in order to ensure all members' knowledge and competence stay up to date, as well as FHMs self-monitoring their own management skills. Doing so includes ensuring preceptorship is supported in care settings, continuing learning is managed, revalidation requirements for registrants are met and maintaining a learning culture in their practice setting. Funding for CPD is also briefly explored, followed by accentuating the importance of, and ways of, learning from patient safety incidents (PSIs).

Managing Team Members' Continuing Learning

Every healthcare professional, of necessity, has to engage in CPD to ensure their practice is evidence-informed, safe, effective and person-centred. More broadly, CPD is a part of lifelong learning (Gopee, 2001; Davis et al., 2014); that is, continuing to learn throughout one's career and life. The FHM's duties incorporate supporting continuing learning (e.g. NHS Employers, 2019a) for team members, which can be undertaken through formal studies and non-formal methods; that is, through attending structured training and education programmes or more informal learning respectively.

Learning has motivational function as it is associated with personal growth (Maslow, 1987; Herzberg, 2003). While formal learning is associated with attending accredited courses, non-formal learning occurs through much shorter but structured learning events, and includes short courses held in the care organisation's post-graduate education centre or in-service training department, for example. Learning can also be partially structured or 'incidental' or 'opportunistic'; that is, more informal. All healthcare providers have staff development strategies in their annual business plans. Staff development can enable achievement of IDPR objectives and personal development plans as indicated in the NHS KSF (NHS Employers, 2019b).

Particularly noteworthy, though, is that substantial knowledge and competence acquisition by learners occurs while engaged in clinical activities. Consequently, the care setting and its general work ethos should reflect an environment where learning is promoted. Facilitating learning and the acquisition of knowledge and competence in care settings is also a feature of professionalism, as indicated by the NMC (2018a).

The next section on managing team members' CPD encompasses managing structured preceptorship programmes for NRHPs, which incorporates orientation and induction in the healthcare setting, then enabling registrants to meet revalidation requirements, which includes different forms of practice-related or work-based learning.

Managing structured preceptorship programmes

Following several years of attempts at implementation of preceptorship for NRHPs, this mechanism is now generally well implemented by most healthcare organisations in the UK who employ newly qualified registrants. As a NRHP and a frontline manager, the FHM is initially a preceptee, and approximately a year after qualifying, their responsibilities start to include managing transition and preceptorship for NRHPs joining the team. Preceptorship is a mechanism that has been instituted for all newly registered nurses, midwives, nursing associates and AHPs.

In its 'Principles of preceptorship', which essentially comprise good practice of this mechanism, the NMC (2020a) indicates that preceptorship mustn't be seen as a substitute for formal induction or for mandatory training, nor is it a way to re-test or repeat any knowledge and skills that a professional will have already acquired through pre-registration programmes; nor does it replace IDPRs.

The FHM may be required to undertake preparation for the preceptor role, which can take many forms to enable them to become competent supervisors of NRHPs' learning, including online or blended learning modes. However, preceptors are not accountable for preceptees' actions or omissions, because all registrants are accountable in their own right for their own practice, but their role does include providing preceptees with feedback on good performance, and honest, constructive and objective feedback, and support on performance that needs improvement.

Alternatively, the DH's (2010b) framework for implementation of preceptorship for all care professions includes a reminder of the principles of the NHS Constitution, and then provides further details on the attributes of effective preceptors, the implementation of preceptorship, the content and design of preceptorship programmes and outcome measures, as well as organisational investment and continual evaluation of their effectiveness.

Evidence of effectiveness of preceptorship includes an integrative systematic review of the impact of preceptorship on NRNs by Edward et al. (2017), who found that the factors that influence their work readiness depend on a positive working relationships between preceptors and NRNs, preparation and support for the preceptor role, using a model to guide preceptorship, and adequate clinical exposure for developing clinical competence. These provisions improve the competence and self-confidence of NRHPs, their job satisfaction, critical thinking, and reduces their stress and anxiety, and therefore recommend that such structured support should be provided to all NRHPs.

As for models of preceptorship, this refers to whether one named preceptor is allocated to one (or more) NRHPs, or more than one named preceptor for each NRHP (because some preceptors work part-time, or can be transferred to another care setting for the shift because of their specialist competence, etc.), or support from any registrant who is on duty. Whether registrants are formally prepared for the role and whether they have protected time for the role also form part of these models.

Preceptorship programmes incorporate learning to form working relationships with preceptees, agreeing on intended outcomes, which can be documented as a learning contract, etc., and also initiating NRHPs into taking personal responsibility for keeping up to date. However, there can be issues related to effectiveness of preceptorship, which can be due to poor staffing levels, lack of time to precept, or unclear criteria to measure progress against, which is one of the reasons for preceptorship programmes having to be formally structured and fully supported by healthcare organisations.

Additionally, a preceptorship toolkit for preparation of preceptors that include tools to gauge level of organisational support, managerial support, supernumerary time and local culture of support, and which can be adapted for use locally, is presented by Owen et al. (2020) – see details in Further Reading section at the end of this chapter.

Professional regulation and team members' revalidation requirements

All healthcare professions in the UK that come under the aegis of one of the professional regulatory bodies (e.g. HCPC) now require its registrants to undertake a specified minimum amount of relevant learning regularly.

Revalidation as evidence of CPD has been in force for some years now for the majority of healthcare professions including doctors, dentists, etc. For nurses and midwives, revalidation requirements have been established and published by the NMC (2019a); for doctors, by the GMC (e.g. GMC, 2021), for AHPs, by the HCPC (e.g. HCPC, 2017), etc. There are specific requirements stipulated by each regulatory body, which registrants have to meet to show that they have updated their knowledge and competence, and then self-declare to the regulatory body that they have done so, resulting in the registrant being allowed to remain on the register and to practise in that capacity.

As the regulatory body for nurses, midwives and nursing associates, the NMC indicates that its prime role is ensuring safety and protection of the public by monitoring the knowledge and competence of its registrants, and revalidation is one way in which it does so. The NMC's mechanism for revalidation is consistent with the Department of Health's (2008b) *Principles for Revalidation*, which include revalidation should be carried out in such a way that it is: transparent, addresses accountability, is proportionate, is consistent and is targeted, which also means action is taken when revalidation requirements are not met by the registrant.

The requirement to revalidate for doctors by the GMC started in 2012 and lasts for five years; for nurses, midwives and nursing associates with the NMC it started in 2015 and lasts for three years, etc. Consequently, every NMC registrant has to apply for revalidation every three years, and for successful NMC revalidation there are eight requirements for the registrant to fulfil to keep their name on the NMC's live register, and therefore to be able to practise legally. These requirements span the preceding three years, and they are:

1. 450 practice hours or 900 hours if revalidating as both nurse and midwife;
2. 35 hours of CPD including 20 hours of participatory learning;
3. Five pieces of practice-related feedback;
4. Five written reflective accounts;
5. Reflective discussion (with reflective discussion partner);
6. Health and character declaration;
7. Professional indemnity arrangement; and
8. Confirmation (by a Confirmer).

The NMC's revalidation process is closely linked to the NMC's (2018b) code of practice, and the NMC (2019b) provides substantial details of ways in which registrants can demonstrate that they have met these requirements; and as part of the revalidation application the NMC's annual fee is also payable. Having accumulated all required evidence beforehand, at the three-yearly cycle the registrant completes the online forms on the NMC website, and declares that they have engaged in the required CPD. Registrants are expected to keep evidence of the achievement of the eight revalidation requirements in a personal portfolio, and a sample of registrants are selected by the NMC periodically to provide evidence of having met the revalidation requirements shortly after the event.

Additionally, the NMC provides details of the format of portfolios, which includes a number of templates. A wide variety of means of updating and advancement of knowledge and skills can be included as evidence for meeting revalidation requirements. Attending a university course is only one of multiple ways of meeting them, which can include assessment of attendees' knowledge and competence through academic assignments (discussed later).

ACTION POINT 10.1
How to meet revalidation requirements.

Just as a reminder, consider the following queries:

- Do you have a portfolio, as an e-portfolio as well as paper-form information for certificates, preliminary notes, etc.?
- Is the portfolio carefully divided into sections so that they can be easily extracted for (a) revalidation requirements and (b) for a job application?
- Can you cite at least two models of structured reflection, and are aware of the components of each model?
- Can you state the four themes in the NMC's code of practice?

A survey conducted by Osborne (2015) revealed that more than 30% of nurses do not keep a portfolio of evidence of their continuing learning. However, in the NMC's (2019b) revalidation document mentioned earlier, there are some very useful publications that provide further advice to registrants on how to collate all requirements in readiness for the revalidation event, which the FHM could draw on to advise team members, for example the RCN's (2017c) *Guide to Revalidation for Employers*. The HCPC, GMC and other regulatory bodies also provide further guidance on revalidation that is freely available via their websites. Individuals can also discuss the evidence required for revalidation at IDPR meetings with their line managers or clinical supervisors.

With regards to reflective accounts, the registrant can choose from various published structured frameworks such as Gibbs' model of reflection (1988), or use the NMC's guidelines on this. The reflection also needs to state the ways in which they address one or more of the four themes in the NMC's (2018b) code of practice. However, neither reflective accounts, nor most of the other evidence required, need to be uploaded to the NMC website by the registrant, but registrants have to keep all components addressing revalidation safe for potential auditing purposes. On the other hand, it is a resource-intensive task for the NMC to audit the portfolio of every one of the 732,000 or so registrants on its register.

Informal learning that meets revalidation requirements

Non-academic learning can take multifarious forms and those discussed here are practice-based or work-based learning, peer learning and reflective practice learning.

Work-based learning

It is widely recognised that one of the most effective ways of learning clinical skills is through learning-by-doing in work settings, which is often referred to as practice-based learning or as work-based learning (WBL). In pre-registration healthcare programmes, WBL occurs during practice placements, and generally for post-graduate programmes it is referred to as internships or work placement, which involves the student spending a pre-determined number of hours developing competence and gaining knowledge through their observation and supervised practice in an appropriate organisation, locally or abroad.

The Quality Assurance Agency for Higher Education (2018: 1) asserts that WBL 'involves learning through work, learning for work and/or learning at work [and] consists of authentic structured opportunities for learning which are achieved in a workplace setting'. The word 'authentic' in this context mean learning that potential employers consider relevant for the workplace. WBL can also be perceived as learning that takes place in the workplace, learning that is based on the workplace and learning for the workplace. 'Workplace' sometimes refers to a specific specialist area of work, and at other times it signifies workplaces in general.

Thus, as with students' on practice placements, WBL usually occurs in a tri-partite partnership between the student, placement provider and the HEI, and it is facilitated principally by work-based learning supervisors. The effectiveness of WBL can be enhanced through the use of learning contracts (or learning agreements), with specific learning objectives identified for the duration of the WBL.

The learning activity is predominantly situated learning and is incorporated into the widely implemented healthcare apprenticeships programmes, HSWs on NVQ courses, for learning management skills in the practice setting and for facilitating learning for NRHPs during precepteeship. Because WBL is founded on learning in the work setting, it enhances the likelihood of individuals' 'fitness for practise' on qualifying, and for career-long learning.

Peer learning and social capital

As noted in Table 2.1 in Chapter 2, peer learning represents individuals learning knowledge or skills informally from each other; that is, from someone of equal professional status and of similar age. Accessing the internet with work colleagues in the care setting's resource room or the staffroom for informal social learning, or in the organisation's education and training department locating critically appraised research literature are instances of informal peer learning.

Another mode of peer learning is from informal social networks of healthcare professionals. However, learning through electronic social networking websites needs to be approached with scepticism because of the risk of incorrect information being passed on to peers in an unmonitored environment. The NMC (2016) has therefore published advice on the use of social networking sites on the internet, where it primarily indicates that the NMC's (2018b) code of practice also applies to communicating through social networking sites (such as maintaining patient confidentiality).

Another form of peer learning occurs through partnering first-year and third-year student nurses for clinical practice sessions as a formal peer learning strategy and an educational model that results in positive learning experiences for both groups of students, according to research by Stenberg and Carlson (2015) and Zwedberg et al. (2021). The studies found that students shared skills, experience, ideas, thoughts and knowledge as equals and took responsibility for their peers' learning in care settings.

Also increasingly recognised as a vehicle for peer learning and peer support is human and social capital, which comprises the *ad hoc*, non-formal learning and support that individuals provide and/or receive from peers, friends, colleagues and even families in relation to their formal education. In this context, 'capital' refers to knowledge and skills imparted, and 'social capital' refers to time, patience, knowledge and teaching that individuals 'invest' in each other in small social groups or in twos.

The influence of care colleagues, co-students and personal relations on learning is thus very significant and valuable. Human and social capital is consistent with the basis of social learning theory and learning and teaching input by care practitioners have considerable effect on individuals' learning.

On reviewing the literature on human and social capital, Royal (2012) found that with nurse education located in higher education, there has been an increase in human capital; that is, in time and effort that individuals invest in their own education and skill acquisition. However, appreciation of ways of benefiting from social capital remains limited, according to Gopee (2002) and Taylor (2012), who recommend that such activity should be further supported and strengthened.

Furthermore, on examining the concept social capital, Hofmeyer (2013) concludes that it enhances team relationships between nurses and can have a positive impact on patient outcomes. Social capital thrives in settings that reflect the features of learning organisations, which is discussed later in this chapter.

Peer learning, however, requires an atmosphere of trust and openness, a collaborative, non-competitive learning environment at all levels of the organisation for it to function freely and benefit patient care. It can be enhanced further by reflection on clinical experiences' mechanisms.

Reflective practice learning

Another medium for learning is through structured reflection on unanticipated events and incidents that develop in care settings. Such events, including problem situations, decision-making dilemmas and conflict situations, can be highly beneficial for learning as they provide an opportunity to consider alternative solutions for if they recur. Reflective practice learning, therefore, is a further dimension of WBL, and its benefits through reflective discussion, journalling or narratives are widely appreciated and accepted in care professions (e.g. GMC, 2021).

Structured reflection can take place through reflective discussion with a facilitator, or individual reflection-on-action, which is more effective when a structured framework such as Gibbs' (1988) model of reflection is applied. Without reflection, there is always a risk of reductionist descriptions (i.e. seen as simply tasks) of clinical interventions and, therefore, to overlook the extensive theoretical knowledge and rationales that underpin these interventions.

The Gibbs' (1988) model of structured reflection comprises a cyclical sequence of six components:

1. Description: what happened?
2. Feelings: how do you feel deep down about the event/situation?
3. Evaluation: what was good or bad about the experience?
4. Analysis: what sense can you make of the situation overall?
5. Conclusion: what else could you have done (that is new learning)?
6. Action Plan: what will you do next time?

Various other models or frameworks of reflection in healthcare are available to choose from. In its revalidation guidance document, the NMC (2019b: 28), for example, indicates that at revalidation the registrant must declare that they have written at least five reflective accounts in the preceding three years, and reflected on them with a 'reflective discussion partner', and explained how they have changed or improved their practice as a result. The NMC's framework for writing reflective accounts constitutes of (p. 47):

1. What was the nature of the CPD activity and/or practice-related feedback and/or event or experience in your practice?
2. What did you learn from the CPD activity and/or feedback and/or event or experience in your practice?
3. How did you change or improve your practice as a result?
4. How is this relevant for at least one of the themes of the Code: Prioritise people – Practise effectively – Preserve safety – Promote professionalism and trust?

Continuing Professional Development for Everyone

All healthcare professionals of necessity have to engage in CPD because healthcare being a science (and art), evidence for new or improved ways of caring for individuals with health problems is continuously emerging. This section now explores CPD for team members as one of the responsibilities of FHMs, including learning through formal programmes as well as non-formal and informal work-based learning and reflective learning. Continuing learning for FHMs themselves encompasses management training and leadership development programmes, in addition to ongoing development of evidence-based clinical competence.

Several policy documents have over the years recognised the importance of, and advocated, CPD for all throughout our professional careers, including *Working Together – Learning Together* (DH, 2001) and *Continuing Professional Development and Your Registration* (HCPC, 2017). The HCPC (2017: 5) defines CPD as follows: 'CPD is the way in which registrants continue to learn and develop throughout their careers so they keep their skills and knowledge up to date and are able to practise safely and effectively.'

Much continuing learning and development are achieved at the workplace, and the FHM's role is crucial in leading and managing these learning activities. CPD also enhances the learning ethos and culture in care settings, leading to improved care for service users. Learning activities in healthcare settings is firmly endorsed by the NHS Constitution for England (DHSC, 2019a), which under the section 'Staff: your rights and NHS pledges to you' indicates that the NHS pledges to provide staff with personal development, access to appropriate education and training for their jobs and line management support to enable them to fulfil their potential.

Professional development programmes that are university based tend to be referred to as continuing professional education, and a popular article by Gopee (2002) in the Further Reading section of this chapter provides guidance on academic writing to support assignment writing for when attending HEI-based CPD programmes.

Career-long continuing learning

One of the main purposes of continuing learning is to ensure practitioners' fitness to practise. Consequently, profession-related learning throughout one's career is an inevitable feature of being a healthcare professional, and FHMs' duties include managing their own learning as well as learning for all individual team members.

Learning to lead effectively, and to manage effectively, can occur in various ways, and from different good leaders. The clinical skills learnt by healthcare professionals can be perceived as both a science and an art. Benner (2001) referred to 'expert' practice as artistry, which is the result of all the training and knowledge base acquired through several years of learning and experience. However, to become an expert as a leader or manager, there needs to be some formal training together with learning from one's own and others' experience.

Learning encompasses informal day-to-day learning through reflection-in-action as well as reflection-on-action, 'mandatory learning', that is, learning that has to be undertaken to meet the employer's mandatory training requirements (e.g. fire procedures), as well as continuing learning for the purpose of revalidation. Continuing learning can also be triggered by clinical supervision meetings, and formally at IDPR meetings, both noted in Chapter 2. Other informal means of professional development include peer-mentoring, action learning sets, peer reviews, reading and researching professional journals and learning communities.

Continuing learning has also increasingly become an essential ingredient for delivering high-quality patient care, and therefore employers and employees need to be aware of, and nurture, all informal opportunities and the formal structures that enable learning. Several mechanisms and opportunities for learning for healthcare professionals have become available over time, which include not only the substantial number of short courses provided by employers and the longer courses run at universities, but also:

Learning events at profession-based national or international conferences.

Online learning offered by professional journals and other specialist organisations, which sometimes include post-learning assessments.

Learning events organised locally, regionally or nationally by professional forums.

Inter-professional informal teaching and learning.

Practice-based teaching by medical staff, clinical leads, medical device agencies, etc.

Learning through visits or internships in other care settings.

ACTION POINT 10.2
Learning opportunities at your workplace

Several instances of learning in healthcare settings has been mentioned in this section. Specifically reflecting on learning opportunities at your workplace and the employing healthcare organisation, list at least five learning opportunities that have been accessible to team members recently.

Under the current overarching ethos of efficiency with the meticulous monitoring of funding for healthcare, teaching and learning can risk being overlooked, and therefore FHMs have to make a concerted effort to ensure that opportunities for the acquisition of knowledge and skills are seized as they occur, and maximised when feasible. Additionally, 'personal and people development', as one of the six dimensions of the NHS KSF (NHS Employers, 2019b), is a requirement that implies frontline managers have to support team members' CPD.

Management training and development programmes for frontline managers

The NHS KSF (NHS Employers, 2019b; DH, 2004) categorises all the duties and roles of healthcare professionals, including those of FHMs, in the form of the seven dimensions (including leadership as the seventh); the HEE (2015: 53) groups them as four policy areas; and NHS Scotland (2018) as clinical practice, management/leadership, education and research. Continual updating of clinical skills generally occur through practice-based learning and attending bespoke learning events, as healthcare professionals develop their clinical competence and knowledge throughout their careers as they progress from being competent to proficient, and eventually experts (see also Figure 10.1).

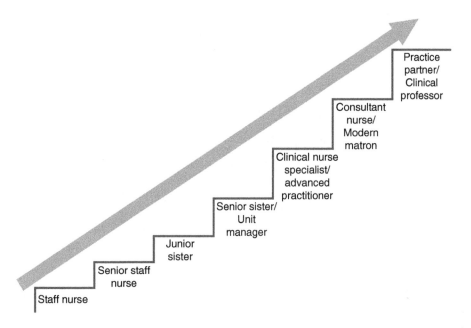

Figure 10.1 The potential career progression of registrants

As for developing management skills further, the FHM's career can progress to next level management positions such as charge nurse, ward manager, etc. Furthermore, from senior sister or unit manager level post, the healthcare professional can decide whether the future of their career stays in clinical practice (as for example clinical nurse specialist), or go towards higher management posts, or start to pursue working in education (hospital-based or university-based, etc.), or a combination of these.

For management posts, staff normally also enter the management pay scale (as different from Band 7, 8, etc.). However, for NRHPs, despite having been exposed substantially to management and leadership duties during pre-registration programmes and care management skills during practice placements, FHMs benefit further from guidance and structured learning that may be available to them post-qualifying.

As for teaching students and learners in clinical settings, the frontline manager will also have acquired some teaching skills during their pre-registration programmes but developed further subsequently. For research skills, these can also be developed further post-qualifying through attending specific courses and completing assignments, joining special interest groups, and sometime later even conducting research under the guidance of a research supervisor if they choose to pursue these further.

In addition to the six core dimensions of most NHS posts stated in the NHS KSF (NHS Employers, 2019b), including FHM posts, the optional seventh dimension is 'leadership and management'. Each dimension lists a number of skills, knowledge and behaviours that essentially comprise a competence framework for managerial posts, and these components can form the basis for managerial skill development.

ACTION POINT 10.3
Developing your own management skills

Reflecting on your own managerial and leadership skills development so far as a registrant, think of the different ways and sources from which you learned and developed your care setting management skills to be able to perform them competently. Think also of other first-line managers who you know, and how they developed their management and leadership skills. How much of these skills have been learned from:

a. Knowledge gained during your pre-registration programme?
b. Attending workshops or study days since qualifying?
c. Trial and error?
d. Advice sought from own line manager?
e. Other methods?

It is recognised that nursing careers take different forms, in that while some healthcare professionals choose increasing responsibility, many choose a more lateral career journey, moving to different specialism or care settings (HEE, 2015: 53). The HEE also recognises that management and leadership competence is one of the areas of the 'nursing career framework'. Multiple leadership and management training and education courses based in the UK and abroad are advertised by education institutions and other providers on the internet, as well as work-based management coaching and mentoring for trainee managers.

FHMs tend to learn management skills from their own line managers, or more senior managers, either through direct advice or through reflective conversations. Management preparation learning can be complemented by attending in-house or external short workshops, which generally are centred on decision-making and problem-solving activities and acquiring knowledge of policies and legislation.

On the other hand, the healthcare manager may have attended more substantial management courses leading to academic awards, which may have included role play or discussing scenarios, the learning from which they later apply to work settings under supervision. However, a survey of over 4,000 employees across healthcare and other sectors in the UK by the Chartered Management Institute [CMI] (2013: 4) revealed that employers in health and social care tend to prefer to offer in-house or on-the-job management training, rather than through formal qualification courses, despite the latter being seen as more effective. The survey also found that more than a third of respondents considered their line manager to be ineffective, which results in low employee engagement.

Furthermore, in a systematic review of literature on the management role of the ward manager, Pegram et al. (2014) conclude that the ward manager's role lacks clarity, educational development of the role as a skill-set before appointment to the post and during (ongoing education) tenure is erratic, and that it is imperative for the role to become more evidence-informed.

Additionally, structured management coaching is another systematic means of acquiring management skills. Structured coaching prevails in various arenas, such as in sports coaching, life coaching and executive coaching. In addition, 'leadership coaching', as professional development for healthcare professionals, are individually tailored programmes that also increase individual motivation, feelings of empowerment, etc., with subsequent positive effects on service users' health. The development of leadership skills can be enhanced further by facilitated self-awareness of personal values and beliefs, and assessment.

However, on exploring the factors that influence how senior healthcare professionals who attend leadership coaching programmes acquire and integrate their learning into their day-to-day practice, Rafferty and Fairbrother (2015) found that leadership coaching remains a problematic area as some programme participants wholeheartedly utilise the newly acquired skills while others were reluctant to do so. These different outcomes were dependent upon the 'courage, commitment and motivation' of participants to do so, as well as on their pre-programme perceptions of leadership coaching, and on the organisational support that they receive.

The Chartered Institute of Personnel and Development (CIPD) (2020) provides wide-ranging coaching and mentoring courses for line managers, while indicating that these are development techniques based on the use of one-to-one discussions to enhance an individual's skills, knowledge or work performance. The CMI (2021), on the other hand, work with management education and training providers to accredit their courses, and thereby provide them with nationally recognised qualifications (in addition to diplomas or degrees). The education provider institution can itself be 'recognised' as an 'Approved Centre' for example.

A number of strategies have been suggested to enable the FHM to reflect upon and self-assess their effectiveness as a manager. The categories of frontline managers' roles suggested in Figure 4.1 is one, Mintzberg's (2011) role theory is another, and yet another is Fayol's (2012) groups of management activities (or functions). Effective management practice comprises being proficient in the roles identified in Figure 4.1 as they are extracted from contemporary management practice. This section provides you with the opportunity to gauge your own effectiveness as a manager.

ACTION POINT 10.4
Enhancing your managerial effectiveness

Reflect on the managerial roles identified in Table 4.1 in Chapter 4 in response to Action point 1.1 and Figure 4.1. Based on these role components of effective managers, think of the management requirements of your role, and identify how you can apply what you have learnt about management and leadership in this book to your everyday management practice.

This Action point enables you to identify your current managerial strengths and development needs using the format presented on Table 10.1, where you can rate your skill level on each item as excellent, average or weak.

Brief suggestions for 'Resource manager' are given as an example for guidance on how an action plan could be constituted. You may find it helpful to compile a full action plan for yourself.

On completion of the activity suggested in Action point 10.4, you should have developed further insights into your own areas of strengths as a manager, as well as those of deficit, and those in which you wish your management role to develop further and develop self-confidence. Personal objectives can be constituted and an action plan to achieve them. In the context of particular objectives, and action to improve competence in that area, you may add some specific review dates and achieve-by-dates.

Managing funding for learning

As noted in Chapter 5 of this book, Handy (1984) suggests that staff should be treated as assets, not costs, and that the workplace should invest in this asset by supporting continuing education for staff. Some of the continuing learning activities identified so far in this chapter require payment of course fees, while others may be performed without any cost except one's time. Learning for team members are usually based on FHMs' awareness of the skill needs of the care setting for the delivery of safe and effective care, and, when required, informing the organisation's management of any potential skill deficiency that seems imminent.

Table 10.1 Self-assessment and action plan for managerial role development

Managerial role development area	Level of relevance to my current post	Skill rating	Objectives & action to improve my competence in this area	Resources that should help
Resource manager	Highly relevant	Weak	1) Develop competence in the conduct of IDPRs a) Attend in-house course for preparation as reviewer b) Discuss opportunities to conduct IDPRs with line manager 4) Complete a reflective account of an IDPR I have completed 2) Interviewing for staff vacancies a) ...	• Line manager • Reading about IDPRs • Attend workshop on staff interviews
Care co-ordinator and communication hub				
Health and safety monitor				
Care quality overseer				
Evidence-informed clinician				
Teamwork facilitator				
Leader and role model				
Learning supervisor and teacher				
Staff wellbeing promoter				
Decision-maker and problem-solver				

Continuing learning can be self-selected by registrants or determined mutually through their IDPRs. However, the CPD interests of the individual employee has to be matched with the skill needs of the practice setting. Nonetheless, there are various factors that can instigate or hinder learning in care settings, and therefore learning and teaching have to be managed and resourced.

Health Education England (2020b) has responsibility to determine and distribute funding for pre-registration education, training and CPD for healthcare workers, both clinical and non-clinical. HEE operates through eight regional centres. However, until 2022, it will also continue to operate through 13 Local

Education and Training Boards (LETBs), including as examples Health Education England South London, and South London LETB (Londonwide LMC, 2021).

The amount of funds allocated for CPD have fluctuated over the years. However, according to the RCN (2019d: 2), 'A nurse's education doesn't finish on graduation … ongoing training and development for a registered nurse is not an optional extra, but a basic professional requirement', because CPD enhances healthcare professionals' competence and, consequently, service users benefit from better quality of care.

Health Education England (2019) indicates that funding for CPD will increase by approximately £200m for 2020/21 budget year, of which £50m is to be mobilised through the NHS People Plan (NHSE, 2020a). This is partly because the UK Government has pledged £1000 for CPD for every nurse, midwife and AHP providing NHS services in England to be spread over three years to meet revalidation requirements. However, it is unclear given the current time pressures on the workforce, whether staff will have to complete structured learning in their own personal time, rather than during paid working hours (NHSE, 2020a: 37), especially as employers have to absorb backfilling staff time.

In addition to HEE and LETBs, Local Workforce Action Boards have been established specifically to co-ordinate and to support the workforce requirements for ICS model of health-social care. They operate in collaboration with healthcare service providers such as NHS trusts and primary care, and social care providers, while LETBs work with service providers (e.g. NHS trusts), CCGs and education providers (e.g. universities), and they are accountable to HEE for their decision-making and activities.

To a good extent, healthcare workers' continuing learning is determined by the local education and training strategy for healthcare trusts' employees in primary, secondary and community care, thereby ensuring supply of a competent health and care workforce locally. Nonetheless, healthcare staff can also apply for scholarship from other sources to support their learning (e.g. from the Florence Nightingale Foundation, some charity organisations, etc.). The next section explores teaching duties towards students during practice placements and the care setting's learning culture.

Managing Supervision of Students' Practice Learning

As noted in the introduction of Chapter 1, FHMs' duties and responsibilities can be grouped as: (1) organising care; (2) care and treatment activities; (3) managing staff and other resources; (4) teaching and educating; (5) engaging with research; and (6) leadership. For the teaching and educating role, this is every registrant's responsibility and for many they include supervision of students' practice-based learning and maintaining a learning culture in the care setting. It involves supervision of learning in order to ensure that everyone in the care setting is competent, safe and effective at all times.

ACTION POINT 10.5
Teaching responsibilities in your care setting

Frontline healthcare managers' teaching responsibilities extend to all colleagues, peers and learners. Pause momentarily and make a list of all different professions whose students have had placement in your care setting over the last year or two.
   Then reflect of the different teaching skills required to facilitate learning for:

a. different members of staff/peers;
b. student nurses, and other healthcare students;
c. other learners such as HSWs;
d. service users.

Registrants will have had some experience of teaching during their pre-registration programme, especially during the final placement when they focused mostly on management and leadership skills. Health profession students normally arrive in your care setting with identified objectives and competencies to be achieved, and FHMs have to decide on a daily basis which learner to allocate to which registrant for supervision of their learning.

Supervising students' learning

All registrants are in a position to teach students after completing their preceptorship programme and feeling competent and confident as healthcare professionals, according to the NMC (2018c). Other healthcare regulatory bodies may have specific training requirements in teaching before their registrants can teach health profession pre-registration students. It is also the registrant's responsibility to familiarise themselves with the student's course requirements for the placement, especially the competencies that need to be achieved while on the placement, or the 'standards of proficiency' that their students have to achieve as set out by their regulatory body.

For nurses, the student's three-year course curriculum is based on the NMC's (2018a) *Standards of Proficiency for Registered Nurses*, for example, and for supervising learning, FHMs need to acquaint themselves with the content of these documents for the relevant healthcare professions, in addition to the specific placement competencies that have to be achieved. Practice-based teachers and practice supervisors of students also have to know about the set standards for student supervision, which for nurses, midwives and nursing associates is identified in the NMC's (2018c) publication *Standards for Student Supervision and Assessment*.

Ample details of practice-based education supervisor role are provided by the NMC (2018c), and an extensive analysis of practice supervisors' and practice assessors' roles in care settings is presented in Gopee's (2018) book entitled *Supervision and Mentoring in Healthcare*. A condition of being a supervisor of learning is for the healthcare professional to be a good role model (e.g. NMC, 2018a platform 5: 19), which was discussed in the context of FHMs' leadership duties in healthcare settings.

Beside the 'practice supervisor' (NMC, 2018c) role that FHMs fulfil towards pre-registration healthcare profession students who are on placement in their care setting, their teaching role is quite wide-ranging as it also covers teaching all other qualified and unqualified team members, as well as service users, and their carers and relatives (in the form of health education). The management of team members' learning needs is another essential role of managers, whereupon the learning needs are often identified first by the individual, and second by frontline managers.

A learning culture in healthcare organisations

For students and all other members of staff to continue to develop their clinical skills, a learning culture is important at the frontline level as well as at organisational level. The term culture itself refers to a 'way of life, especially the general customs and beliefs of a particular group of people at a particular time' (Cambridge University Press, 2021: 1). It is explored in fair detail in Chapter 8 of this book, in the context of creating and maintaining a quality-conscious culture in care settings.

At a broader level, an organisational culture refers to 'shared values, beliefs and norms which influence the way employees think feel and act towards others inside and outside the organisation' according to Buchanan and Huczynski (2019: 798). This definition clearly suggests recognising enduring local attitudes and practices that are transmitted through members of staff who have been based in the particular setting for some time, and yet are open-minded and their practice is evidence-based.

A learning culture thrives in care settings where practice is evidence-informed and where an effective learning environment prevails, an environment that fosters a culture within which team members appreciate, value and are committed to continuous learning for all as essential. Numerous research studies have reported their findings on the characteristics of care settings that are effective learning environments, from one of the earliest landmark studies conducted by Fretwell (1980) to those published much more recently (e.g. Cunningham, 2020). Due to limited space in this textbook, it is advisable to refer to Chapter 4 of the book

Supervision and Mentoring in Healthcare (Gopee, 2018) for a detailed analysis of a range of studies on clinical settings as learning environments.

A learning culture, furthermore, is fundamental for an organisation to be perceived as a 'learning organisation', which the NHSE (2015a: 23) asserts is essential for the NHS to become 'the world's largest learning organisation with a new culture of learning'. A learning organisation, therefore, implies that a positive attitude to learning prevails in the organisation's forward planning, as well as amongst frontline staff, including when challenges surface in care settings.

Concluding from a systematic review of organisational learning in public sector organisations, Rashman et al. (2009) suggest that intra- and inter-organisational learning can be achieved by two-way knowledge sharing between team members, and through interaction within a trusting relationship. An organisational culture that supports learning is essential, as also is a comprehensive infrastructure of staff and supplies (e.g. computer software, protocols and clinical guidelines, consumables, etc.).

ACTION POINT 10.6
Inter-professional learning in your care setting

Precisely when, and in which situations, does inter-disciplinary learning occur in your care setting? Think of examples of instances of their occurrence.

Team learning is an essential feature of collaborative inter-disciplinary teamwork and collaborative learning that supports safe, effective and compassionate care for service users, and of effective learning environments for staff. These are features of learning culture in care settings, and of the wider organisational learning, which is an aspect of social learning theory, which, in turn, indicates that a vast range of learning occurs in social environments, such as care organisations, through interaction with other professionals.

Moreover, as is obvious from the foregoing discussion, learning must not be a superficial add-on activity neither, as it is an inherent day-to-day activity that forms the basis for ensuring well-informed best-quality care being delivered. Staff development strategies are often already built-in into healthcare organisations' annual business plans.

Managing Issues Linked to Learning and Development

This section on managing issues related to staff competence and learning briefly addresses management of poor practice and uncivil behaviour elicited by healthcare professionals or by students, and then it moves on to learning from patient or staff incidents.

Managing poor practice

Frontline managers' duties include supervising all team members, including inter-disciplinary staff, to ensure all interventions are performed competently. When unsafe or ineffective practice does occur, it is up to the frontline manager to question the staff member, and advise them as appropriate, or take any corrective action deemed necessary. A supportive questioning stance is necessary because it provides the team member the opportunity to explain or elaborate on the clinical activity. The FHM can then assess how closely the relevant clinical guidelines have been followed, and then ask for any reason for any divergence, which might reveal gaps in knowledge or competence.

Issues in managing learning have recently also highlighted the occasional occurrence of uncivil behaviour by students, and even by staff members. Uncivil behaviour goes even further than such unprofessional behaviour as bullying and harassment and could take the form of abusive language and physical threats.

From the literature review of the triggers of incivility within healthcare teams, Keller et al. (2020) conclude that perpetrators of such behaviour tend to be seen as having a difficult personality, and the predictors of higher incivility levels tend to be based on high workload, communication or co-ordination issues, patient safety concerns, lack of support and poor leadership. With regards to guidance on management of unprofessional behaviour, the NMC (2021) recommends assessing whether the behaviour constitutes a risk to anyone if the person continues to behave the way they are, and after initial questioning, consider which steps to take, including:

- competence assessments;
- supervision;
- referral to occupational health or another healthcare professional;
- formal training or retraining;
- role changes; or
- in rare cases, suspension.

A realistic and achievable plan needs to be constituted for the benefit of both the professional and the care setting for the individual to follow to address the risks, followed by deep reflection and learning from the situation by both parties (see also conflict management in Chapter 7 of this book). All steps that have been taken to address the concerns must be clearly documented.

Learning from patient safety incidents

There are several benefits in working in teams as opposed to working in groups or individually, and in healthy organisations, one of the benefits of inter-disciplinary teamwork is that healthcare professionals learn from each other within the team, both informally and formally. Learning within teams can occur in various formal and informal ways, a number of which were examined under career-long continuing learning earlier in this chapter.

Sources of learning might also include 'critical incidents' in the workplace, including patient safety incidents (PSIs) such as near misses. Despite the UK having one of the best health services in the world, reports of malpractice and failures to provide safe and effective care still tend to surface now and again, and some of these are exposed on national television through BBC's *Panorama* programme, for example. Instances of individual malpractice when reported are managed by the regulatory body such as the NMC or GMC, but when mistakes or failures occur team-wide or organisation-wide they tend to get discovered later, often after complaints from service users (which include their families) have been received.

One extreme instance of malpractice is when multiple complaints were received about very poor quality of care and treatment at a UK NHS Foundation Trust (Francis, 2013), which resulted in the eventual closure of the main hospital and transfer of services to other sites. On investigating complaints by several service users at the Trust over a number of years, the investigators identified a number of warning signs of failures to achieve expected standards across the trust, which should have been detected and actions take to resolve them, as well as learn to prevent future recurrence. Very poor communication between various parties and staff reneging responsibility for quality of care meant service users continued to be at risk of harm.

Such dangerous modes of service provision and unhealthy local cultures are often the consequence of 'dysfunctional leadership', which is another reason for requiring training programmes for healthcare professionals in leadership positions. Hundreds of recommendations for changes health service-wide ensued from the inquiry into the above-mentioned example, including a fundamental change in culture, ensuring openness, transparency, candour about matters of concern, and accountability at both individual level and organisational level. A strong emphasis was placed on compassionate care, on standards and safety, and a monthly report of ward staffing levels, as well as continuing training and education for staff.

Reporting of PSIs is an integral component of quality management, as it includes monitoring lapses in standards that cause adverse events and near misses. Frontline managers have a responsibility to ensure that team members report any such incident. According to NHS Improvement (2018d), patient safety incidents are any unintended or unexpected incident which could have, or did, lead to harm for one or more patients receiving healthcare. Incidents can be reported by healthcare professionals or the public.

Furthermore, the CQC (2018b: 1) identifies 'never events', which it states are 'serious, largely preventable safety incidents that should not occur if the available preventative measures are implemented'. As a concept that is also supported by

NHS Improvement (2018d), the CQC indicates that never events include wrong site surgery or foreign objects left in a person's body during an operation, of which 469 cases had been provisionally reported between April 2017 and March 2018 – incidents that can cause further harm to the patient, and to the healthcare provider's reputation.

The costs of PSIs occur in human terms as well as financial, as also found by research conducted by Haxby and Shuldham (2018). However, at times, care staff have felt incident reporting are bureaucratic activities that deprive service users of their time and attention, and sometimes no preventive or corrective action seems to have been taken following reporting.

However, in their qualitative research on how hospital culture and climate impact on nurses actively reporting medical errors in the interest of patient safety in the USA, Levine et al. (2020) found that nurses do perceive and understand the benefits, as well as the barriers, to reporting such errors when they occur. Levine et al. also note that the barriers including inefficient reporting systems and organisational influences of the perceived consequences of reporting on the person makes reporting prohibitive and recommend that frontline managers should endeavour to effect change of this culture to one that is more positive by promoting organisational commitment to reporting. Almost identical issues have been reported from research in primary care elsewhere, and similar recommendations made (Vázquez-Sánchez, 2020), which suggest that reporting of PSIs currently remains an issue.

Some of the mechanisms in place contemporarily to facilitate healthcare professionals to report PSIs, never events and near misses without being incriminated for reporting them include incident forms to be completed and forwarded to management of the organisation. This can be in paper-form or as computer software for ease of reporting such as by using the Local Care Direct Reporter Form (D1F1) (Datix, 2017). Another is the National Reporting and Learning System (NRLS) which is now managed by NHS Improvement (2018d), and also normally completed online, and is due to be replaced by a more staff-friendly *Learn from Patient Safety Events Service* in 2022.

To strengthen PSI reporting further, the Patient Safety Incident Response Framework is being piloted, and due to be implemented in full in 2022. Healthcare sites where it is being piloted are currently using the 'Serious Incident Framework'.

The NMC and GMC (2019: 1) jointly identify specific steps that the healthcare professional should take when they do make a mistake, which are:

Tell the patient (or, where appropriate, the patient's advocate, family or carer) when something has gone wrong.

Apologise to the patient (or the patient's family or carer).

Offer an appropriate remedy or support to put matters right (if possible).

Explain fully to the patient (or the patient's family or carer) the short- and long-term effects of what has happened.

ACTION POINT 10.7
Learning from patient safety incidents

Visit the NHSE+I (2019) website and view the 2018 'Learning from patient safety incidents' document. Then follow the links to 'Patient safety review and response report October 2018 to March 2019' (https://webarchive. nationalarchives.gov.uk/20200501113026/https://improvement.nhs.uk/doc-uments/5988/2019.09.23_PS_Review_and_Response_Report_Oct_2018_-_March_2019_FINAL.pdf) which has reports of patient incidents and the health service's response to the incident, and includes learning from the incident. The site includes reports on pulse oximetry, mental health, etc. Feel free to read the whole document, but examine in particular the learning and actions that ensued from the reporting of the incident.

Alternatively, search on the internet for the investigation report of a nationally publicised healthcare major incident, and again feel free to read the whole document, but examine in particular the learning and actions that ensued from the reporting of the incident.

Consider what you can learn from this and how you can apply the learning to your practice as a FHM to safeguard quality and patient safety, and ensure that you are working within the code of practice for your profession.

Learning by the healthcare team is paramount in the interest of providing highest quality care (discussed in Chapter 8 of this book) and to prevent similar incidents. As to the actions that follow after the incident form has been completed, there is a danger that they can just become a statistic, rather than being actioned to prevent recurrence and learning from them. For example, Moore (2017) reports on NHS trusts where healthcare professionals meet each morning and form 'patient safety huddles' to discuss any PSI event that might have occurred during the preceding 24 hours. Huddles are usually approximately ten-minute-long brief meetings by multidisciplinary frontline team members (including relevant non-clinical staff) that occur every day, and that focus on one or more agreed patients most likely to be at risk of harm (e.g. falls), and actions are agreed (NHS Improvement, 2019a).

Another form of reporting PSIs is referred to as whistleblowing, which occurs when a recurring aspect of poor standard of care is reported more publicly, for example reported in a newspaper, thereby escalating the concern. Instances of whistleblowing include unsafe working conditions, lack of (or poor) response to reported PSIs, bullying or harassment, suspected fraud, etc. and lack of training for temporary workers.

In 2020, a news item reported that whistleblowing cases have risen 70% in one year, and that nurses are the most likely healthcare professionals to raise concerns in this way (Stephenson, 2020), probably because it enables staff to exercise their duty of candour. Additionally, the NMC (2021) indicates that when concern is raised regarding suspected malpractice, then employers should take into account the local context (staffing levels, etc.) before referring the individual to the regulatory body.

Thus, as with all healthcare professionals, the duty of candour (also noted in Chapter 2 of this book) is another stance that FHMs have to have in their armoury of knowledge and competence to discharge their role safely and effectively, and thereby strive for highest quality of care.

It is generally acknowledged that failure in care setting is usually unintentional, and that there is often more than one explanation particularly with major failures, as also identified some years ago by the DH (2000a). A failure can be treated as a problem, and multiple reasons for failure can be identified by performing a root cause analysis (see Chapter 7 for details). However, learning from mistakes to prevent their recurrence is an imperative for all healthcare professionals (e.g. NHSE+I, 2019; CQC, 2020a).

Guidance for Managing Team Members' Continuing Development

The following comprises good practice guidelines for managing all team members' and learners' continuing development.

- Access management training and development programmes for frontline healthcare managers to further develop your competence in this area.
- Review your own leadership and management abilities and performance at formal and safe opportunities when they arise.
- Manage team members' continuing learning but ensuring they are based on the care setting's needs and on the career aspirations of the individual, as well as for revalidation requirements.
- Harness and promote all modes of learning including in-house training and university-based education to facilitate team members' professional development, including facilitation of practice-based preceptorship.
- Recognise and support informal and peer learning where they occur, and ascertain whether all staff have equal opportunities for attending professional development activities.
- Support professional development activities that comprise evidence of safe and effective practice for team members' revalidation requirements.
- Ensure an inter-disciplinary learning culture prevails and endures in your workplace, and that all learners' learning needs are attended to, including those of service users.
- Identify and apply learning from patient safety incidents, failures in health services and 'near misses', and manage poor practice according to the organisation's procedures, and ensure learning occurs from all incidents for all concerned.

Chapter Summary

Engaging with continuing learning is no doubt an indispensable activity for healthcare professionals, and FHMs' duties include supporting, recommending, facilitating and reinforcing continuing learning and education. Consequently, this chapter has addressed:

- Cognisance of ways in which frontline managers manage and facilitate team members' continuing professional development, starting with managing structured preceptorship development programmes for NRHPs, then covering professional regulation and team members' revalidation requirements, which also takes into account various non-formal practice-based learning methods;
- Enabling team members to appreciate the significance and ways of engaging in continuing learning, followed by focus on management training and development programmes for frontline managers as well as funding for staff development;
- Supervision of students' practice learning while maintaining a learning culture in care settings as learning organisations; and
- Management of issues related to learning and development, including management of poor practice and clinical incidents as sources of further learning.

Further Reading

- For details of a preceptorship toolkit for preparation of preceptors that include an organisational support tool, a managerial support framework, a supernumerary time tool and a local culture of support tool, and can be adapted for use locally – see: Owen P, Whitehead B, Beddingham E, Simmons M (2020) A preceptorship toolkit for nurse managers, teams and healthcare organisations. *Nursing Management*, 27(4): 20–25.
- Patient Safety Incidents have been managed by NHS Improvement (2018b), and will be replaced by *Learn from Patient Safety Events Service* in due course. PSIs are normally completed online, one of the programs for this being Datix – Incident Reporting System. For more details see, for example: Central and North West London NHS Foundation Trust (2020) *Incident Reporting*. Available at: www.rcpsych.ac.uk/docs/default-source/improving-care/nccmh/reducing-restrictive-practice/resources/incident-reporting.pdf?sfvrsn=2932a4bf_2. Accessed Date: 20 July 2020.
- For information and full details on revalidation, visit the NMC's dedicated website: Revalidation | The Nursing and Midwifery Council (nmc.org.uk)
- For guidance on how you can demonstrate knowledge, critical analysis and synthesis in academic assignments, see: Gopee N (2002) Demonstrating critical analysis in academic assignments. *Nursing Standard*, 16(35): 45–52. Also published in: *Cancer Nursing Practice*, 1(7): 32–38; *Learning Disability Practice*, 5(7): 29–36.

Glossary

Several management and leadership terminologies are defined or explained in this book in the section where they are actually discussed, and most can be located from the Index, which is the final component of the book after the References section. Several of the terminologies explained in this Glossary are those not defined in the book.

Budget – A budget is a statement of revenues and costs in financial terms that are anticipated and identified in advance of a period of time for spending on specific activities that reflect the agreed policies and strategies for meeting the objectives of the organisation.

Capital expenditure – Funds allocated to finance long-term and investment spending such as for a new building for a new department for a specific group of service users, for example, or for costly equipment or technology.

Effectiveness – The achievement of expected health recovery and patient outcomes following planned care interventions.

Efficiency – The achievement of set goals at minimum financial costs, in the minimum amount of time, but to the required standard.

Health and Wellbeing Boards (HWBs) – A forum in which key leaders from the local health-social care system work together to improve the health and wellbeing of their local population, working collaboratively with local authorities with adult social care and public heath responsibilities.

Healthcare support worker (HSW) – Healthcare staff who are not registered with a professional regulatory body. Also known as healthcare assistant, and includes nursing support worker.

Integrated Care Systems (ICSs) – ICSs bring together NHS, local authority and third sector bodies to take on collective responsibility for the resources and the health of the population of a defined geographical area, with the aim of delivering integrated health-social care for patients, and thereby there is shared commitment to deliver services, manage resources, and the inherent quality monitoring arrangements.

Lean methods – The least wasteful ways to provide equivalent or better and safer healthcare to service users, within the same timescale.

Operational planning – Care and treatment plans and goals usually set for one financial year.

Primary Care Networks (PCNs) – Geographically based networks of GP Practices covering 30,000 –50,000 patients each, which have come together as part of NHS LTP to deliver 'national service specifications', including structured medication reviews, enhanced health in care homes, anticipatory care (with community services), personalised care, supporting early cancer diagnosis, cardiovascular disease case-finding and locally agreed action to tackle inequalities.

Productivity – The number of units of output (e.g. number of patients seen by a community nurse) resulting from each unit of input (time in hours, and other resources). The ratio or relationship between one or more outputs to one or more inputs, and the quality of the outputs.

Qualitative research – A method used mainly in social sciences to obtain an in-depth understanding of a social issue or concept, often using a smaller number of participants, while applying research methods that include individual interviews, case studies, etc. to collect data and then draw general conclusions.

Quantitative research – A systematic empirical investigation that incorporates measurement and statistical testing, and often aims to find or show co-relation between components of the study, including 'cause and effect' of interventions, and possible generalisation of the findings to the larger population.

Reflection-on-action – Making time to stop and think about a clinical event by describing it in detail and thinking of alternative ways of managing such events if they recur. However, reflection-in-action entails thinking about micro-decisions just made while performing clinical interventions.

Relational leadership theory – The interpersonal relationship between leadership and team members, which views leadership as a social influence process through which change (e.g. new approaches, values, attitudes, behaviours, ideologies) is constructed and produced.

Risk assessment – A structured mechanism for assessing the potential dangers that a novel intervention might pose.

Root cause analysis (RCA) – A structured method used to analyse serious adverse events to identify both active errors and latent errors that contribute to the adverse event.

Service providers – Organisations that provide care and treatment, e.g. hospitals, care homes, GP practices, etc.

Skill mix – The numbers and ratio, capability and experience of qualified and unqualified staff, which in the case of nursing are required for the delivery of safe and effective care.

Span of duty – A shift or duration of time that the staff member is on duty on any particular day, which in healthcare involves working in hours that are outside the traditionally acknowledged hours between 9am and 5pm. It might involve early hours, night hours, longer hours and other patterns.

Strategic planning – The organisation's planning for the forthcoming three, five or ten years; different from operational planning, which in turn usually refers to planning for one financial year.

Sustainability and Transformation Partnership (STP) – Partnership between NHS, local authority and other health-social care organisations to collaboratively determine the future of their health and care system with the aim of providing integrated health and social care.

Urgent care centre (UCC) – Along with 'urgent treatment centres (UTCs), same day emergency care (SDEC) are new models of healthcare developed under the *NHS Long Term Plan*.

References

Adair J (2005) *Effective Leadership Development*. London: Chartered Institute of Personnel and Development.

Agile-Mercurial (2019) *Tuckman's Model – 5 Stages of Team Development and Practical Limitations*. Available at: https://agile-mercurial.com/2019/04/16/tuckmans-model-5-stages-of-team-development-and-practical-limitations/. Accessed Date: 6 July 2020.

Alkhawaldeh J M A, Soh K L, Mukhtar F B M, Ooi C P (March 2020) Effectiveness of stress management interventional programme on occupational stress for nurses: A systematic review. *Journal of Nursing Management*, 28(2): 209–220.

Almost J (2006) Conflict within nursing work environments: Concept analysis. *Journal of Advanced Nursing*, 53(4): 444–453.

Anastas T, Waddell E N, Howk S, Remiker M, Horton-Dunbar G, Fagnan L J (2019) Building behavioural health homes: Clinician and staff perspectives on creating integrated care teams. *Journal of Behavioral Health Services & Research*, 46(3): 475–486.

Anderson C (2018) Exploring the role of advanced nurse practitioners in leadership. *Nursing Standard*, 33(2): 29–33.

Andrews A, St Aubyn B (2015) 'If it's not written down; it didn't happen …'. *Journal of Clinical Nursing*, 29(5): 20–22.

Aritzeta A, Swailes S, Senior B (2007) Belbin's team role model: Development, validity and applications for team building. *Journal of Management Studies*, 44(1): 96–118.

Armstrong M, Taylor S (2020) *Armstrong's Handbook of Human Resource Management Practice* (15th edn). London: Kogan Page.

Arnold J, Coyne I, Randall R, Patterson F (2020) *Work Psychology – Understanding Human Behaviour in the Workplace* (7th edition). Harlow (UK): Pearson Education Limited.

Association of Project Management (2020) *What is Project Management?* Available at: www.apm.org.uk/resources/what-is-project-management/. Accessed Date: 31 March 2020.

Baird B (2020) *Primary Care Networks Explained*. Available at: www.kingsfund.org.uk/publications/primary-care-networks-explained. Accessed date: 13 May 2021.

Baldwin A, Mills J, Birks M, Budden L (2014) Role modelling in undergraduate nursing education: An integrative literature review. *Nurse Education Today*, 34(2014): e18–e26.

Bass B M (1990) *Bass and Stogdills Handbook of Leadership: Theory, Research and Managerial Applications* (3rd edn). New York: Free Press.

Bass B M, Riggio R E (2006) *Transformational Leadership*. London: Lawrence Erlbaum Associates.

BBC News (17 August 2020) *Coronavirus: Public Health England 'to be replaced'*. Available at: www.bbc.co.uk/news/health-53799854. Accessed Date: 20 August 2020.

BBC One *Panorama* (2019) *Undercover Hospital Abuse Scandal. Broadcasted on Wednesday 22 May 2019*. Available at: www.bbc.co.uk/programmes/m00059qb. Accessed date: 9 February 2020.

Beattie M, Shepherd A, Howieson B (2012) Do the Institute of Medicine's (IOM's) dimensions of quality capture the current meaning of quality in health care? – An integrative review. *Journal of Research in Nursing*, 18(4) 288–304.

Beckhard R and Harris R T (1987) *Organisational Transitions: Managing Complex Change* (2nd edn). Reading, MA: Addison-Wesley.

Belbin Associates (2020) *The Nine Belbin Team Roles*. Available at: www.belbin.com/about/belbin-team-roles/. Accessed Date: 21 August 2020.

Benner P (2001) *From Novice to Expert: Excellence and Power in Clinical Nursing Practice*. London/Menlo Park, CA: Addison-Wesley.

Berlin J M, Carlstrom E D, Sandberg H S (2012) Models of teamwork: ideal or not? A critical study of theoretical team models. *Team Performance Management*, 18(5/6): 328–340.

Best C (2020) Is there a place for servant leadership in nursing? *Practice Nursing*, 31(3): 128–132.

Bianchi M, Bagnasco A, Bressan V, Barisone M, Timmins F, Rossi S, Pellegrini R, Aleo G, Sasso L. (2018) A review of the role of nurse leadership in promoting and sustaining evidence-based practice. *Journal of Nursing Management*, 26(8): 918–932.

Blake R and McCanse A (1991) *Leadership Dilemmas – Grid Solutions*. Houston: Gulf Publishing Company. [Also Available at: www.bumc.bu.edu/facdev-medicine/files/2010/10/Leadership-Matrix-Self-Assessment-Questionnaire.pdf. Accessed Date: 27 May 2020].

Boamah S (2018) Linking nurses' clinical leadership to patient care quality: The role of transformational leadership and workplace empowerment. *Canadian Journal of Nursing Research*, 50(1): 9–19.

Boedker C (2012) *The rise of the compassionate leader: Should we be cruel to be kind?* University of New South Wales Australia Business School. Available at: The rise of the compassionate leader - SmartCompany. Accessed Date: 1 December 2020.

Bonner G, McLaughlin S (2014) Leadership support for ward managers in acute mental health inpatient settings. *Nursing Management*, 21(2): 26–29.

Brewer K C, Oh K M, Kitsantas P, Zhao X (2020) Workplace bullying among nurses and organizational response: An online cross-sectional study. *Journal of Nursing Management*, 28(1): 148–156.

Briner R B, Denyer D, Rousseau D M (2009) *Evidence-Based Management: Concept Clean-up Time?* Available at: www.cebma.org/wp-content/uploads/Briner-Denyer-Rousseau-Evidence-based-management-Concept-cleanup-time.pdf. Accessed Date: 2 June 2020.

British Association for Counselling and Psychotherapy (2018) *Ethical Framework for the Counselling Professions*. Available at: www.bacp.co.uk/media/3103/bacp-ethical-framework-for-the-counselling-professions-2018.pdf. Accessed Date: 15 September 2020.

British Association of Social Workers (2020) *Professional Capabilities Framework*. Available at: www.basw.co.uk/professional-development/professional-capabilities-framework-pcf/the-pcf/social-worker. Accessed date: 17 May 2020.

British Broadcasting Corporation (2020) *BBC Documentary Follows Nurses at Queen's and King George Hospitals*. Available at: www.time1075.net/159566-2-bbc-nurse-documentary-queens-king-george-hospitals/. Accessed Date: 24 June 2020.

British Standards Institute (2020) *BS 13500 Code of Practice for Delivering Effective Governance of Organizations*. Available at: www.bsigroup.com/en-GB/bs-13500-Organizational-governance/. Accessed Date: 29 September 2020.

Brookes J (2011) Engaging staff in the change process. *Nursing Management*, 18(5): 16–19.

Brown P (1998) 'Endangered species'. *The Times*, 29 October 1998, p. 2.

Buchanan D A, Huczynski A (2019) *Organisational Behaviour* (10th edn). London: Pearson.

Byrne G (2007) Unlocking potential – coaching as a means to enhance leadership and role performance in nursing. *Journal of Clinical Nursing*, 16(11): 1987–1988.

Calpin-Davies F (2000) 'Nurse manager, change thyself'. *Nursing Management*, 6(9): 16–20.

Cambridge University Press (2021) *Cambridge Dictionary* (online). Available at: https://dictionary.cambridge.org/dictionary/english/. Accessed Date: 23 May 2021.

Care Quality Commission (CQC) (2015) *Regulation 20: Duty of Candour, Information for All Providers: NHS Bodies, Adult Social Care, Primary Medical and Dental Care, and Independent Healthcare.* Available at: www.cqc.org.uk/sites/default/files/20150327_duty_of_candour_guidance_final.pdf. Accessed on 16 August 2020.

Care Quality Commission (CQC) (2018a) *Statement on CQC's Role and Responsibilities for Safeguarding Children and Adults.* Available at: www.cqc.org.uk/sites/default/files/20190621_SC121706_CQC_statement_February_2018_v3_0.pdf. Accessed date: 16 September 2020.

Care Quality Commission (CQC) (2018b) *Learning from Never Events.* Available at: www.cqc.org.uk/news/stories/learning-never-events. Accessed Date: 15 August 2020.

Care Quality Commission (CQC) (2020a) *What We Do – The five key questions we ask.* Available at: www.cqc.org.uk/what-we-do/how-we-do-our-job/five-key-questions-we-ask. Accessed Date: 25 August 2020.

Care Quality Commission (CQC) (2020b) *Surveys.* Available at: www.cqc.org.uk/publications/surveys/surveys. Accessed Date: 25 August 2020.

Carlin A, Duffy K (2013) Newly qualified staff's perceptions of senior charge nurse roles. *Nursing Management*, 20(7): 24–30.

Centre for Advancement of Interprofessional Education (2020) *About CAIPE.* Available at: www.caipe.org/about-us. Accessed Date: 20 July 2020.

Chartered Global Management Accountant (2015) *CGMA Tools – Lean Management Techniques.* Available at: www.cgma.org/Resources/Tools/DownloadableDocuments/lean-management-techniques.pdf. Accessed Date: 2 May 2020.

Chartered Institute of Personnel and Development (2020) *Coaching and Mentoring – Factsheet.* Available at: Coaching and Mentoring | Factsheets | CIPD. Accessed Date: 11 January 2021.

Chartered Management Institute (2013) *A Management and Leadership Health-Check – A diagnosis of management and leadership development needs in the health and social care sector.* Available at: www.managers.org.uk/wp-content/uploads/2013/11/4779-MLD-Healthcare-Report-White-Paper-NOV-2013.pdf. Accessed Date: 8 February 2021.

Chartered Management Institute (2021) *2020 Annual Reports and Account.* Available at: www.managers.org.uk/wp-content/uploads/2020/08/CMI-Annual-Report-2020.pdf. Accessed Date: 8 February 2021.

Chartered Society for Physiotherapy (2018) *Service improvement: An introduction.* Available at: www.csp.org.uk/professional-clinical/improvement-and-innovation/improving-and-transforming-your-service/intro. Accessed Date: 10 September 2020.

Chin R J (2015) Examining teamwork and leadership in the fields of public administration, leadership, and management. *Team Performance Management*, 21(3/4): 199–216.

Clarke C, Mantle R (2016) Using risk management to promote person-centred dementia care. *Nursing Standard*, 30(28): 41–46.

Clegg S, Kornberger M (2003) *Modernism, postmodernism, management and organization theory*. Available at: www.researchgate.net/publication/295472957_MODERNISM_POSTMODERNISM_MANAGEMENT_AND_ORGANIZATION_THEORY. Accessed Date: 22 May 2020.

Cole E (2020) Supporting Gen Y and Z: What it takes to retain newly qualified nurses. *Nursing Standard*, 35(3): 14–17.

Collins (2021) *Collins Dictionary*. Available at: Collins Online Dictionary | Definitions, Thesaurus and Translations (collinsdictionary.com). Accessed Date: 6 March 2021.

Collins E, Owen P, Digan J, Dunn F (2020) Applying transformational leadership in nursing practice. *Nursing Standard*, 35(5): 59–66.

Council of Deans of Health (2014) *Care Transformed: The Impact of Nursing, Midwifery and Allied Health Professional Research*. Available at: www.councilofdeans.org.uk/wp-content/uploads/2014/12/Care-Transformed-web-version-1.pdf. Accessed date: 20 August 2020.

Covey S R (2006) *The 8th Habit – from Effectiveness to Greatness*. London: Simon & Schuster UK.

Cripps M (2018) *Leadership Q&A: NHS RightCare*. Available at: www.hsj.co.uk/leadership-qanda/leadership-qanda-nhs-rightcare/7021633.article. Accessed Date: 6 April 2020.

Cunningham S (2020) Clinical learning environments. In: Cunningham S (ed.) *Dimensions on Nursing Teaching and Learning* (Chapter 3). Cham (Switzerland): Springer Nature.

Cziraki K, McKey C, Peachey G, Baxter P, Flaherty B (2014) Factors that facilitate registered nurses in their first-line nurse manager role. *Journal of Nursing Management*, 22(8): 1005–1014.

Datix Ltd (2017) *Local Care Direct Reporter Form (D1F1)*. Available at: https://datix.localcaredirect.org/datix/live/index.php. Accessed Date: 16 August 2020.

Davies A, James W, Griffiths L (2020) Implementing a quality improvement programme in a locality mental health service. *Nursing Management*, 27(1): 27–32.

Davis L, Taylor H, Reyes H (2014) Lifelong learning in nursing: A Delphi study. *Nurse Education Today*, 34(3): 441–445.

Dawson P, Andriopoulos C (2021) *Managing Change, Creativity and Innovation* (4th edn). London: Sage Publications.

Dean, E (2012) Building resilience: Nurses are vulnerable to burnout, but with support they can learn how to bounce back. (CARE CAMPAIGN). *Nursing Standard*, 26(32): 16–18.

Dellefield M E, Verkaaik C (2021) Using the Observational Teamwork Assessment in Surgery Instrument to Measure RN Teamwork During Cardiac Surgery – Lessons Learned. *Journal of Nursing Care Quality*, 36(2): 162–168.

Department of Health (DH) (2000a) *An Organisation with Memory – Report of an Expert Group on Learning from Adverse Events in the NHS Chaired by the Chief Medical Officer*. Available from: www.igt.hscic.gov.uk/KnowledgeBaseNew/DH_An%20organisation%20with%20a%20memory.pdf. Accessed Date: 16 August 2020.

Department of Health (DH) (2000b) *The NHS Plan: A Plan for Investment, a Plan for Reform*. Available at: http://webarchive.nationalarchives.gov.uk/20130107105354/http://www.dh.gov.uk/prod_consum_dh/groups/dh_digitalassets/@dh/@en/@ps/documents/digitalasset/dh_118522.pdf. Accessed date: 28 January 2020.

Department of Health (DH) (2001) *Working Together – Learning Together. A Framework for Lifelong Learning for the NHS*. Available at: https://dera.ioe.ac.uk/13612/1/

Working%20together%20-%20learning%20together%20dept.%20of%20health.pdf. Accessed Date: 9 January 2021.

Department of Health (DH) (2004) *NHS Knowledge and Skills Framework.* Available at: http://webarchive.nationalarchives.gov.uk/+/www.dh.gov.uk/en/publicationsand-statistics/publications/publicationspolicyandguidance/dh_4090843. Accessed date: 5 May 2020.

Department of Health (DH) (2006) *Our Health, Our Care, Our Say: A New Direction for Community Services.* Available at: https://webarchive.nationalarchives.gov.uk/+/http://www.dh.gov.uk/en/Publicationsandstatistics/Publications/PublicationsPolicyAnd-Guidance/DH_4127453. Accessed date: 28 January 2020.

Department of Health (DH) (2008a) *High Quality Care For All – NHS Next Stage Review Final Report (Darzi Report).* Available at: www.gov.uk/government/uploads/system/uploads/attachment_data/file/228836/7432.pdf. Accessed date: 28 January 2020.

Department of Health (DH) (2008b) *Principles for Revalidation: Report of the Working Group for Non-medical Revalidation; Professional Regulation and Patient Safety Programme.* Available at: http://webarchive.nationalarchives.gov.uk/20130107105354/http://www.dh.gov.uk/en/Publicationsandstatistics/Publications/PublicationsPolicy-AndGuidance/DH_091111. Accessed date: 2 June 2016.

Department of Health (DH) (2010a) *Equity and Excellence: Liberating the NHS.* Available at: https://assets.publishing.service.gov.uk/government/uploads/system/uploads/attachment_data/file/213823/dh_117794.pdf. Accessed date: 3 February 2020.

Department of Health (DH) (2010b) *Preceptorship Framework – for Newly Registered Nurses, Midwives and Allied Health Professionals.* Available at: Preceptorship Framework for Newly Registered Nurses, Midwives and Allied Health Professionals (nationalarchives.gov.uk). Accessed date: 12 January 2021.

Department of Health (DH) (2012) *Compassion in Practice – Nursing, Midwifery and Care Staff Our Vision and Strategy.* Available at: www.england.nhs.uk/wp-content/uploads/2012/12/compassion-in-practice.pdf. Accessed date: 1 March 2020.

Department of Health (DH) (2016) *The Government's Mandate to NHS England for 2016–17.* Available at: at: https://assets.publishing.service.gov.uk/government/uploads/system/uploads/attachment_data/file/600604/NHSE_Mandate_2016-17.pdf. Accessed Date: 18 April 2020.

Department of Health and Social Care (DHSC) (2016a) *Care Act 2014 – Care and Support Statutory Guidance: Changes in March 2016.* Available at: www.gov.uk/government/publications/care-act-2014-part-1-factsheets. Accessed Date: 4 April 2020.

Department of Health and Social Care (DHSC) (2016b) *Operational Productivity and Performance in English NHS Acute Hospitals: Unwarranted Variations (Carter Review).* Available at: www.gov.uk/government/publications/productivity-in-nhs-hospitals. Accessed Date: 18 April 2020.

Department of Health and Social Care (DHSC) (2019a) *The NHS Constitution for England* (last updated 2015). Available at: www.gov.uk/government/publications/the-nhs-constitution-for-england/the-nhs-constitution-for-england. Accessed date: 24 January 2019.

Department of Health and Social Care (DHSC) (2020a) *The Government's Revised 2019–20 Accountability Framework with NHS England and NHS Improvement* [DHSC] statutory Mandate to NHSE]. Available at: https://assets.publishing.service.gov.uk/government/uploads/system/uploads/attachment_data/file/875716/The_government_s_revised_2019-20_Accountability_Framework_with_NHS_England_and_NHS_Improvement.pdf. Accessed date: 10 April 2020.

Department of Health and Social Care (DHSC) (2020b) *Care Act 2014: Supporting Implementation – Care and Support Statutory Guidance*. Available at: www.gov.uk/government/publications/care-act-statutory-guidance/care-and-support-statutory-guidance. Accessed Date: 6 April 2020.

Department of Health and Social Care (DHSC) (2020c) *Funding Boost for Artificial Intelligence in NHS to Speed up Diagnosis of Deadly Diseases (Press release)*. Available at: www.gov.uk/government/news/funding-boost-for-artificial-intelligence-in-nhs-to-speed-up-diagnosis-of-deadly-diseases. Accessed Date: 30 August 2020.

Department of Health and Social Care (2021) *Health and Care Bill: Integrated Care Boards and Local Health and Care Systems*. Available at: www.gov.uk/government/publications/health-and-care-bill-factsheets/health-and-care-bill-integrated-care-boards-and-local-health-and-care-systems. Accessed date: 18 November 2021.

Department of Health and Social Care and Public Health England (2019) *Handbook to the NHS Constitution for England*. Available at: www.gov.uk/government/publications/supplements-to-the-nhs-constitution-for-england. Accessed date: 26 January 2020.

Dinibutun S R (2020) Leadership: A comprehensive review of literature, research and theoretical framework. *Journal of Economics and Business*, 3(1): 44–64.

Donabedian, A (2005) Evaluating the quality of medical care. *The Milbank Quarterly*, 83(4): 691–729.

Donohoe C (2019) An exploration of NHS clinical staff perceptions of changes to clinical products and their procurement. *Nursing Management*, 21(1): 26–33.

Driscoll J, Stacey G, Harrison-Dening K, Boyd C, Shaw T (26 April 2019) Enhancing the quality of clinical supervision in nursing practice. *Nursing Standard*, 34(5): 43–50.

Drucker P F (2007) *The Practice of Management* (The Classic Drucker Collection edition). Oxford: Butterworth-Heinemann.

Duygulu S, Kublay G (2011) Transformational leadership training programme for charge nurses. *Journal of Advanced Nursing*, 67(3): 633–642.

Dyess S M, Sherman R O, Pratt B A, Chiang-Hanisko L (2016) Growing nurse leaders: Their perspectives on nursing leadership and today's practice environment. *Online Journal of Issues in Nursing*, 21(1): 1–7.

Edward K, Ousey K, Playle J, Giandinoto J (2017) Are new nurses work ready – The impact of preceptorship. An integrative systematic review. *Journal of Professional Nursing*, 33(5): 326–333.

Ekstrom L, Idvall E (2015) Being a team leader: Newly registered nurses relate their experiences. *Journal of Nursing Management*, 23(1): 75–86.

Ellis P, Abbott J (2011) Strategies for managing conflict within the team. *Journal of Renal Nursing*, 3(1): 40–43.

Emerald Works (2020) *Team Effectiveness Assessment – How Good is Your Team?* Available at: www.mindtools.com/pages/article/newTMM_84.htm. Accessed Date: 18 July 2020.

England Centre for Practice Development (2021) *About the Centre*. Available at: www.canterbury.ac.uk/medicine-health-and-social-care/england-centre-for-practice-development/about-the-centre/about-the-centre.aspx. Accessed Date: 26 January 2021.

Fayol H (2012) *Five Functions of Management*. Available at: www.businessmate.org/Article.php?ArtikelId=228. Accessed date: 12 August 2016.

Feary S (2012) Barriers to managing and improving quality. *Nursing Times*, 108(10): 12–14.

Felstead I S, Springett K (2016) An exploration of role model influence on adult nursing students' professional development: A phenomenological research study. *Nurse Education Today*, 37 (February): 66–70.

Fernandez R, Johnson M, Tran D, Miranda C (2012) Models of care in nursing: A systematic review. *International Journal of Evidence-Based Healthcare*, 10(4): 324–337.

Fiedler F (1967) *A Theory of Leadership Effectiveness*. London: McGraw-Hill Education.

Fischer S A (2016) Transformational leadership in nursing: A concept analysis. *Journal of Advanced Nursing*, 72(11): 2644–2653.

Forde-Johnston C (2017) Developing and evaluating a foundation preceptorship programme for newly qualified nurses. *Nursing Standard*, 31(42): 42–52.

Francis R (2013) *Report of the Mid-Staffordshire NHS Foundation Trust Public Inquiry*. Available at: www.gov.uk/government/organisations/mid-staffordshire-nhs-foundation-trust-public-inquiry. Accessed date: 27 July 2020.

Fretwell J E (1980) An inquiry into the ward learning environment. *Nursing Times*, 26 June, pp. 69–75.

Gage W (2013) Using service improvement methodology to change practice. *Nursing Standard*, 27(23): 51–57.

Gardner G, Gardner A, O'Connell J (2014) Using the Donabedian framework to examine the quality and safety of nursing service innovation. *Journal of Clinical Nursing*, 23(1–2): 145–155.

General Medical Council (2021) *Continuing Professional Development*. Available at: Continuing professional development - GMC (gmc-uk.org). Accessed Date: 14 January 2021.

Gibbs G (1988) *Learning by Doing: A Guide to Teaching and Learning Methods*. Oxford: Further Education Unit, Oxford Polytechnic.

Gluyas H (2015) Effective communication and teamwork promotes patient safety. *Nursing Standard*, 29(49): 50–57.

Goodrich J, Fitzsimons B (2019) Capturing patient experience to improve healthcare services. *Nursing Standard*, 34(8): 24–28.

Gopee G (2018) *Going Nowhere? Lead Yourself!: If you don't lead yourself, others will lead your life*. London: Austin Macauley Publishers.

Gopee N (2001) Lifelong learning in nursing – perceptions and realities. *Nurse Education Today*, 21(8): 607–615.

Gopee N (2002) Human and social capital as facilitators of lifelong learning in nursing. *Nurse Education Today*, 22(7): 608–616.

Gopee N (2010) *Practice Teaching in Healthcare*. London: Sage Publications.

Gopee N (2018) *Supervision and Mentoring in Healthcare* (4th edn). London: Sage Publications.

Gopee N, Galloway J (2017) *Leadership and Management in Healthcare* (3rd edn). London: Sage Publications.

Gov.uk (2016) *NHS Foundation Trusts: Documents and Guidance*. Available at: www.gov.uk/government/collections/nhs-foundation-trusts-documents-and-guidance. Accessed Date: 4 April 2020.

Griffiths P, Maben J (2009) The metrics of care. *Nursing Standard*, 23(20): 62–63.

Griffiths P (2021) Why safe and nurse effective staffing is more than just a number. *Nursing Times*, 117(3): 26–28.

Hackett K (2020) *Nurse whistleblowing cases up almost 70% (News)*. Available at: https://rcni.com/nursing-standard/newsroom/news/nurse-whistleblowing-cases-almost-70-156886. Accessed Date: 14 November 2021.

Hamm R M (1988) Clinical intuition and clinical analysis: expertise and the cognitive continuum. In: Dowie J and Elstein A (eds) *Professional Judgement: A Reader in Clinical Decision Making*. Milton Keynes: Open University Press.

Handy C (1985) *The Future of Work: A Guide to a Changing Society*. Oxford: Blackwell Publications.

Handy C (1993) *Understanding Organizations* (4th edn). Harmondsworth: Penguin Books.

Harrington A (2019) Chairing and managing formal workplace meetings: Skills for nurse leaders. *Nursing Management*, 26(5): 36–41.

Hatler C, Sturgeon P (2013) Resilience building: A necessary leadership competence. *Nurse Leader*, 11(4): 32–34, 39.

Havyer R D, Wingo M T, Comfere N I, Nelson D R, Halvorsen A J, McDonald F S, Reed D A (2014) Teamwork assessment in internal medicine: A systematic review of validity evidence and outcomes. *Journal of General Internal Medicine*, 29(6): 894–910.

Hawkins P, McMahon A (2020) *Supervision in the Helping Professions* (5th edn). Maidenhead: Open University Press.

Haxby E, Shuldham C (2018) How to undertake a root cause analysis investigation to improve patient safety. *Nursing Standard*, 32(20): 41–46.

Health and Care Professions Council (HCPC) (2013) *Standards of Proficiency – Dietitians*. Available at: www.hcpc-uk.org/globalassets/resources/standards/standards-of-proficiency—dietitians.pdf. Accessed date: 3 February 2020.

Health and Care Professions Council (HCPC) (2016) *Standards of Conduct, Performance and Ethics*. Available at: www.hcpc-uk.org/standards/standards-of-conduct-performance-and-ethics/. Accessed Date: 22 February 2021.

Health and Care Professions Council (HCPC) (2017) *Continuing Professional Development and Your Registration*. Available at: www.hcpc-uk.org/globalassets/resources/guidance/continuing-professional-development-and-your-registration.pdf?v=637106442760000000. Accessed Date: 9 January 2021.

Health and Care Professions Council (HCPC) (2018) *Standards of Proficiency – The Professional Standards all Registrants Must Meet in Order to Become Registered, and Remain on the Register – What is the Role of the Standards of Proficiency*. Available at: standards-of-proficiency—physiotherapists.pdf (hcpc-uk.org). Accessed Date: 18 May 2021.

Health and Safety Executive (2008) *Safe Use of Work Equipment. Provision and Use of Work Equipment Regulations 1998. Approved Code of Practice and Guidance*. Available at: www.hse.gov.uk/work-equipment-machinery/puwer.htm. Accessed date: 18 April 2020.

Health and Safety Executive (2020) *Managing Risks and Risk Assessment at Work*. Available at: www.hse.gov.uk/simple-health-safety/risk/steps-needed-to-manage-risk.htm. Accessed Date: 19 August 2020.

Health Education England (HEE) (2015) *Raising the Bar – Shape of Caring: A Review of the Future Education and Training of Registered Nurses and Care Assistants*. Available at: www.hee.nhs.uk/sites/default/files/documents/2348-Shape-of-caring-review-FINAL.pdf. Accessed date: 11 January 2021.

Health Education England (HEE) (2016) *Values Based Recruitment Framework*. Available at: www.hee.nhs.uk/sites/default/files/documents/VBR_Framework%20March%202016.pdf. Accessed Date: 17 October 2020.

Health Education England (HEE) (2019) *Health Education England Welcomes Funding Boost for 2020/21*. Leeds: HEE.

Health Education England (HEE) (2020a) *HEE Star – User Guide*. Available at: HEE Star user guide v2.0.pdf. Accessed Date: 22 March 2021.

Health Education England (HEE) (2020b) *Annual Report and Accounts 2019-20*. Available at: HEE Annual Report and Accounts 2019–20_3.pdf. Accessed Date: 17 January 2021.

Health Education England, NHS Improvement & NHS England (2017) *Multi-Professional Framework for Advanced Clinical Practice in England*. Available at: www.hee.nhs.uk/sites/default/files/documents/multi-professionalframeworkforadvancedclinical-practiceinengland.pdf. Accessed Date: 26 October 2021

Health Foundation (2013) *Measuring Patient Experience*. Available at: www.health.org.uk/sites/default/files/MeasuringPatientExperience.pdf. Accessed Date: 28 September 2020.

Health Foundation (2019) *NHS Long Term Plan Announcement: A Welcome Commitment But Trade-Offs are Inevitable*. Available at: www.health.org.uk/news-and-comment/news/nhs-long-term-plan-announcement-response. Accessed date: 30 January 2020.

Heriot Watt University (2020) *Records Management: Terminology and definitions*. Available at: www.hw.ac.uk/uk/services/information-governance/manage/records-management-terminology-definitions.htm. Accessed Date: 26 June 2020.

Heron J (1989) *Six Category Intervention Analysis. Human Potential Research Project* (2nd edn). Guildford: University of Surrey.

Herzberg F (2003) One more time: How do you motivate employees? *Harvard Business Review*, 81(1): 87–96.

HM Treasury (2020) *Budget 2020*. Available at: Budget 2020 – GOV.UK (www.gov.uk). Accessed Date: 14 November 2021.

Hofmeyer A T (2013) How can a social capital framework guide managers to develop positive nurse relationships and patient outcomes? *Journal of Nursing Management*, 21(5): 782–789.

Holly C, Igwee G (2011) A systematic review of the influence of transformational leadership style on nursing staff in acute care hospitals. *International Journal of Evidence-Based Healthcare*, 9(3): 301.

Home Office (2010) *The Equality Act 2010*. Available at: www.legislation.gov.uk/ukpga/2010/15/contents. Accessed date: 12 August 2016.

Horner D L, Bellamy M C (2012) Care bundles in intensive care. *Continuing Education in Anaesthesia Critical Care & Pain*, 12(4): 199–202.

Hossain M A, Uddin M K, Hasan M R, Hasan M F (2018) Conflict management on the organizational performance: A synthesis of literature. *Journal of Innovation and Development Strategy*, 12(1): 56–67.

House of Commons (2011) *Health and Social Care Bill*. Available at: https://publications.parliament.uk/pa/cm201011/cmbills/132/11132.i-v.html. Accessed date: 8 February 2020.

Huber P, Schubert H (2019) Attitudes about work engagement of different generations – A cross-sectional study with nurses and supervisors. *Journal of Nursing Management*, 27(7): 1341–1350.

Humphries R (2019) *Health and Wellbeing Boards and Integrated Care Systems*. Available at: www.kingsfund.org.uk/publications/articles/health-wellbeing-boards-integrated-care-systems. Accessed Date: 15 November 2021.

Hurst K (2010) Evaluating the strengths and weaknesses of NHS workforce planning methods. *Nursing Times*, 106(40): 10–14.

Institute for Healthcare Improvement (IHI) (2020a) *The IHI Triple Aim*. Available at: www.ihi.org/Engage/Initiatives/TripleAim/Pages/default.aspx. Accessed date: 5 February 2020.

Institute for Healthcare Improvement (IHI) (2020b*)* *Plan-Do-Study-Act (PDSA) Worksheet*. Available at: www.ihi.org/resources/pages/tools/plandostudyactworksheet.aspx. Accessed date: 30 July 2020.

Institute of Medicine (2001) *Crossing the Quality Chasm: A New Health System for the 21st Century*. Washington, DC: National Academy Press. Also available at: https://pubmed.ncbi.nlm.nih.gov/25057539/. Accessed Date: 24 September 2020.

Investopedia (2020) *Total Quality Management (TQM)*. Available at: www.investopedia.com/terms/t/total-quality-management-tqm.asp. Accessed Date: 13 September 2020.

ITV News (2020) *Shrewsbury maternity scandal: Mothers were blamed for the death of their baby* (11 December). Available at: www.itv.com/news/2020-12-10/shrewsbury-maternity-scandal-mothers-were-blamed-for-the-death-of-their-baby. Accessed Date: 11 December 2020.

Jaffray L, Bridgman H, Stephens M, Skinner T (2016) Evaluating the effects of mindfulness-based interventions for informal palliative caregivers: A systematic literature review. *Palliative Medicine*, 30(2): 117–131.

Jennings B M, Scalzi C C, Rodgers J D, Keane A (2007) Differentiating nursing leadership and management competencies. *Nursing Outlook*, 55(2007): 169–175.

Johansen M L (2012) Performance potential. Keeping the peace: Conflict management strategies for nurse managers. *Nursing Management*, 43(2): 50–54.

Johansson C, Aström S, Kauffeldt A, Helldin L, Carlström E (2014) Culture as a predictor of resistance to change: A study of competing values in a psychiatric nursing context. *Health Policy*, 114(2/3): 156–162.

Johnston S, Heneghan P, Daniels P (2020) Mentoring initiative to retain community-based registered nurses in palliative care. *British Journal of Community Nursing*, 25(7): 335–339.

Jones-Berry S (2016) Study urges anti-burnout aid for intensive care nurses. *Nursing Standard*, 30(47): 10.

Jones-Berry S (2018) Survey confirms failure to tackle attrition rates, *Nursing Standard*, 33(6): 19–22.

Jung T, Scott T, Davies H, Bower P, Whalley D, Mcnally R, Manion R (2009) Instruments for exploring organizational culture: A review of the literature. *Public Administration Review*, (October) 69(6): 1087–1096.

Karimi L, Leggat S G, Donohue L, Farrell G, Couper G E (2014) Emotional rescue: The role of emotional intelligence and emotional labour on well-being and job-stress among community nurses. *Journal of Advanced Nursing*, 70(1): 176–186.

Kaya G K, Ward J R, Clarkson P J (2019) A framework to support risk assessment in hospitals. *International Journal for Quality in Health Care*, 31(5): 393–401.

Keller S, Yule S, Zagarese V, Henrickson Parker S (2020) Predictors and triggers of incivility within healthcare teams: A systematic review of the literature. *BMJ Open*, 10(2020): 1–15 / e035471.

Kim J (2018) Relationship between incivility experiences and nursing professional values among nursing students: Moderating effects of coping strategies. *Nurse Education Today*, 65(June 2018): 187–191.

King's Fund (2016a) *Health and Wellbeing Boards (HWBs) Explained*. Available at: Health and wellbeing boards (HWBs) explained | The King's Fund (kingsfund.org.uk). Accessed Date: 25 July 2021.

King's Fund (2016b) *A Programme with NHS Improvement to Support Culture Change through Collective Leadership.* Available at: www.kingsfund.org.uk/projects/changing-culture-collective-leadership. Accessed date: 2 January 2021.

King's Fund (2016c) *Improving Quality in the English NHS A strategy for action.* Available at: www.kingsfund.org.uk/sites/default/files/field/field_publication_file/Improving-quality-Kings-Fund-February-2016.pdf. Accessed Date: 18 September 2020.

King's Fund (2017) *Making the Case for Quality Improvement: Lessons for NHS Boards and Leaders.* Available at: www.kingsfund.org.uk/publications/making-case-quality-improvement#:~:text=The%20term%20'quality%20improvement'%20refers,Healthcare%20Improvement's%20Model%20for%20Improvement.. Accessed Date: 10 July 2020.

King's Fund (2018) *The Health Care Workforce in England – Make or Break?* Available at: www.kingsfund.org.uk/sites/default/files/2018-11/The%20health%20care%20work-force%20in%20England.pdf. Accessed Date: 11 April 2020.

King's Fund (2019a) *Key Facts and Figures about the NHS.* Available at: www.kingsfund.org.uk/audio-video/key-facts-figures-nhs. Accessed Date: 7 January 2020.

King's Fund (2019b) *How the NHS is Funded.* Available at: www.kingsfund.org.uk/projects/nhs-in-a-nutshell/how-nhs-funded. Accessed Date: 20 June 2020

King's Fund (2019c) *Closing the Gap: Key Areas for Action on the Health and Care Workforce.* Available at: www.kingsfund.org.uk/publications/closing-gap-health-care-workforce. Accessed date: 17 January 2020.

King's Fund (2021) *The NHS Budget and How it has Changed.* Available at: www.kingsfund.org.uk/projects/nhs-in-a-nutshell/nhs-budget. Accessed Date: 2 April 2021.

Kneafsey R, Brown S, Sein K, Chamley C, Parsons J (2016) A qualitative study of key stakeholders' perspectives on compassion in healthcare and the development of a framework for compassionate interpersonal relations. *Journal of Clinical Nursing,* 25(1–2): 70–79.

Kotter J P (2009) What leaders really do. *Harvard Business Review,* 68(3): 103–111. Also available at: What Leaders Really Do (researchgate.net). Accessed Date: 3 March 2021.

Kotter, J P (2012) *Leading Change* (with a new preface). Boston: The Harvard Business School Press.

Kouzes J M, Posner B Z (2017) *The Leadership Challenge* (6th edn). San Francisco, CA: Jossey-Bass.

Kramer M (1974) *Reality Shock: Why Nurses Leave Nursing.* St Louis, MO: Mosby.

Kumaran S, Carney M (2014) Role transition from student nurse to staff nurse: Facilitating the transition period. *Nurse Education in Practice,* 14(6): 605–611.

Kwok A Y T, Mah A P Y, Pang K M C (2020) *Our First Review: An Evaluation of Effectiveness of Root Cause Analysis Recommendations in Hong Kong Public Hospitals. Health Economics and Outcomes Research.* Available at: www.researchsquare.com/article/rs-15698/v2. Accessed date: 2 September 2020.

Labrague L J, De los Santos J A A (2020) Transition shock and newly graduated nurses' job outcomes and select patient outcomes: A cross-sectional study. *Journal of Nursing Management,* 28(5): 1070–1079.

Labrague L J, Hamdan Z A, McEnroe-Petitte D M (2018) An integrative review on conflict management styles among nursing professionals: Implications for nursing management. *Journal of Nursing Management,* 26(8): 902–917.

Lacobucci G (2019) A&E doctors urge NHS not to abandon four hour target. *BMJ,* 364(2019): 1455.

Lacobucci G (2020) GPs in UK report more stress and the time pressure than international peers. *BMJ,* 368(8237): 392.

Lang N (1976) *Issues in Quality Assurance Nursing*. Kansas City, KS: American Nurses Association.

Lay K (2020) NHS seeks teenagers to join as cadets. *The Times*, 4 July 2020, p. 2.

Legislation.gov.uk (2012) *Health and Social Care Act 2012*. Available at: www.legislation. gov.uk/ukpga/2012/7/contents/enacted. Accessed date: 12 February 2020.

Legislation.gov.uk (2014) *Care Act 2014*. Norwich: The Stationery Office.

Levine K J, Carmody M, Silk K J (2020) The influence of organisational culture, climate and commitment on speaking up about medical errors. *Journal of Nursing Management*, 28(1) 130–138.

Lewin K (1951) *Field Theory in Social Science*. London: Harper Row.

Lister S, Hofland J, Grafton H (eds) (2020) *The Royal Marsden Manual of Clinical Nursing Procedures* (Royal Marsden Manual Series) (10th edn). Hoboken, NJ: Wiley-Blackwell.

Liu H, Wang I, Chen N, Chao C (2020) Effect of creativity training on teaching for creativity for nursing faculty in Taiwan: A quasi-experimental study. *Nurse Education Today*, 85.

Lomas C (2012) The burden of bureaucracy. *Nursing Standard*, 26(30): 22–24.

Londonwide LMC (2021) *London's three LETBs: Direct links and information*. Available at: www.lmc.org.uk/article.php?group_id=5317. Accessed Date: 29 January 2021.

Lucas B (2019) Developing the personal qualities required for effective nurse leadership. *Nursing Standard*, 34(12): 45–50.

Lv C, Zhang L (2017) How can collective leadership influence the implementation of change in health care? *Chinese Nursing Research*, 5(2017): 182–185.

Magnusson C, Allan H, Horton K, Johnson M, Evans K, Ball E (2017) An analysis of delegation styles among newly qualified nurses. *Nursing Standard*, 31(25): 46–53.

Marquis B L, Huston C J (2021) *Leadership Roles and Management Functions in Nursing* (10th edn). Philadelphia, PA: Wolters Kluwer.

Marsh T (NHS Confederation) (2018) *How devolution is delivering change in Greater Manchester*. Available at: www.nhsconfed.org/blog/2018/03/greater-manchester-devo-lution. Accessed date: 21 February 2020.

Maslow A H (1987) *Motivation and Personality* (3rd edn). London: Harper & Row.

Maxwell R (1984) Quality assessment in health. *British Medical Journal*, 288(6428): 1470–1472.

May R (2019) Collective leadership – why it's our direction of travel. *Nursing Standard*, 34(6): 51–52.

McCarthy J, Rose P (2010) *Values-Based Health & Social Care: Beyond Evidence-Based Practice*. London: Sage Publications.

McDonald J, Jayasuriya R, Harris M F (2012) The influence of power dynamics and trust on multidisciplinary collaboration: A qualitative case study of type 2 diabetes mellitus. *BMC Health Services Research*, 12(63): 1–10.

McGregor D (1987) *The Human Side of Enterprise*. Harmondsworth: Penguin.

Menzies I E (1960) A case study in the functioning of social systems as a defence against anxiety: A report of a study of nursing services of a general hospital. *The Tavistock Institute of Human Relations*, 13(2): 95–121.

Mintzberg H (2011) *Managing*. San Francisco, CA: Berrett-Koehler Publishers.

Mishoe S C, Tufts K A, Diggs L A, Blando J D, Claiborne D M, Hoch J, Walker M L (2018) Health professions students' teamwork before and after an interprofessional education co-curricular experience. *Journal of Research in Interprofessional Practice and Education*, 8(1): 1–16.

Moore A (2017) All ideas welcome – Empowering staff to affect and sustain change. *Nursing Standard*, 32(9): 19–21.

Moore Z E H, Patton D (2019) *Risk assessment tools for the prevention of pressure ulcers. Cochrane Database of Systematic Reviews.* Available at: www.cochranelibrary.com/cdsr/doi/10.1002/14651858.CD006471.pub4/full. Accessed Date: 23 July 2020. https://doi.org/10.1002/14651858.CD006471.pub4.

Muller-Heyndyk R (2019) *Employers Report Changing Employee Expectations.* Available at: www.hrmagazine.co.uk/article-details/employers-report-changing-employee-expectations. Accessed Date: 26 February 2020.

Mullins L J (2019) *Organisational Behaviour in the Workplace* (12th edn). Harlow (UK): Pearson Education Limited.

National Archives (2010) *What is Records Management? (Guide 1).* Available at: www.nationalarchives.gov.uk/documents/information-management/rm-code-guide1.pdf. Accessed Date: 26 June 2020.

National Audit Office (NAO) (2012) *Healthcare across the UK: A comparison of the NHS in England, Scotland, Wales and Northern Ireland.* Available at: www.nao.org.uk/report/healthcare-across-the-uk-a-comparison-of-the-nhs-in-england-scotland-wales-and-northern-ireland/. Accessed Date: 18 April 2020.

National Audit Office (NAO) (2018a) *A Review of the Role and Costs of Clinical Commissioning Groups.* Available at: www.nao.org.uk/wp-content/uploads/2018/12/Review-of-the-role-and-costs-of-clinical-commissioning-groups.pdf. Accessed Date: 21 February 2020.

National Institute for Health and Care Excellence (NICE) (2014) *NICE Safe Staffing Guideline: Safe Staffing for Nursing in Adult Inpatient Wards in Acute Hospitals.* Available at: www.nice.org.uk/guidance/sg1/resources/resource-impact-commentary-pdf-11947789. Accessed Date: 15 April 2020.

National Institute for Health and Care Excellence (NICE) (2020) *NICE Pathways – Everything NICE says on a topic in an interactive flowchart.* Available at: https://pathways.nice.org.uk/. Accessed Date: 21 January 2021.

National Quality Board (2016) *Shared Commitment to Quality from the National Quality Board.* Available at: www.england.nhs.uk/wp-content/uploads/2016/12/nqb-shared-commitment-frmwrk.pdf. Accessed Date: 3 September 2020.

NHS Confederation (2021) *What are Clinical Commissioning Groups?* Available at: www.nhsconfed.org/articles/what-are-clinical-commissioning-groups. Accessed Date: 14 November 2021.

NHS Digital (2020a) *NHS Outcomes Framework Indicators – May 2020 release* [NS]. Available at: www.gov.uk/government/statistics/nhs-outcomes-framework-indicators-may-2020-release-ns. Accessed Date: 10 July 2020.

NHS Digital (2020b) *Our Role and Remit in the Health Service.* Available at: https://digital.nhs.uk/about-nhs-digital/our-work/our-role-and-remit-in-the-health-service. Accessed Date: 29 August 2020.

NHS Digital (2020c) *Systems and Services.* Available at: https://digital.nhs.uk/services. Accessed Date: 29 August 2020.

NHS Education for Scotland (2021) *Preceptorship.* Available at: www.nes.scot.nhs.uk/our-work/preceptorship/. Accessed Date: 11 March 2021.

NHS Employers (2013) *Tackling Bullying & Harassment in the NHS.* Available at: www.nhsemployers.org/~/media/Employers/Publications/NHS%20Bullying%20Infographic.pdf. Accessed Date: 17 April 2020.

NHS Employers (2018) *Workforce Health and Wellbeing Framework*. Available at: file:///C:/Users/lgope/Downloads/NHS%20Workforce%20HWB%20Framework_updated%20July%2018.pdf. Accessed Date: 23 March 2020.

NHS Employers (2019a) *Advanced Clinical Practice*. Available at: www.nhsemployers.org/articles/advanced-clinical-practice#:⊠:text=As%20part%20of%20the%20framework,and%20management%2C%20education%20and%20research. Accessed Date: 22 July 2021.

NHS Employers (2019b) *Simplified Knowledge and Skills Framework (KSF)*. Available at: www.nhsemployers.org/SimplifiedKSF. Accessed date: 24 April 2020.

NHS Employers (2019c) *NHS Staff Survey 2018*. Available at: www.nhsemployers.org/retention-and-staff-experience/staff-engagement/the-nhs-staff-survey/nhs-staff-survey-2018. Accessed Date: 21 March 2020.

NHS Employers (2020) *Risk Assessments for Staff*. Available at: www.nhsemployers.org/covid19/health-safety-and-wellbeing/risk-assessments-for-staff. Accessed Date: 2 July 2020.

NHS England (NHSE) (2014a) *Five-Year Forward View*. Available at: www.england.nhs.uk/wp-content/uploads/2014/10/5yfv-web.pdf. Accessed Date: 30 January 2020.

NHS England (NHSE) (2014b) *Understanding the NHS*. Available at: www.nhs.uk/NHSEngland/thenhs/about/Documents/simple-nhs-guide.pdf. Accessed Date: 16 February 2020.

NHS England (NHSE) (2014c) *Health and Social Care Leaders Set Out Plans to Transform People's Health and Improve Services Using Technology*. Available at: www.england.nhs.uk/2014/11/leaders-transform/. Accessed Date: 13 February 2021.

NHS England (NHSE) (2015a) *Delivering the Forward View: NHS Planning Guidance 2016/17 – 2020/21*. Available at: www.england.nhs.uk/wp-content/uploads/2015/12/planning-guid-16-17-20-21.pdf. Accessed Date: 17 February 2020.

NHS England (NHSE) (2015b) *The Forward View into Action – New Care Models: Support for the Vanguards*. Available at: www.england.nhs.uk/wp-content/uploads/2015/12/acc-uec-support-package.pdf. Accessed Date: 17 March 2020.

NHS England (NHSE) (2016) *Leading Change, Adding Value – A Framework for Nursing, Midwifery and Care Staff*. Available at: www.england.nhs.uk/wp-content/uploads/2016/05/nursing-framework.pdf. Accessed Date: 14 February 2020.

NHS England (NHSE) (2017a) *Next Steps on The NHS Five Year Forward View*. Available at: www.england.nhs.uk/wp-content/uploads/2017/03/NEXT-STEPS-ON-THE-NHS-FIVE-YEAR-FORWARD-VIEW.pdf. Accessed Date: 30 January 2020

NHS England (NHSE) (2017b) *Culture of Care Barometer – a Guide to the Barometer*. Available at: www.england.nhs.uk/wp-content/uploads/2017/03/ccb-barometer-rep-guide.pdf. Accessed Date: 9 September 2020.

NHS England (NHSE) (2019a) *NHS Long Term Plan*. Available at: www.england.nhs.uk/long-term-plan/. Accessed Date: 16 January 2020.

NHS England (NHSE) (2019b) *NHS Long Term Plan Implementation Framework*. Available at: www.longtermplan.nhs.uk/wp-content/uploads/2019/06/long-term-plan-implementation-framework-v1.pdf. Accessed Date: 27 February 2020.

NHS England (NHSE) (2020a) *We are the NHS: People Plan for 2020/2021 – Action for us all*. Available at: We-Are-The-NHS-Action-For-All-Of-Us-FINAL-March-21.pdf (england.nhs.uk). Accessed Date: 15 April 2021.

NHS England (NHSE) (2020b) *About NHS England – What do we do?* Available at: www.england.nhs.uk/about/about-nhs-england/. Accessed Date: 18 August 2020.

NHS England (NHSE) (2020c) *Integrated Care Systems*. Available at: www.england.nhs. uk/integratedcare/integrated-care-systems/. Accessed Date: 14 February 2020.

NHS England (NHSE) (2020d) *Change Model*. Available at: www.england.nhs.uk/sus-tainableimprovement/change-model/. Accessed Date: 17 June 2020.

NHS England (NHSE) (2021) *Project Management: An Overview*. Available at: NHS England » Quality, service improvement and redesign (QSIR) tools by stage of project. Accessed Date: 22 May 2021.

NHS England and NHS Improvement (2020a) *NHS Operational Planning and Contracting Guidance 2020/21*. Available at: www.england.nhs.uk/wp-content/ uploads/2020/01/2020-21-NHS-Operational-Planning-Contracting-Guidance.pdf. Accessed date: 7 April 2020.

NHS England and NHS Improvement (2020b) *Risk Assessments for At-Risk Staff Groups*. Available at: www.england.nhs.uk/coronavirus/wp-content/uploads/sites/52/2020/06/ C0625-risk-assessments-for-at-risk-staff-groups-letter.pdf. Accessed Date: 2 July 2020.

NHS England and NHS Improvement (2019) *Patient Safety Review and Response Report October 2018 to March 2019*. Available at: 2019.09.23_PS_Review_and_Response_ Report_Oct_2018_-_March_2019_FINAL.pdf (nationalarchives.gov.uk). Accessed Date: 3 January 2021.

NHS England Survey Co-ordination Centre (2020) *NHS Staff Survey 2019 National Results Briefing*. Available at: ST19 National briefing (nhsstaffsurveys.com). Accessed Date: 7 April 2021.

NHS Improvement (NHSI) (2018a) *SBAR Communication Tool – Situation, Back-ground, Assessment, Recommendation*. Available at: https://improvement.nhs.uk/docu-ments/2162/sbar-communication-tool.pdf. Accessed Date: 18 July 2020.

NHS Improvement (NHSI) (2018b) *Root Cause Analysis – Using Five Whys*. Avail-able at: https://improvement.nhs.uk/resources/root-cause-analysis-using-five-whys/. Accessed Date: 8 May 2020.

NHS Improvement (NHSI) (2018c) *Plan, Do, Study, Act (PDSA) Cycles and The Model for Improvement*. Available at: https://improvement.nhs.uk/resources/pdsa-cycles/. Accessed Date: 8 August 2020.

NHS Improvement (NHSI) (2018d) *Learning from Patient Safety Incidents*. Available at: https://improvement.nhs.uk/resources/learning-from-patient-safety-incidents/. Accessed Date: 27 July 2020

NHS Improvement (NHSI) (2019) *How Can I Make Safety Huddles Work in My Area?* Available at: https://improvement.nhs.uk/documents/1140/SLIDES_B3_W_Safety_ huddles.pdf. Accessed Date: 29 July 2020.

NHS Improvement (NHSI) (2020a) *What We Do*. Available at: https://improvement.nhs. uk/about-us/what-we-do/. Accessed Date: 30 April 2020.

NHS Improvement (NHSI) (2020b) *Quality, Service Improvement and Redesign (QSIR) Tools*. Available at: NHS England Quality, service improvement and redesign (QSIR) tools. Accessed Date: 21 May 2021.

NHS Improvement and NHS Employers (2018) *Start Well: Stay Well – a model to support new starter*. Available at: file:///C:/Users/lgope/AppData/Local/Packages/Microsoft. MicrosoftEdge_8wekyb3d8bbwe/TempState/Downloads/CUH-case-study-Final— June-2018%20(1).pdf. Accessed Date: 22 March 2020.

NHS Improvement and NHS Employers (2019) *The National Retention Programme: Two Years on*. Available at: https://improvement.nhs.uk/resources/national-retention-pro-gramme-two-years-on/. Accessed date: 18 February 2020.

NHS Improvement and NHS England (2016) *Freedom to Speak Up: Raising Concerns (Whistleblowing) Policy for the NHS*. Available at: https://improvement.nhs.uk/documents/27/whistleblowing_policy_final.pdf. Accessed Date: 30 October 2020.

NHS Leadership Academy (2012) *Clinical Leadership Competency Framework Self-assessment Tool*. Available at: CLCF Self Assessment_Layout 1 (leadershipacademy.nhs.uk). Accessed Date: 4 April 2021.

NHS Leadership Academy (2021) *Healthcare Leadership Model – The nine dimensions of leadership behaviour*. Available at: www.leadershipacademy.nhs.uk/resources/healthcare-leadership-model/nine-leadership-dimensions/. Accessed Date: 4 April 2021.

NHS News (2021) *NHS Achieves Key Long Term Plan Commitment to Roll Out Integrated Care Systems Across England*. Available at: www.england.nhs.uk/2021/03/nhs-achieves-key-long-term-plan-commitment-to-roll-out-integrated-care-systems-across-england/. Accessed Date: 10 May 2021.

NHS Providers (2020) *About Us*. Available at: https://nhsproviders.org/about-us. Accessed Date: 1 May 2020.

NHS Scotland (2018) *Advanced Nursing Practice Toolkit (Definitions: Beyond the clinical domain)*. Available at: Advanced Practice Toolkit (scot.nhs.uk). Accessed Date: 11 January 2021.

NHS.UK (2018) *Ten stress busters*. Available at: www.nhs.uk/conditions/stress-anxiety-depression/reduce-stress/. Accessed Date: 29 March 2020.

NHS.UK (2019) *5 Steps to Mental Wellbeing*. Available at: www.nhs.uk/conditions/stress-anxiety-depression/improve-mental-wellbeing/. Accessed Date: 3 February 2021.

NHSX (2021a) *Records Management Code of Practice 2020*. Available at: Records Management Code of Practice 2020 – NHSX. Accessed Date: 11 January 2021.

NHSX (2021b) *NHSX – What we do*. Available at: www.nhsx.nhs.uk/about-us/what-we-do/. Accessed Date: 12 February 2021.

Nibbelink, C W, and Brewer, B B (2018) Decision-making in nursing practice: An integrative literature review. *Journal of Clinical Nursing*, 27(5-6), 917–928.

Nightingale A (2020) Implementing collective leadership in healthcare organisations. *Nursing Standard*, 35(5): 53–57.

Nuffield Trust (2014) *The Four Health Systems of the UK: How Do They Compare*. Available at: www.nuffieldtrust.org.uk/research/the-four-health-systems-of-the-uk-how-do-they-compare/. Accessed Date: 18 April 2020.

Nuffield Trust (2019) *The NHS Workforce in Numbers*. Available at: www.nuffieldtrust.org.uk/resource/the-nhs-workforce-in-numbers. Accessed Date: 16 April 2020.

Nuffield Trust (2020) *Health and Social Care Explained*. Available at: www.nuffieldtrust.org.uk/health-and-social-care-explained/nhs-reform-timeline. Accessed Date: 26 April 2020.

Nursing and Midwifery Council & General Medical Council (2019) *Guidance on the professional duty of candour – Joint guidance with the General Medical Council on the duty of candour*. Available at: www.nmc.org.uk/standards/guidance/the-professional-duty-of-candour/. Accessed date: 16 August 2020.

Nursing and Midwifery Council (NMC) (2015) *NMC response to Secretary of State's statement to the House of Commons*. Available at: www.nmc.org.uk/news/press-releases/2015/nmc-response-to-secretary-of-states-statement-to-the-house-of-commons/. Accessed Date: 29 March 2020.

Nursing and Midwifery Council (NMC) (2016) *Social Media Guidance – Our Guidance on the Use of Social Media*. Available at: social-media-guidance.pdf (nmc.org.uk). Accessed date: 3 February 2021.

Nursing and Midwifery Council (NMC) (2018a) *Future Nurse: Standards of Proficiency for Registered Nurses.* London: NMC. Also available at: www.nmc.org.uk/globalassets/sitedocuments/standards-of-proficiency/nurses/future-nurse-proficiencies.pdf. Accessed Date: 16 July 2020.

Nursing and Midwifery Council (NMC) (2018b) *The Code: Professional Standards of Practice and Behaviour for Nurses, Midwives and Nursing Associates.* Available at: www.nmc.org.uk/globalassets/sitedocuments/nmc-publications/nmc-code.pdf. Accessed Date: 1 March 2020.

Nursing and Midwifery Council (NMC) (2018c) *Realising Professionalism: Standards for Education and Training – Part 2: Standards for Student Supervision and Assessment.* Available at: student-supervision-assessment.pdf (nmc.org.uk). Accessed Date: 7 January 2021.

Nursing and Midwifery Council (NMC) (2018d) *Standards Framework for Nursing and Midwifery Education.* Available at: www.nmc.org.uk/globalassets/sitedocuments/standards-of-proficiency/standards-framework-for-nursing-and-midwifery-education/education-framework.pdf. Accessed Date: 21 July 2020.

Nursing and Midwifery Council (NMC) (2019a) *Revalidation – Your step-by-step guide through the process.* Available at: http://revalidation.nmc.org.uk/. Accessed Date: 9 January 2021.

Nursing and Midwifery Council (NMC) (2019b) *How to Revalidate with the NMC Requirements for Renewing Your Registration.* Available at: www.nmc.org.uk/globalassets/sitedocuments/revalidation/how-to-revalidate-booklet.pdf. Accessed Date: 12 January 2021.

Nursing and Midwifery Council (NMC) (2020a) *NMC publishes principles of preceptorship.* Available at: www.nmc.org.uk/news/press-releases/principles-preceptorship/. Accessed Date: 18 December 2020.

Nursing and Midwifery Council (NMC) (2020b) *Health and Care Leaders celebrate incredible contributions of Nursing Associates on one year anniversary of the role.* Available at: www.nmc.org.uk/news/press-releases/health-and-care-leaders-celebrate-incredible-contributions-of-nursing-associates-on-1-year-anniversary-of-the-role/. Accessed Date: 22 February 2020.

Nursing and Midwifery Council (NMC) (2021) *Managing Concern Locally.* Available at: www.nmc.org.uk/employer-resource/managing-concerns/managing-concerns-locally/. Accessed Date: 17 February 2021.

Nursing Standard (2020) *Search 'patient safety'.* Available at: https://rcni.com/nursing-standard/search?search_api_views_fulltext=patient%20safety&sort_by=search_api_relevance&f%5B0%5D=created%3A2020&page=18. Accessed date: 27 November 2021.

Nursing Standard News (2009) Staff bamboozled and alienated by metrics jargon. *Nursing Standard,* 23(40): 11.

Odiorne S (1979) *MBO II: A System of Managerial Leadership for the 80s.* Belmont, CA: Fearon Pitman Publishers.

Office for National Statistics (ONO) (2020) *Overview of the UK Population: August 2019.* Available at: www.ons.gov.uk/peoplepopulationandcommunity/populationandmigration/populationestimates/articles/overviewoftheukpopulation/august2019. Accessed Date: 9 February 2020.

Olden P C (2016) Contingency management of health care organizations: It depends. *Health Care Management,* 35(1): 28–36.

Oosterholt R I, Simonse L W L, Boess S U, Vehmeijer S B W (2017) Designing a care pathway model – A case study of the outpatient total hip arthroplasty care pathway. *International Journal of Integrated Care,* 17(1): 1–14.

Oreg S, Bayazıt M, Arciniega L (2008) Dispositional resistance to change: Measurement equivalence and the link to personal values across 17 nations. *Journal of Applied Psychology*, 93(4): 935–944.

Osborne K (2015) Are nurses ready for revalidation? *Nursing Standard* 29(3): 22–23.

Ovretveit J (1992) *Health Service Quality: An introduction to quality methods for health services.* Oxford: Blackwell Publishing.

Owen P, Whitehead B, Beddingham E, Simmons M (2020) A preceptorship toolkit for nurse managers, teams and healthcare organisations. *Nursing Management*, 27(4): 20–25.

Parish C (2006) 'Being nice is not enough' for good leadership on the wards. *Nursing Standard*, 20(41): 6.

Parliamentary and Health Service Ombudsman (2015) *Complaints About Acute Trusts 2014-15.* Available at: NHS_Complaint_stats_report_2014-15.pdf (ombudsman.org.uk). Accessed Date: 3 January 2021.

Peek S (2020) *Human relations management theory basics.* Available at: www.business.com/articles/human-relations-management-theory-basics/. Accessed Date: 20 September 2020.

Peerally M F, Carr S, Waring J, Dixon-Woods M (2017) The problem with root cause analysis. *BMJ Quality and Safety*, 26(5): 417–422.

Pegram A M, Grainger M, Sigsworth J, While A E (2014) Strengthening the role of the ward manager: A review of the literature. *Journal of Nursing Management*, 22(6): 685–696.

Perneger T V, Peytremann-Bridevaux I, Combescure C (2020) Patient satisfaction and survey response in 717 hospital surveys in Switzerland: A cross-sectional study. *BMC Health Services Research*, 20(158): 1–8.

Petersen A, Bunton R (eds) (1997) *Foucault, Health and Medicine.* New York: Routledge.

Pfeffer J, Sutton R I (2006) Evidence-based management. Available at: https://hbr.org/2006/01/evidence-based-management. Accessed Date: 18 January 2022.

Phillips B C, Morinand K, Valiga T M T (2021) Clinical decision making in undergraduate nursing students: A mixed methods multisite study. *Nurse Education Today*, 97 (February): 1–6.

Phillips C, Esterman A, Kenny A (2015) The theory of organisational socialisation and its potential for improving transition experiences for new graduate nurses. *Nurse Education Today*, 35(1): 118–124.

Proctor B (2001) Training for the supervision alliance attitude, skills and intention! In: Cutcliffe J, Butterworth T and Proctor B (eds) *Fundamental Themes in Clinical Supervision* (Chapter 3). London: Routledge.

Proctor T (2020) Creative problem-solving techniques, paradigm shift and team performance. *Team Performance Management*, 26(7/8): 451–466.

Professional Standards Authority for Health and Social Care (2020) *How We Work.* Available at: www.professionalstandards.org.uk/about-us/how-we-work. Accessed Date: 15 March 2020.

Project Management Institute (2020) *What is Project Management?* Available at: www.pmi.org/about/learn-about-pmi/what-is-project-management. Accessed Date: 28 July 2020.

Quality Assurance Agency for Higher Education (2018) *UK Quality Code for Higher Education: Advice and Guidance – Work-based Learning.* Available at: www.qaa.ac.uk/docs/

qaa/quality-code/advice-and-guidance-work-based-learning.pdf?sfvrsn=f625c181_2. Accessed Date: 13 November 2021.

Radecki, B, Keen A, Miller J, McClure J, Kara A (2020) Innovating fall safety – engaging patients as experts. *Journal of Nursing Care Quality*, 35(3): 220–226.

Radford M (2019) *Meeting the Staffing Challenge (Blog)*. Available at: www.england.nhs. uk/blog/meeting-the-staffing-challenge/. Accessed Date: 16 April 2020.

Raeissi P, Zandian H, Mirzarahimy T, Delavari T, Moghadam Z, Rahimi G (2019) Relationship between communication skills and emotional intelligence among nurses. *Nursing Management*, 26(2): 31–35.

Rafferty R, Fairbrother G (2015) Factors influencing how senior nurses and midwives acquire and integrate coaching skills into routine practice: A grounded theory study. *Journal of Advanced Nursing*, 71(6): 1249–1259.

Rashman L, Withers E, Hartley J (2009) Organisational learning and knowledge in public service organisations: A systematic review of the literature. *International Journal of Management Reviews*, 11(4): 463–494.

Reed J E, Card A J (2016) The problem with Plan-Do-Study-Act cycles. *BMJ Quality and Safety*, 25(3): 147–152.

Resuscitation Council (UK) (2021) *2021 Resuscitation Guidelines*. Available at: www.resus. org.uk/library/2021-resuscitation-guidelines. Accessed Date: 20 May 2021.

Richards A (2020) Exploring the benefits and limitations of transactional leadership in healthcare. *Nursing Standard*, 35(12): 46–50.

Rogers C, Freiberg H J (1994) *Freedom to Learn* (3rd edn). Upper Saddle River, NJ: Pearson Education.

Rogers E and Shoemaker F (1971) *Communication of Innovations: A Cross Cultural Report* (2nd edn). New York: The Free Press.

Rogers S, Redley B, Rawson H (2021) Developing work readiness in graduate nurses undertaking transition to practice programs: An integrative review. *Nurse Education Today*, 105 (October): 1–6.

Rowson T, McSherry W (2018) Using the Care Excellence Framework to benchmark and improve patient care. *Nursing Management*, 25(3): 22–28.

Royal College of Nursing (RCN) (2015a) *Bullying and Harassment: Good Practice Guidance for Preventing and Addressing Bullying and Harassment in Health and Social Care Organisations*. Available at: www.rcn.org.uk/professional-development/publications/ pub-004969. Accessed Date: 17 April 2020.

Royal College of Nursing (RCN) (2015a) *Stress and You: A Short Guide to Coping with Pressure and Stress*. Available at: www.rcn.org.uk/professional-development/publications/pub-004966. Accessed Date: 18 May 2021.

Royal College of Nursing (RCN) (2015b) *Nursing morale has "dropped through the floor" - RCN research*. Available at: https://healthwatchtrafford.co.uk/news/nursing-staff-morale-has-dropped-through-the-floor-say-royal-college-of-nursing/. Accessed Date: 18 May 2021.

Royal College of Nursing (RCN) (2017a) *Accountability and Delegation – A Guide for the Nursing Team*. Available at: www.rcn.org.uk/professional-development/publications/ pub-006465 Accessed Date: 24 April 2020.

Royal College of Nursing (RCN) (2017b) *Record Keeping – The Facts*. Available at: https:// www.rcn.org.uk/professional-development/publications/pub-006051. Accessed Date: 24 April 2020.

Royal College of Nursing (RCN) (2017c) *RCN Guide to Revalidation for Employers: Mitigating the Risks to Your Business.* Available at: www.rcn.org.uk/professional-development/revalidation. Accessed Date: 16 January 2021.

Royal College of Nursing (RCN) (2019a) *RCN Comments ahead of NHS Long Term Plan.* Available at: www.rcn.org.uk/news-and-events/press-releases/rcn-comments-ahead-of-nhs-long-term-plan. Accessed Date: 23 April 2020.

Royal College of Nursing (RCN) (2019b) *Quality Improvement.* Available at: www.rcn.org.uk/clinical-topics/clinical-governance/quality-improvement. Accessed Date: 6 September 2020.

Royal College of Nursing (RCN) (2019c) *Clinical Governance: Five Key Themes.* Available at: www.rcn.org.uk/clinical-topics/clinical-governance/five-key-themes. Accessed Date: 7 August 2020.

Royal College of Nursing (RCN) (2019d) *Continuing Professional Development in England – Member Briefing.* London: RCN.

Royal College of Nursing (RCN) (2020a) *RCN Leadership.* Available at: Leadership programme | Royal College of Nursing (rcn.org.uk). Accessed Date: 16 December 2020.

Royal College of Nursing (RCN) (2020b) *Clinical Governance: Leadership.* Available at: www.rcn.org.uk/clinical-topics/clinical-governance/leadership. Accessed Date: 9 December 2020.

Royal College of Nursing (RCN) (2020c) *Staffing for Safe and Effective Care in the UK.* Available at: www.rcn.org.uk/employment-and-pay/safe-staffing/staffing-for-safe-and-effective-care. Accessed Date: 7 July 2020.

Royal College of Nursing (RCN) (2021) *Statements: How to write them.* Available at: www.rcn.org.uk/get-help/rcn-advice/statements. Accessed Date: 21 March 2021.

Royal J (2012) Evaluating human, social and cultural capital in nurse education. *Nurse Education Today,* 32(5): e19–e22.

Ruane S (2019) Integrated care systems in the English NHS: A critical view. *Archives of Disease in Childhood,* 104(2019): 1024–1026.

Sarre S, Robert G, Maben J, Griffiths P, Chable R (2020) Productive Ward: Lessons from a quality-improvement programme. *Nursing Times,* 116(3): 27–29.

Scally G, Donaldson L J (1998) Looking forward: Clinical governance and the drive for quality improvement in the new NHS in England. *BMJ,* 317: 61–65.

Scaria M K (2016) Role of care pathways in interprofessional teamwork. *Nursing Standard,* 30(52): 42–47.

Scott G (2015) This staffing model is great news for nursing. *Nursing Standard,* 29(39): 3.

Sebire S J, Toumpakari Z, Turner K M, Cooper A R, Page A S, Malpass A, Andrews R C (2018) 'I've made this my lifestyle now': A prospective qualitative study of motivation for lifestyle change among people with newly diagnosed type two diabetes mellitus. *BMC Public Health,* 18(1): 1–10.

Sfantou D F, Laliotis A, Patelarou A E, Sifaki-Pistolla D, Matalliotakis M, Patelarou E (2017) Importance of leadership style towards quality of care measures in healthcare settings: A systematic review. *Healthcare (Basel),* 5(4): 1–17.

Shahid S, Thomas S (2018) Situation, Background, Assessment, Recommendation (SBAR) communication tool for handoff in health care – A narrative review. *Safety in Health,* 4(7): 1–9.

Skills for Health (2019) *What is 'National Early Warning Scores 2 (NEWS2)'?* Available at: www.skillsforhealth.org.uk/news/blog/item/805-what-is-national-early-warning-scores-2-news2. Accessed Date: 30 June 2020.

Skills for Health (2020) *Six Steps Methodology to Integrated Workforce Planning.* Available at: https://visual.ly/community/Infographics/health/six-steps-methodology-integrated-workforce-planning. Accessed Date: 22 March 2020.

Skills for Health (2021) *Person Centred Care Meaning & Implications.* Available at: Person Centred Care Meaning & Implications (skillsplatform.org). Accessed Date: 23 February 2021.

Smyth C (2020) A&E four-hour waiting limit at risk of axe 'saves 15,000 lives'. *The Times,* 18 January 2020. Available at: www.thetimes.co.uk/article/a-amp-e-four-hour-waiting-limit-at-risk-of-axe-saves-15-000-lives-dhzgjbv25. Accessed Date: 13 November 2021.

Social Work England (2020) *Professional Standards.* Available at: www.socialworkengland.org.uk/media/3074/professional-standards-guidance-designed_april-final.pdf. Accessed Date: 17 May 2020.

South Warwickshire Clinical Commissioning Group (2020) *About South Warwickshire CCG.* Available at: www.southwarwickshireccg.nhs.uk/About-Us/About-South-Warwickshire-CCG. Accessed Date: 10 December 2020.

Southworth P, Roberts L (2020) Captain Tom Moore's 100th birthday: War veteran hails British public as fundraising effort tops £32m. *The Telegraph,* 30 April 2020. Available at: www.telegraph.co.uk/news/2020/04/30/captain-tom-moore-birthday-colonel-flypast-raf-spitfire/. Accessed Date: 3 May 2020.

Stenberg M, Carlson E (2015) Swedish student nurses' perception of peer learning as an educational model during clinical practice in a hospital setting – an evaluation study. *BMC Nursing,* 14(1): 1–7.

Stephenson J (2020) Whistleblowing cases up 70% in year under guardians scheme. *Nursing Times.* Available at: www.nursingtimes.net/news/reviews-and-reports/whistleblowing-cases-up-70-in-year-under-guardians-scheme-19-03-2020/. Accessed Date: 30 October 2020.

Stewart R (1993) *The Reality of Organisations.* London: Macmillan Press.

Stewart R (2018) *Evidence-based Management: A Practical Guide for Health Professionals.* (eBook). London: CRC Press (Taylor & Francis Group).

Taylor R (2012) Social capital and the nursing student experience. *Nurse Education Today* 32(3) 250–254.

The Times Budget (2020) Balancing the Books (12 March 2020, p. 16).

Timmins N (2015) *The Practice of System Leadership – Being Comfortable with Chaos.* London: King's Fund. Also available at: www.kingsfund.org.uk/publications/practice-system-leadership. Accessed Date: 3 July 2020.

Tomey A M (2009) *Guide to Nursing Management and Leadership* (8th edn). St. Louis, MO: Mosby.

Toode K, Routasalo P, Helminen M, Suominen T (2015) Hospital nurses' work motivation. *Scandinavian Journal of Caring Sciences,* 29(2): 248–257.

Traynor M, Knibb W (2020) What it's like to be the first nursing associates. *Nursing Standard,* 35(8): 26–28.

Trueland J (2019) 'We value your feedback'_ What patient experience really tells us. *Nursing Standard,* 34(1): 20–22.

Tuckman B W, Jensen M A C (1977) Stages of small-group development revisited. *Group & Organization Studies,* 2(4): 419–427.

UK Health Security Agency (UKHSA) (2022) *What the UK Health Security Agency Does.* London, UKHSA.

UNISON (2020) *Risk Assessment*. Available at: www.unison.org.uk/get-help/knowledge/health-and-safety/risk-assessment/. Accessed Date: 2 July 2020.

University of Leicester (2018) *Guidance for Writing Reports*. Available at: www2.le.ac.uk/offices/staff-development/docs/minutes/guidelines-report-writing. Accessed Date: 21 March 2021.

Valentine M, Nembhard I M, Edmondson A C (2015) Measuring teamwork in health care settings: A review of survey instruments. *Medical Care*, 53(4): e16–e30.

Vaughn V M, Saint S, Krein S L, Forman J H, Meddings J, Ameling J, Winter S, Townsend W, Chopra V (2019) Characteristics of healthcare organisations struggling to improve quality: Results from a systematic review of qualitative studies. *BMJ Quality and Safety*, 28(1): 74–84.

Vázquez-Sánchez M A, Jiménez-Arcos M, Aguilar-Trujillo P, Guardiola-Cardenas M, Damián-Jiménez F, Casals C (2020) Characteristics of recovery from near misses in primary health care nursing: Prospective descriptive study. *Journal of Nursing Management*, 28(8): 2007–2016.

Wain, A (2017) Examining the lived experiences of newly qualified midwives during their preceptorship. *British Journal of Midwifery*, 25(7): 451–457.

Walshe K (2016) Evidence-based management: A critical appraisal. In: Walshe K, Smith J (eds) *Healthcare Management*, Chapter 2 (3rd edn). London: McGraw Hill Education.

Waterman H (2011) Principles of 'servant leadership' and how they can enhance practice. *Nursing Management*, 17(9): 24–26.

West M, Dawson J, Adamaschew L, Topakas A (2011) *NHS Staff Management and Health Service Quality*. Lancaster University Management School and The Work Foundation, Aston Business School. Available at: https://assets.publishing.service.gov.uk/government/uploads/system/uploads/attachment_data/file/215455/dh_129656.pdf. Accessed Date: 19 July 2020.

West M, Eckert R, Collins B, Chowla R (2017) *Caring to Change – How Compassionate Leadership Can Stimulate Innovation in Healthcare*. Available at: Caring_to_change_Kings_Fund_May_2017.pdf. Accessed Date: 15 December 2020.

West M, Eckert R, Steward K, Passmore B (2014) *Developing Collective Leadership for Health Care*. Available at: www.ctrtraining.co.uk/documents/DevelopingCollective-Leadership-KingsFundMay2014.pdf. Accessed Date: 16 November 2020.

Whitby P (2018) Role of front-line nurse leadership in improving care. *Nursing Standard*, 33(8): 30–34.

Whitehair L, Hurley J, Provost S (2018) Envisioning successful teamwork: An exploratory qualitative study of team processes used by nursing teams in a paediatric hospital unit. *Journal of Clinical Nursing*, 27(23–24): 4257–4269.

Wilson C B, Slade C, Wong W Y A, Peacock A (2020) Health care students experience of using digital technology in patient care: A scoping review of the literature. *Nurse Education Today*, 95 (December 2020): 1–8. https://doi.org/10.1016/j.nedt.2020.104580.

Wise J (2015) Substandard care at 'dysfunctional' Morecambe Bay maternity unit led to unnecessary deaths. *BMJ*, 350(2015): h1221.

Wong C A, Cummings G G, Ducharme L (2013) The relationship between nursing leadership and patient outcomes: A systematic review update. *Journal of Nursing Management*, 21(5): 709–724.

World Health Organization (2010) *Framework for Action on Interprofessional Education and Collaborative Practice*. Available at: www.who.int/hrh/resources/framework_action/en/. Accessed Date: 21 July 2020.

World Health Organization (2012) *Being an Effective Team Player*. Available at: www. who.int/patientsafety/education/curriculum/course4_handout.pdf Accessed Date: 22 July 2020.

Yan S, Wu S, Zhang G (2016) Impact of connective leadership on employees; goal commitment during M & A (mergers and acquisitions) integration. *Leadership & Organization Development Journal*, 37(6): 789–801.

Yau C W H, Leigh B, Liberati E, Punch D, Dixon-Woods M, Draycott T (2020) Clinical negligence costs: Taking action to safeguard NHS sustainability. *BMJ*, 368(8237): 411–413.

Yun C (2020) Early innovation adoption: Effects of performance-based motivation and organizational characteristics. *Public Performance & Management Review*, 43(4): 790–817.

Zoutman D E, Ford B D (2017) Quality improvement in hospitals: barriers and facilitators. *International Journal of Health Care Quality Assurance*, 30(1): 16–24.

Zulch B (2014) Leadership communication in project management. *Procedia – Social and Behavioural Sciences*, 119(2014): 172–181.

Zwedberg S, Alnervik M, Barimani M (2021) Student midwives' perception of peer-learning during their clinical practice in an obstetric unit: A qualitative study. *Nurse Education Today*, 99(April 2021): 1–6. https://doi.org/10.1016/j.nedt.2021.104785.

Index